MILTON AND MATERNAL MORTALITY

All too often, childbirth in early modern England was associated with fear, suffering, and death, and this melancholy preoccupation weighed heavily on the seventeenth-century mind. This landmark study examines John Milton's life and work, uncovering evidence of the poet's engagement with maternal mortality and the dilemmas it presented. Drawing on both literary scholarship and up-to-date historical research, Louis Schwartz provides an important new reading of Milton's poetry, including *Paradise Lost*, as well as a wide-ranging survey of the medical practices and religious beliefs that surrounded the perils of childbirth. The reader is granted a richer understanding of how seventeenth-century society struggled to come to terms with its fears, and how one of its most important poets gave voice to that struggle.

Louis Schwartz is Associate Professor of English at the University of Richmond, Virginia.

MILTON AND MATERNAL MORTALITY

LOUIS SCHWARTZ
University of Richmond

CAMBRIDGE
UNIVERSITY PRESS

CAMBRIDGE UNIVERSITY PRESS
Cambridge, New York, Melbourne, Madrid, Cape Town, Singapore, São Paulo, Delhi

Cambridge University Press
The Edinburgh Building, Cambridge CB2 8RU, UK

Published in the United States of America by Cambridge University Press, New York

www.cambridge.org
Information on this title: www.cambridge.org/9780521896382

First published 2009

Printed in the United Kingdom at the University Press, Cambridge

A catalogue record for this publication is available from the British Library

ISBN 978-0-521-89638-2 hardback

This book is dedicated to the memory of my grandfathers,

Louis Schwartz (1903–1959)
and
Moe Ash (1912–1971).

Contents

Acknowledgments

I owe thanks, first, to William Flesch and to Mary Nyquist, in whose classrooms my interest in Milton's life and work was first nurtured; to Mita Giacomini, for bringing the materials of medical history to my attention, and for suggesting that they might be relevant to the poetry; and to Gardner Campbell, who taught me to see Milton with new eyes at a crucial stage in the development of the project – much of what I have to say here was first inspired by conversation and correspondence with him. I would also like to thank Anthony Russell for his learning, his incisive comments, and his irritating habit of being almost always right. My thinking also would lack a good deal of whatever sharpness it has without the conversation and friendship of Terryl Givens.

John Shawcross read over a draft of the manuscript with great care, pointing me in a number of fruitful directions and saving me from a number of embarrassing errors. He is a model of scholarly generosity, and I am indebted to him in countless ways. John Rumrich also offered lengthy comments on a draft of the manuscript, and has been unfailingly helpful and supportive over the years. Roy Flannagan published an early version of Chapter 7, the first piece of this project to see print, in *Milton Quarterly* in 1993. His encouragement at that time pushed me to explore the topic more deeply. I would also like to thank Albert Labriola, whose sharp editorial eye helped give the material on Sin and Death some much-needed rhetorical force and concision when it first appeared in *Milton Studies*. I have also received helpful comments, suggestions, and important encouragement from Diane McColley, John Leonard, Stephen Fallon, Dennis Danielson, Robert Entzminger, Margaret Thickstun, Heather Dubrow, Stuart Clark, Sidney Watts, Elizabeth Hodgson, Kathy Hewett-Smith, Susan McDonald, Wendy Furman, Richard DuRocher, Raphael Falco, Lynne Greenberg, John Hale, Edward Jones, Shari Zimmerman, James Fleming, Elizabeth Sagasser, Kent Lenhnof, David Urban, Debrah Raschke, Kathryn MacPherson, Amy Boesky, and Alice Berghof. Thanks also to Ray Ryan at

Cambridge University Press for believing in the project (and for seeing that it could be shorter), and to the anonymous readers at Cambridge University Press, who offered many detailed comments and suggestions. Whatever flaws remain are, of course, my own.

Special thanks must also go to Charles Durham, Kristin Pruitt, Kevin Donovan, and everyone else responsible for the Conference on John Milton in Murfreesboro. Not only did parts of Chapters 5 and 8 first appear in volumes edited by Charley and Kris, but most of what I say in the book as a whole had its first public airing in the generous atmosphere of the conference. They have done important work for the community of Milton scholars, and their warmth and encouragement have meant the world to me. A special thanks also must go to Kevin Creamer for creating another space (this one virtual) for the exchange of ideas. The world of Milton scholarship would be a far less lively place without Milton-l.

The University of Richmond provided important financial and institutional support at all stages. I owe particular thanks to Andy Newcombe, Dona Hickey, David Leary, Barbara Griffin, Ray Hilliard, and Louis Tremaine, for their friendship, collegiality, and administrative support. Ray also offered a number of important stylistic suggestions after reading an early draft of Part I. The Faculty Research Committee provided generous funding for travel and research. Wendy Levy, Kathy Zacher, and Toni Blanton all gave countless hours to the tasks of proofreading, copying, and mailing, and my research would have been impossible without the help of Noreen Cullen, Jeri Townsend, and Nancy Vick in the interlibrary loan office. I also owe thanks to Marcia Whitehead for keeping the Milton collection at the Boatwright Memorial Library up to date, and for helping me track down some difficult-to-find materials. Sophie Pufahl provided careful and sensitive copy-editing, and Katherine Peters was a tremendous help with final proofreading and citation checking.

Finally, I want to thank my parents, Arthur and Cynthia Schwartz, for their love and support, and above all my wife, Donna Perry, for her love, her patience, and her clear-eyed and sensible partnership over the too many years it has taken me to finish this book. I also owe her thanks for helping me to understand whatever I have been able to understand about maternal experience, and for lessons in selflessness that I can only hope to live up to. These things, though quiet, shall not go unrecorded.

Abbreviations

CP	*Complete Prose Works of John Milton*, gen. ed. Don M. Wolfe, 8 vols. (New Haven, CT: Yale University Press, 1953–1982)
DNB	*Oxford Dictionary of National Biography*, online edn. (Oxford University Press, 2008), www.oxforddnb.com
KJV	The Bible: Authorized King James version, eds. Robert Carroll and Stephen Prickett (Oxford University Press, 1997)
OED	*Oxford English Dictionary*, online edn. (Oxford University Press, 2000), www.oed.com
Parker	William R. Parker, *Milton: A Biography*, 2nd edn., rev. and ed. Gordon Campbell, 2 vols. (Oxford: Clarendon Press, 1996)

Citations to Milton's poetry employ standard abbreviations and are taken from *The Complete English Poetry of John Milton*, ed. John T. Shawcross (New York, NY: Anchor Books, 1963). These citations appear parenthetically in the body of the text. Notes will be used for other references, with each chapter's initial citation of any given work provided in full.

Introduction

MILTON'S POETRY AND THE BURDEN OF FEMALE SUFFERING

This study is an attempt to uncover an aspect of Milton's poetry that has been obscured by the vagaries of history: its part in the dramatic spiritual, intellectual, and psychological struggle that so many men and women of his era had to wage in coming to terms with the suffering and death of women in childbirth. The reproductive imagery of the poetry has, of course, been studied in some detail, especially by feminist critics, who have revealed a good deal about Milton's sometimes vexed relationship with sexual and reproductive life, especially as it was embodied in the women he knew and imagined. It is only very recently, however, that literary scholars have paid much attention to the *material* conditions that Milton would have experienced when it came to childbirth, conditions that over the past twenty years have been explored in some detail by social historians and historians of medicine. Milton was, in fact, deeply concerned with such material conditions. Indeed, during two particularly important periods of his poetic career, his work is marked by a struggle to create a poetic mode capable of offering what he thought of as a theologically and affectively adequate consolation in the face of them. In attempting to do so, Milton was trying to bridge a gap that had opened between literary convention and the highly complex discourses about childbirth that had begun to appear in the medical and religious writings of the era.

Placing Milton in this historical context – one that has only recently been pieced together in enough detail by historians to make it of much use to literary scholars – forces us to rethink a number of the venerable warhorses of Milton criticism. The past twenty years or so of sensitive and searching work on Milton and gender has to some extent laid to rest the old caricature of Milton as a dour misogynist. Most scholars today have a reasonably clear view of what is and what is not "progressive" about Milton in twenty-first-century terms, and this clarity has allowed us to see where the strangeness and intensity of Milton's poetry often exceeds and overwhelms the unexamined pieties, customs, and prejudices of his age. But it has also allowed us to see more clearly what remains tied to them. Such studies, along with the important work that has been done on Milton's life records since the initial publication of Parker's monumental biography in 1968, have allowed us to make much finer distinctions and judgments than we were able to make before, giving our accounts of Milton's relations with the historical conditions and conflicting ideas of his time more nuance.

A brief anecdote will explain more clearly the sort of nuanced distinction I mean. At a conference a few years ago, I was discussing the implications of a paper I had just given on the reproductive imagery at work in Milton's representation of chaos with a well-known feminist scholar.[1] After musing for a while on what I had argued, she said that she thought it was true that while Milton did not really care about women's *oppression*, he did care about women's *suffering*. I think that this formulation gets it exactly right, and the fine distinction at its heart is of tremendous importance to the argument I mean to present. The "oppression" of women is not a category that would have even occurred to Milton, certainly not in the modern sense of the term. He did, however, as I will demonstrate, have a pained feeling that women bore a greater burden of suffering for original sin than men. He also had an acute and uneasy sense of the seeming injustice of this fact. The curses of Adam and Eve, he realized, were, in important ways, asymmetrical. While they seemed to neatly prescribe two complementary areas of human endeavor (a division of labors, as it were, and hence two equal modes of suffering that dovetailed in a shared mortality), in practical experience they were never quite so "separate but equal." It was true that men suffered in the work that they did, that some died trying to earn bread by the sweat of their brows, and that women suffered – and all too often died – in childbirth, trying to bring new human beings into the world. It was also true, however, that women have never been exempt from productive labor over and above the processes of reproduction, and the domestic labor that followed from it, in a patriarchal society like that of early modern England. Milton himself made sure that his own daughters all learned a productive trade (in this case embroidery), and they all worked at their trade in their adult lives. While it was true that men might, in some circumstances, be called upon to care for children (although this was rare in the seventeenth century), it was also true

[1] This was at the 1999 International Milton Symposium at the University of York, and the scholar in question was Jackie di Salvo. I am deeply grateful to her for the formulation.

that men obviously could not give birth to them, and it was in birth that women met what the culture took to be their most characteristic form of suffering. The only experience that in most circumstances mirrored the gendered exclusivity of childbed suffering was warfare, but in warfare, while soldiers might suffer extravagantly, and while women did not traditionally serve as soldiers, many non-combatants suffered as well. Given the destructiveness that could be unleashed by a group of men set free to loot, burn, rape, and kill in a conquered city, and given the fate of many a woman left behind by a husband or father who died in battle (not to mention the suffering of women who lost children and other relatives), it was clear that women were hardly exempt from the suffering caused by war. The example itself, in fact, suggests a whole host of other ways in which women suffered due to a hierarchy of authority that Milton may not have objected to in principle, but that he knew could be and often was abused. In fact, that hierarchy, ripe for abuse, had also been laid on women as part of their curse, and warfare was not mentioned specifically in God's words to Adam at all.

If men abused their authority and women suffered from that, the fault would have seemed to Milton to lay with the men, not with their God-given authority, and he would have expected women to accept male authority properly exercised. Suffering in childbirth, however, had been ordained directly, and the sheer awfulness of such suffering under contemporary conditions caused Milton, along with many other men and women of his age, to think long and hard about how to approach it within the religious frameworks offered by reformed Christianity. Such thought was especially important given the new importance that Protestantism, along with a host of socio-economic changes in English life, had begun to give to marriage, human reproduction, and the inward experiences of the individual believer.

In the chapters that follow, I will explore the implications that such trends in religious thought and social change had for Milton as he set about trying to fit his sense of the seeming injustice of childbed suffering with his vision of a just and good divinity. He would have been committed to the notion that it only *seemed* unjust, that if the right framework could be found, if the right theology could be articulated, God's ways to Eve and her daughters could be shown to be as justifiable as any of his ways to men. The traditional, and traditionally misogynistic, explanations for the disparity between the two fateful curses laid on Eve and Adam were not satisfying to him, as they were not for a small but still surprising number of writers in the period. Most people accepted that God was right to punish Eve more than Adam because her sin was the first, and because she was guilty of seducing him to follow her. But the theological traditions were not univocal on this matter, many blaming Adam more for having fallen undeceived, while Eve's guilt was, at least to some extent, mitigated by the fact that the serpent had tricked her. As many commentators have noted, on the face of it, nothing in Genesis suggests anything but the sequence of events. She ate the fruit, then she gave some to him, and he also ate. Milton took that sequence and did some remarkable things with it, often making use of traditional sources but also giving his imagination a certain amount of free rein. He refused to make his Eve a deliberate seductress (whatever effect her sexual allure had on Adam is clearly rooted in his responses, not in her behavior). He also has God clearly make the fact that Eve was deceived by Satan the reason for humankind's redeemability (the rebel angels, who were not deceived, are, in contrast, damned eternally), and he gives Eve the crucial role of reconciler. In Book 10 of *Paradise Lost*, she is the first human being to engage in *imitatio Christi*, and it is the self-sacrificial love behind her gesture that causes Adam's heart to relent towards her, making him commiserate with her for the first time since the Fall, and ensuring that there will, in fact, be a human future to be redeemed by the divine act she unconsciously imitates (*PL*, 10.914–46).

The poem contains a good deal of rhetoric in favor of gender hierarchy, some of it in the words of some pretty authoritative figures (including the Son at 10.147–56), but it is also marked by a counter-discourse that complicates any easy characterization of Milton's views on women. As we will see, in the course of constructing his sometimes ambivalent characterization of Eve, and in the way he treats central female figures at several other points in his work, Milton struggled to identify the proper theological function of the suffering many women experienced in childbirth. As we will also see, many of his decisions, not the least of which was making Eve the original human imitator of Christ, were designed to place that suffering in a context that could offer consolation while still giving full recognition to its peculiar intensity, the power such experiences had, in fact, to mark the limitations of conventional religiosity.

MILTON'S PARTICULAR EXPERIENCES

Milton confronted the death in childbirth of women he knew (or knew of) at, at least, three important moments in his career. The first confrontation concerned a somewhat distant event that struck him at the time, and for various reasons, as a good subject for poetry. On the other two occasions, he was intimately involved. In his early years as a poet, after hearing of the death in childbirth of a gentlewoman who was connected in various ways with people he knew at Cambridge, Milton thought he could dictate to both men and women, in elegant poetic form, the theological sense he found he could make of such an experience. However, in later life, after the deaths of his first two wives due to complications arising in childbirth, he found he needed to approach the subject in a humbler, more inconclusive manner. Although this is essentially a book about the poetry he produced in the wake of these events, and although the questions I will be asking and trying to answer are essentially literary ones, it is also a book centrally concerned with the suffering of these three women: Lady Jane Paulet, Mary Powell, and Katherine Woodcock. The first was an aristocrat from a prominent Catholic family close to royal circles. She made an advantageous marriage with Lord John Paulet, fifth Marquis of Winchester, in 1622, and died about nine years later while giving birth to her second son. Milton was among about a half-dozen poets (they included Ben Jonson and William Davenant) who were motivated to compose elegies for her. The other two women were Milton's first and second wives. They were both members of downwardly mobile families of the lower gentry (both married Milton, perhaps, at least in part, to help their families' social and economic standings), and both died due to complications in childbirth, Mary three days after giving birth to her fourth child, and Katherine of a consumption probably contracted in the childbed about three months after giving birth to her first. In both cases, about one month later, a child died (John Jr., Mary's one-year-old son, in the first case, and the newborn infant named for her mother in the second). Milton probably wrote Sonnet 23 sometime shortly after Katherine's death, but as many have felt, and as I will argue, the poem reflects the impact of both deaths.

These three women wrote no poetry themselves (at least nothing survives – there is some evidence that Lady Jane did write); they also left no diaries or letters, and our grasp on their specific historical circumstances is relatively weak. Only the smallest scattering of documentary evidence exists to attest to their ever having lived and breathed at all. Bits of their personalities and bits of the texture of their everyday lives emerge here and there, but it is often hard to tell fact from conventional idealization or, in the case of Mary, from the negative implications of circumstances we only imperfectly grasp. However, because among the documents that survive are the two poems I have already mentioned, as well as a broadly distributed set of puzzling and deeply moving passages in Milton's works, whose pattern can be traced from the early 1630s until at least the late 1660s, these three women have inhabited – with varying degrees of vividness – the minds of Milton's readers for more than three-and-a-half centuries.

Some of these poems and passages have been studied in detail, but they have never been given the systematic attention they deserve as a set. The three women have also never been thought of together in terms of what their experiences and fates might have meant to the poet whose works and biography links them. I have therefore attempted to gain access, imaginatively and intellectually, to the childbirth experiences of these three women, and those of any number of women like them in the early years of the seventeenth century, providing for the first time a comprehensive and historically informed gloss on Milton's scattered but purposeful allusions to childbed suffering, and demonstrating the impact that such suffering had on his imagination.

I will argue that the deaths of Katherine, Mary, and to a lesser extent Lady Jane need to be counted among the constellation of causes, not only for the sonnet and "An Epitaph on the Marchioness of Winchester" (hereafter "An Epitaph"), but for *Paradise Lost* itself, which some biographers believe Milton began writing in earnest just after or around the time of the deaths of Katherine and her infant daughter. In other words, at a key moment in his life as a poet, Milton found himself engaged in two struggles: one with the composition of an epic, the other with a personal loss that painfully echoed both an earlier loss and an earlier artistic achievement. The two struggles dovetailed, the latter being among the forces driving the former, and they marked the poem he finally produced with a strange and unconventional network of figures.

MILTON AND THE POETRY OF CHILDBED SUFFERING

The fact that Milton wrote as he did about death in childbirth is a stranger thing than might at first appear. Women of the upper and middle classes in the rapidly growing cities and towns of the era, especially in London, were dying in childbed at a rate approaching one in every forty births – that is, at a rate some 300 times higher than is common today in the industrialized West, about four or five times higher than is common today in the developing world, and about twice the rate estimated for most of rural England at the time. Poets of sixteenth- and seventeenth-century England, however, who were for the most part from the middling and upper classes, and most of whom were either native to London or spent the majority of their professional lives in or around it, did not by and large concern themselves with this suffering in their work, at least not directly, and certainly not systematically. They had no large storehouse of conventional figures for the description of death in childbirth; the genres of funereal verse were not regularly and conventionally adapted to its occasion. With a few striking exceptions, poets did not see it as their task to provide readers with a way of alleviating the particular anxieties that such deaths inspired (anxieties that, as we shall see, most people in the period lived with as a matter of course). Few poets even tried, tending instead to ignore the subject even when writing occasional verse about women who did die as a consequence of childbirth.

As we shall see, there were many reasons for this. Why Milton, however, should have been one of the few to ignore those reasons and to treat the subject both directly and systematically is a question worth examining in some detail. He was certainly not the only writer to have had experience, both personal and otherwise, with the deaths of women in childbirth. Like other men in the period, he read some of the medical literature concerned with human reproduction; he attended sermons preached on the occasions of churchings, baptisms, and at the funerals of women who had died giving birth. He heard the murmured prayers of the women surrounding his own wives in the birthing chamber, and perhaps also those surrounding his mother and his older sister. In all probability, although he never records it, he prayed along with them from outside the chamber for the safe delivery of these women and for the lives and the health of their infants. He certainly came across prayers composed for such occasions. They commonly appeared in the many works of theology, devotion, and exegesis he studied and used in his work. When he was a young man, however, he had no particular reason to find the subject of specifically *poetic* interest. No more than any other ambitious young poet might. But his attention was, in fact, directed toward the subject, and toward the theological and psychological difficulties it presented, from very early on.

The anomaly of Milton's concern, and the nature of the ambitions it inspired, is worthy of study, in part because it reveals a great deal about why most poets did not concern themselves with the problems of maternal suffering and mortality. This is not to say that the culture at large was silent in the face of such suffering. Indeed, the seventeenth century saw a veritable explosion of writing on the subject, and as I will show later, Milton was certainly familiar with a wide range of these materials, as well as with some of the small number of poems that had, in fact, attempted to engage the subject. Bringing the context of childbirth lore and practice to a study of Milton's poetry allows us, in fact, to explain the way certain literary forms and conventions operating in particular historical circumstances imposed limitations on the ability of poets to engage certain subjects. It also allows us to explore how these limitations could sometimes be overcome for the accomplishment of ends that were in some ways alien to the ostensible purposes of the forms and conventions themselves. It is one of my larger arguments that the striking originality of *Paradise Lost* was to some extent inspired by an attempt to overcome conventional limitations in the face of the particular subject matter of childbed suffering. That attempt is certainly responsible for much of what remains uncanny and fascinating about the poem for modern readers.

At first, in the epitaph for Lady Jane, Milton confronted death in childbirth as an ambitious artist with a clear theological and vocational mandate. He attempted to explain this kind of suffering and to offer consolation by wrestling with the conventions of the funeral elegy until they could address the specific occasion. At the same time, he used images derived from such suffering to heighten the drama of his own self-representation within the poem, the way he represented his own struggle to imagine and compose it. Throughout his early work, he tended to think of that process, in line with conventional Renaissance medicine and psychology, as itself reproductive and fraught with danger. He might, he thought, give birth to monsters, or his aspirations might be aborted; his imagination might prove sterile, or its processes might kill the poems it struggled to bring to birth. Indeed, it is in terms of birth that he struggled – in poems like "On Shakespear" and "On the Morning of Christs Nativity" – with his own developing sense of visionary vocation. In *A Mask*, he tried to find decorous ways of making childbed suffering a part of what he imagined his young female protagonist would face as she passed through puberty and into adult married life. This habit of mind followed him into his later years. However, after his own personal, marital experiences with childbed suffering, he came to approach the subject in less conclusive and confident ways. In his later works, he paid more attention to the physical details of birth. He also came to see the representation of such details as a theological and aesthetic challenge to which he would have to rise in a new way (and with, as we will see, equivocal results).

Theologically, it required a confrontation with passages in Genesis 3 and with questions of divine justice that would ultimately become central to his epic poem. Aesthetically, it continued to force him to mix and alter genres in order to find ways in which they might be made to handle these theological questions more adequately. It also forced him, within the requirements of rhetorical decorum, to find ways of representing the kind of frighteningly grotesque and painful physical experiences that readers of his age (including himself) would have found impossible to deal with mimetically in any direct way. Most importantly, childbed suffering gave a particular shape to both the sense of lost innocence and the search for restoration that pervade *Paradise Lost*. He came to place birth at the heart of his ideal vision of what humanity lost with Eden, and, perhaps even more painfully, at the heart of the only process he believed would allow humanity to return to that paradise. For Milton, human reproduction became both the sword and gate at the entrance to Eden. It stood between the fallen world and what it had lost, suggesting, too, what it might regain, how it might do so, and just how difficult that process could be.

THE SCOPE AND STRUCTURE OF THIS STUDY

The bulk of this study is a detailed examination of "An Epitaph," "On Shakespear," *A Mask*, Sonnet 23, and *Paradise Lost*, but it begins with a sketch of the social history of childbirth in the period. This sketch, which makes up the three chapters of Part I, pays particular attention to what we know and what we do not know about maternal mortality and its larger cultural effects. It also closely examines the role religious discourses played in the management of obstetric anxieties, and concludes with a discussion of what Milton is likely to have known, suggesting where his work fits into the wide array of materials and ideas covered in the section as a whole. Part II of the study then looks at Milton's work in the 1630s, beginning with a discussion of the strange reproductive imagery of his early poem for Shakespeare, moving through an extended discussion of "An Epitaph" and ending with a discussion of *A Mask*. The discussion of "An Epitaph" reads the poem against the backdrop of elegiac conventions in general, while also showing how Milton adapted motifs he may have encountered in childbed prayers, marriage sermons, and a little known elegy by Michael Drayton, which may have been his primary model. The section also discusses how other poets approached the subject (when they paid attention to it at all), why so few of them ventured to do so, and what might have motivated Milton to write about it so elaborately and ambitiously. The concluding section on *A Mask* discusses the network of reproductive images that Milton wove into his text, and how the implications of these images are summed up in the allegorical tableau that he created for the conclusion of its printed version. This tableau strikingly alludes to the conclusion of the epitaph for Lady Jane Paulet, and suggests the importance of married reproductive life in Milton's imagination of Lady Alice Egerton's future.

Part III of the book is devoted to Milton's later poetic work. The first chapter (Chapter 7) offers an extended reading of Sonnet 23 that suggests a new way of understanding both the poem's allusive structure and its complicated relationship to biographical context. I discuss the significance of the poem's allusion to the Churching of Women, a popular Anglican rite that celebrated a woman's survival of childbirth and welcomed her back into the community of worshipers, suggesting a reconsideration of Parker's argument that the poem concerns Mary Powell rather than Katherine Woodcock. The poem, I argue, uses images derived from churching, as well as from mythology and the Bible, as signs of the speaker's complex of mourning and guilt over the deaths of *both* of his late wives in circumstances related to childbirth. Its allusive structure, in some ways a reworking of the one Milton employed in the epitaph for Lady Jane, is remarkable, not only for its attempt to provide an aesthetic conciliation with maternal mortality, but also for its guilt-ridden concentration on men's exemption from the risks women took each time they had sexual intercourse.

The poem's fall back into darkness at its end suggests, however, an ambivalence that Milton felt could not be resolved in fourteen lines. At the end of the chapter, I discuss the fact that Milton echoes the first and last lines of the sonnet in Adam's description of the "birth" of Eve (*PL*, 8.452–90) as well as the fact that this description includes details derived from contemporary medical descriptions of obstetric surgery, as well as iconographic traditions associated with childbirth and caesarian section. The "birth" of Eve is a central moment in the epic, a central marker of Milton's personal investment in the poem, and part of a network of images of reproductive suffering and consolation that Milton distributed throughout its structure. His purpose in doing so, I argue, is to use the machinery of his epic theodicy to resolve the deep ambivalence that he and his culture as a whole felt about childbirth, given the nature of contemporary conditions.

The second chapter of Part III (Chapter 8) extends my analysis of this network to the allegory of Sin and Death (*PL*, 2.629–889), showing how Milton deliberately constructed the episode to emphasize figures of pregnancy, birth, disfigurement, and specifically female states of physical vulnerability. Sin's account of her transforming and torturous births closely follows what most educated Londoners knew about birth from medical and midwifery texts, as well as what they themselves would have frequently experienced or witnessed, not only as fathers or as male obstetric practitioners, but as gossips, midwives, sisters, and especially as mothers themselves. This leads me to revise certain commonly held notions about the function of Milton's allegory, suggesting that it provides a set of positions from which both men and women could contemplate childbed suffering as a figure for the fallen condition itself.

The chapter concludes with a reading of the last three books of the epic, in which I show that Milton found himself in a difficult rhetorical situation, having to set the consoling figure of the Nativity against the mounting reasons to despair offered by Michael's prophetic vision of the history of the world. The problem he faced concerned the difficulty of evoking the painful childbirth experiences figured in the allegory of Sin and Death while building a consolation that was also centered on a figure of birth. This rhetorical problem explains the absence of explicit figures of catastrophic birth in the unfolding of Michael's history. Milton's emphasis on the figure of the Nativity also, however, continues to imply the importance of human procreation, not only to the unfolding of the providential plan of creation as a whole, but to the lives and choices of individual men and women in the course of that unfolding. I argue that the consolatory function of the figure of the Nativity required that Milton, at least on the surface, relinquish the discourse he had created in order to bring a concern with childbed suffering into the epic. However, the fact that Milton has Adam allude to John 16:20 (one of the most important biblical touchstones in discussions of childbirth suffering in the period) during his reconciliation scene with Eve suggests that Milton wanted the final books of the epic to suggest a mode of consolation that did adequately face childbirth pain and loss. In addition, at several moments in the last two books of the epic, partially repressed or occluded images of catastrophic birth do threaten to undermine the repose for which the poem is reaching. I conclude with a discussion of how Milton may have wanted his readers to imagine the instruction that Eve, at the end of the poem, tells us she received in a dream while Adam was given his visions and instruction by the Archangel.

The book's final chapter (Chapter 9) explores the implications my argument has for a new reading of certain aspects of Milton's cosmology. Milton insistently used reproductive images to describe his cosmos. However, because the nature, function, and physical shape of the cosmic realms are never rendered with perfect precision, the full purpose and the implications of his reproductive images have remained unclear. I argue that these images associate Milton's cosmology with the passages I study in the earlier chapters of this book, and they can therefore be interpreted in light of seventeenth-century obstetric conditions. Milton presents both chaos and creation as wombs, the one created from the other. They form a dyad central to the epic's cosmology and ontology, placing images of human reproduction, with its attendant seventeenth-century horrors, at the heart of its double matrix. If I am right that Milton's and his immediate audience's perceptions of reproduction were filtered through a pervasive anxiety, then it should be possible to read the parts of the cosmos of *Paradise Lost* that are described in terms of reproductive imagery as bearing the marks of that anxiety. I conclude with reflections on how closely Milton associated his responses to reproductive trauma with his whole poetic project.

Deaths in childbirth were commonplace in the early seventeenth century, and they produced the need for some kind of conciliation. The culture of the period offered such conciliation in several forms, but imaginative literature was only rarely called upon to provide it, and the instances in which it was have only rarely been discussed. We are now, however, beginning to learn how to look for the ways in which even the most familiar poems of the age may have been doing unfamiliar work. The conflations of genre and allusion in "An Epitaph," the complex of allusions in Sonnet 23, the web of associations touched off in *Paradise Lost* by Milton's echoing of that sonnet in Adam's dream, as well as the complex of obstetric allusions and images that Milton wove into the allegory of Sin and Death and his descriptions of creation and chaos, are evidence of just such an attempt at conciliation. As such, they give us a rare glimpse of (and a method for coming to understand) the ways in which early-modern literary culture could deal with the pains and dangers of childbirth. They also allow us to see a remarkable case in which a literary figure worked, as I said earlier, to bridge a gap that had opened between literary conventions and the discourses about childbirth that emerged in the medical and religious writing of the age. My purpose is to establish that Milton was consciously concerned with this project from very early on in his career, and that it was for him a pervasive, not a local, concern. Attention to the ways in which he dealt with the subject at several key moments in his poetic development allows us to peer into some of the darker corners of his poetry and his age, both making its darkness visible and revealing the attempts the poet made to purge and disperse it.

PART I

Behind the veil: childbirth and the nature of obstetric anxiety in early modern England

CHAPTER I

"Exquisitt torment" and "infinitt grace": maternal suffering and the rites of childbirth

In her memoir, written in her early forties after the death of her husband, Alice Thornton offered the following account of the birth of the fifth of her nine children. The birth had occurred years earlier on December 10, 1657, and Mrs. Thornton recalls that she had recently recovered from a fall she had suffered in her home a few months earlier. She had been worried all during the intervening months that the shock of the fall would cause her to go into early labor and lose the child. She tells us, however, that she finally did carry the child to term, although this did not end her troubles:

> It pleased God, in much mercy, to restore me to strength to goe to my full time, my labour begining three daies; but upon the Wednesday, the ninth of December, I fell into exceeding sharpe travill in great extreamity, so that the midwife did beleive I should be delivered soone. But loe! it fell out contrary, for the childe staied in the birth, and came crosse with his feete first, and in this condition contineued till Thursday morning betweene two and three a clocke, at which time I was upon the racke in bearing my childe with such exquisitt torment, as if each lime [limb] weare divided from other, for the space of two houers; when att length, beeing speechlesse and breathlesse, I was, by the infinitt providence of God, in great mercy delivered. But I having had such sore travell in danger of my life soe long, and the childe comeing into the world with its feete first, caused the childe to be allmost strangled in the birth, only liveing about halfe an houer, so died before we could gett a minister to baptize him, although he was sent for.
>
> ...
>
> This sweete goodly son was turned wrong by the fall I gott in September before, nor had the midwife skill to turne him right, which was the cause of the losse of his life, and the hazard of my owne.

She goes on to recount how she fell into a "consumption" as a result of her weakened condition, and how, having recovered from that, she was plagued in the following months by "losse of blood", due to chronically bleeding hemorrhoids, and a pain in her left knee, which she claimed she "gott in ... labour, for want of the knee to be assisted." It kept her from walking on her left leg for about three months. Despite all of this, she makes sure, in another passage concerning this birth, to conclude with a pious meditation on what she took to be a severe but just spiritual trial: "I trust in the mercys of the Lord for His salvation, He requiring noe more then He gives. And His infinitt grace was to me in sparing my soule from death. Tho' my body was torne in pieces, my soule was miraculously delivered from death." In later life, the memory of this event and others like it caused Mrs. Thornton to contemplate how much more suffering she felt she had actually deserved. Although she claims not to have been guilty of any truly heinous sins, she acknowledges her part in original sin and celebrates God's undeserved goodness toward her. She appends a prayer of thanksgiving.[1]

Although she does not record any details concerning her prayers during the labor itself, it is likely that, at the time, she prayed in a manner not unlike that recommended in the following set prayer, collected by Thomas Bentley in his massive 1582 compendium of devotional materials for women, *The Monument of Matrones*:

> Oh Lord, this daie is a gloomie daie, a bitter time and terrible houre, a daie...of anguish and tribulation, of sorrowe and perturbation, vnto the verie soul of thine hand-maid: for the babe is come vnto the place of the birth, and lo, it seemeth that thou for my sins hast shut vp the dores of my wombe, and caused the babe to stand still like to be stiffled.
>
> ...
>
> ... out alas for the time of this perplexitie, of this sorrowe and griefe, which I now sensiblie feele and endure, both in bodie and mind; for it is like the daie and time of Rachel. My sorowe and trouble may be compared to Phinees wiues trouble, my state and condition seemeth to me and others, to be not much vnlike vnto theirs, I saie; from the which neverthelesse for thy great mercie sake, good Lord, I beseech thee deliuer me, and saue me and my babe from the graue, as my trust is in thee, Amen.[2]

[1] Alice Thornton, *The Autobiography of Mrs. Alice Thornton*, ed. Charles Jackson, Surtees Society (Durham: Andrews and Co., 1875), vol. LXII, pp. 95–7. The prayer was not preserved, and the original manuscript has not survived. For more details, see Raymond A. Anselment, "The Deliverances of Alice Thornton: the Recreation of a Seventeenth-Century Life," *Prose Studies* 19 (1996), 19–36. See also Lucinda McCray Beier, *Sufferers and Healers: The Experience of Illness in Seventeenth-Century England* (London: Routledge and Kegan Paul, 1987), pp. 224–39 and Sharon Howard, "Imagining the Pain and Peril of Seventeenth Century Childbirth: Travail and Deliverance in the Making of an Early Modern World," *Social History of Medicine* 16 (2003), 367–82.

[2] Thomas Bentley, *The Monument of Matrones: Conteining Seuen Seuerall Lamps of Virginity* (London, 1582), pp. 113–16. For more information, see Colin B. and Jo B. Atkinson, "The Identity and Life of Thomas Bentley, Compiler of *The Monument of Matrones* (1582)," *Sixteenth Century Journal* 31 (2000), 323–48 and Charlotte F. Otten, "Women's Prayers in Childbirth in Sixteenth-Century England," *Women and Language* 16 (1993), 18–21.

Another of the prayers in Bentley's collection offers this more general meditation for a mother or those in attendance at a "long and dangerous travell of child":

> In the beginning of the world, O father of heauen, after thou hadst formed man of the slime of the earth, and yet prince ouer all creatures, it pleased thee of thy goodnes to create a woman of his side, aswell for his solace, as for the continuance of his seed: it was thy word vnto them, Increase & multiply. This increase was easie, but mother Eue has made it hard, by passing the bounds of thy will, to all hir posteritie; so that the woman conceiueth and bringeth foorth in great paine, and painefull travell, the fruit of hir wombe. In so great paine, O Lord, in such extreme pangs, that vnlesse thou quench the flame of hir sorrowes with water of comfort, it i[s] impossible for hir to beare that into this vale of miserie, which thou of thy goodnes hast framed, and she conceived.[3]

Mrs. Thornton's account and these two set prayers provide good examples of the way in which the dangers of childbirth were typically confronted in early modern England. Men and women pleaded with God for the mitigation of pain and danger, but also assumed that their experiences should be approached within a religious framework that explained all outcomes – good and bad – in terms of a divine judgment that had to be accepted. To some extent, Mrs. Thornton felt that human actions could make a significant difference (she thought – rightly or wrongly, we do not know – that she would have suffered less and her child might have lived if she had had a more skillful midwife), but for the most part, like the authors of the set prayers, she attributed her plight to the judgment that God passed on Eve, and through Eve on herself. Her survival, as far as she was concerned, was essentially the result of God's decision (miraculous, loving, and undeserved) to spare her despite her sinfulness.

She took for granted that God made that sort of decision. Women died in childbirth all the time, and there was very little that medical ingenuity could do about that sad fact. The religious ingenuity of the time, therefore, concentrated instead on comforting women in the face of their physical plight, while imbuing it with a dramatic, spiritual significance. The religious discourse that governs both the prayers and the memoir I have quoted could give women a way of imagining that they had some control (if they could rectify their lives, for example, God might not see fit to punish them too severely). Failing that (if, for example, they knew themselves to be free of particular sins, and yet found themselves suffering greatly), they could look

[3] Bentley, *Monument*, p. 127.

for an explanation in the general condition of humankind and work to assure themselves of God's ultimate mercy after death.

As we will see later, however, human religious ingenuity in the face of childbed suffering was not exhausted by this particular schema. Religious thought, prayer and meditation in the period exhibited a store of different approaches to childbed consolation, as well as several variants upon the basic one exemplified by the passages I have quoted. Women often freely made analogies between aspects of their experience and central matters of Christian mythos and doctrine. It may not have escaped Alice Thornton's notice, for example, that her particular case was analogous to humankind's in general. She was saved from death by God's "infinitt grace" despite her unworthiness, just as all humankind was offered grace through Christ's sacrifice despite its state of sin. Women also at times imagined themselves as martyrs, as sacrificial offerings, as imitators of Christ both crucified and resurrected. They took their submission to reproductive life within patriarchal marriage as a reflection not only of Eve's curse but also of their own willingness to obey God's primal command to humankind to be fruitful and multiply. That they had to do so in pain and danger was at once their punishment and the mark of a deep, selfless piety that they hoped might win them greater glory in the end. And, although we might today think of their choices as severely limited by both patriarchal ideology and the limits of the contraceptive technology available to them, many women in the period (the married ones, at least) saw their pains as freely chosen in a conscious rejection of an ascetic religious life (this strain of thought was particularly strong among Protestant women), a "free" single life (that such a thing hardly existed mattered little to the self-justifying imagination), or of marriage without the burdens of motherhood. They saw themselves as suffering, anointed vessels for God's creative power, as partners with God in the ongoing creation of human life.

At the same time, women worked very hard at maintaining a complex world of more secular social rituals, which were designed not only to give comfort in the face of childbed pain and danger, but to provide women with ways to imagine not only their place in creation, but also their social roles, positions, and responsibilities, as well as to maintain their physical, mental, and spiritual well-being. In addition, midwives, physicians, and surgeons were all at this time busy learning – with widely varying degrees of success – new things about the way the female body functioned in birth and about how to help it to work in less dangerous and painful ways. Some of these authors were remarkably uninterested in the theological dimensions of birth, their primary concern being physical explanation, whether derived from ancient authorities or from new findings in anatomy and practical experience.[4]

Unbeknownst to women like Mrs. Thornton, or to anyone else at the time for that matter, this was a period in which human technical ingenuity in childbed care underwent a significant improvement that led, over the course of subesequent centuries, to a dramatic drop in cases of maternal mortality. Unfortunately, in the 1650s, when Alice Thornton struggled with the meaning of her own suffering, other factors were making it so that the effects of a number of very important changes (especially the wider availability of sound obstetric information) had little effect on mortality rates, which were at that point on the increase, especially in London, abating only in the early decades of the eighteenth century before dropping even more precipitously over the following two centuries.[5]

Some practitioners were aware that things *could* have been better much sooner. Percival Willughby, for example, a male midwife and obstetric surgeon active in Derby, Stafford, and London from 1621 to 1670, saw himself as an unfortunately ineffective part of this process of change. Like Alice Thornton and the authors of Bentley's collection, he felt that the fate of a woman in childbirth was ultimately in God's hands, but he also believed that training could work wonders, even perhaps restoring what others might have considered an almost Edenic state of affairs. He counseled midwives

> in all their undertakings, ever to desire, That God would bee graciously pleased to inform their judgements, & guide their hands, for the better helping, & saving of their women, and children, and, lastly, with submitting humblenes to implore his gracious mercy for mitigating their punishment [that of the women they treated], which is decreed and pronounced against them "In sorrow thou shalt bring forth children."

He then claims that while "God was displeased with Eve," he never meant for her (or her daughters) to actually die in childbirth. God said, according

[4] Book 24 of Ambroise Paré's *Workes* ("Of the Generation of Man"), for example, hardly mentions religion at all beyond a few prefatory remarks and asides, preferring to offer physical explanations instead: Ambroise Paré, *The Workes of that Famous Chirurgion Ambrose Parey*, trans. Thomas Johnson (London, 1634), pp. 885–960.

[5] Adrian Wilson and Irvine Loudon argue that improvements in the circulation of reliable information and the beginnings of the reduction in maternal mortality rates predated the masculinization of childbirth that took hold toward the end of the eighteenth century. See Adrian Wilson, *The Making of Man-Midwifery: Childbirth in England, 1600–1770* (Cambridge, MA: Harvard University Press, 1995) as well as Loudon's review of that book in *Bulletin of the History of Medicine* 70 (1996), 507–15 and Irvine Loudon, *Death in Childbirth: an International Study of Maternal Care and Maternal Mortality, 1800–1950* (Oxford: Clarendon Press, 1992).

to Willughby, that woman would "In sorrow ... *bring forth children*," but "not that hee would *destroy* her" [my italics]. Midwives should, therefore, "endeavour to mitigate their woman's sorrows, and in no way augment them, by hailing, and pulling their bodies, to help forward, & to increase their sufferings."[6] Over and over again, he recommends gentle techniques for drawing forth an infant, implying – and sometimes claiming outright – that human error, not divine judgment, was the cause of most of the fatalities he witnessed in the course of his years of practice. He even describes in detail procedures for managing malpresentations like the one that befell Mrs. Thornton and her baby, insisting that the proper method for delivery by the feet ("podalic version") was easy enough to learn.[7] We know that most midwives were far better at their jobs than those Willughby portrays in his text (he himself believed that in most cases women were better off in the hands of female midwives rather than male surgeons like himself). He intended to publish his manuscript for the benefit of all practitioners, and certainly believed that if he could just have gotten it into print, many lives would have been saved, and many women spared excessive suffering. He never did, but others from the 1650s on succeeded where he failed, and the gradual improvement in the circulation of technical knowledge toward the end of the seventeenth century was a significant factor in bringing mortality rates down from their high in that century to their relatively low mid nineteenth-century levels.[8]

In this chapter, I do not hope to explain fully what caused the rise in maternal mortality that marks the middle and later seventeenth century (a goal that continues to elude the historians upon whose work I have relied). But because we do have better access now than we have ever had before to an understanding of the conditions themselves, as well as of the rituals, practices, and beliefs that people like Thornton, Willughby, and Bentley took for granted in the face of them, we can begin to produce a nuanced account of how and why the surviving childbed texts took the forms they did. We can then go on to explain how a literary artist like Milton came to poetic terms with similar circumstances. Childbed conditions, beliefs, and practices were important parts of the world that drove Milton to poetry, the world whose contours, obstacles, and crossings he had in mind whenever he set pen to paper or dictated to his amenuenses. It was a world in which

[6] Percival Willughby, *Observations in Midwifery*, ed. Henry Blenkinsop (Warwick: printed by H. T. Cooke, 1863; rpt. Wakefield: S. R. Publishers, 1972), p. 13.

[7] See Willughby, *Observations*, pp. 121, 146–50 for some harrowing cases in which the procedure was botched.

[8] Loudon, *Death in Childbirth*, pp. 160–1.

childbirth was understood by most as a trial, one that could have a happy or an unhappy outcome depending upon how it was faced, a trial in which human medical ingenuity was, at best, of only partial help, while religious mediation and social rituals offered hope, form, and meaning. In what follows, I will try and explain what it was exactly that men and women faced (or thought they faced) and what they feared about it. Most importantly, I hope to explain how many were enabled by various religious ideas and communal rituals to face their fears with some measure of equanimity. We will then be able to see how Milton made literary use of such rituals and ideas as he contemplated and faced such experiences himself.

THE RITES OF CHILDBIRTH

Social historians and historians of medicine are at present still developing a detailed account of the medical conditions, practices, and beliefs of sixteenth- and seventeenth-century England. Much still remains to be done.[9] This is especially true when it comes to the social history of what we sometimes anachronistically refer to today as the "obstetric medicine" of the period. Historians have, however, done enough work on early modern childbirth to give us a rough picture of what a typical birth was like. They have also made significant progress in outlining the statistical data necessary for putting particular experiences in context. It will therefore be useful for us to begin with a survey of current thinking about these matters. We will then pay special attention to the rates of maternal mortality in the period (especially in London), to the causes of this mortality, and to the question of how we are to understand and measure the level of anxiety such deaths inspired. I will conclude with a discussion of the theological discourses and religious practices that people marshalled in the face of their anxieties.

Most historians characterize the various practices surrounding birth, especially those particular to labor and lying-in, as a cohesive sequence of rites. When things worked the way they were supposed to, for most married women of at least modest means, and even for most poorer women, birth unfolded as a coherent sequence of events with marked sacral and

[9] See Andrew Wear, *Knowledge and Practice in English Medicine, 1550–1680* (Cambridge University Press, 2000) and *Medicine in Society: Historical Essays* (Cambridge University Press, 1992); Nancy G. Siraisi, *Medieval and Early Renaissance Medicine: an Introduction to Knowledge and Practice* (University of Chicago Press, 1990); the introduction to Roy Porter's collection, *Patients and Practitioners: Lay Perceptions of Medicine in Pre-Industrial Society* (Cambridge University Press, 1985); Patricia Crawford, "Sexual Knowledge in England, 1500–1750," in *Sexual Knowledge, Sexual Science: the History of Attitudes to Sexuality*, eds. Roy Porter and Mikuláš Teich (Cambridge University Press, 1994); and Beier, *Sufferers and Healers*.

ceremonial characteristics.[10] The rites had a clearly defined narrative shape: a beginning, a middle, and an end, even a kind of climax, or – in the cases in which things went wrong – a catastrophe. When a woman began to labor, she would normally have someone, often her husband, go out and call on a midwife as well as a group of women to attend to her and bear witness to the event. The gossips and midwife were sometimes carefully chosen by the woman, her husband, and/or her family as her caretakers and companions in the rites (usually at least one or two close, female family members were involved), but these groupings could also be much more ad hoc in nature, comprised of whomever was locally available at the time of the labor.[11] The women would arrive and establish a separate space for the mother in the house, and this space was, to whatever extent was possible, enclosed and darkened. Candles were lit, a caudle (a ritual drink) was readied, and the midwife would set about preparing the mother for the birth itself. From this point on, she would normally be surrounded by an exclusively female community that regulated access to her and worked with the midwife to attend to her physical and spiritual needs. This group of women more or less took over the household, shepherding the mother through labor to the crisis of the birth. If all went well, the birth was followed by a kind of denouement, a period of semi-isolation ("lying-in") that could last for several weeks. The woman would remain in her bed and be attended by visiting gossips until the midwife declared she was ready for her "upsitting," an occasion that was itself often celebrated by another social gathering. Gradually, over the course of the next days and weeks, the woman would venture out of the lying-in chamber and receive guests, including men, for perhaps the first time since she went into labor.

The end of this period, and the end of the domestic rite as a whole, was marked by the ecclesiastical rite of "churching," a thanksgiving ceremony enacted in the local parish church. This rite restored the woman to her place in the larger community of worship and brought her symbolically full-circle back to her state prior to pregnancy, ready to take up her household responsibilities again and perhaps reunite sexually with her husband. Churchings themselves were often followed by a final celebration in the

[10] See Wilson, *The Making of Man-Midwifery*, pp. 11–62. See also Wilson's "Participant or Patient? Seventeenth Century Childbirth from the Mother's Point of View," in Porter's *Patients and Practitioners*, pp. 129–44; "The Ceremony of Childbirth and its Interpretation," in *Women as Mothers in Pre-Industrial England: Essays in Memory of Dorothy McLaren*, ed. Valerie Fildes (London: Routledge, 1990), pp. 68–107; and "The Perils of Early Modern Procreation: Childbirth With or Without Fear?," *British Journal for Eighteenth Century Studies* 16 (1993), 1–19. My account is deeply indebted to Wilson's work.

[11] The composition of such groupings, and their purposes, could vary. See Linda Pollock, "Childbearing and Female Bonding in Early Modern England," *Social History* 22(3) (1997), 286–306.

home, and they sometimes entailed customs that echoed those commonly practiced at weddings (the home celebrations might include, for example, the breaking of a "bride-cake," etc.). These customs suggest that the reunion of spouses after lying-in was thought of by some as a second (or third or fourth or fifth, etc.) wedding day or night. Robert Herrick's poem "Julia's *Churching, or Purification*," for example, makes just this association:

> All Rites well ended, with faire Auspice come
> (As to the breaking of a Bride-Cake) home:
> Where ceremonious *Hymen* shall for thee
> Provide a second *Epithalamie.*
> *She who keeps chastity to her husbands side*
> *Is not for one, but every night his Bride*:
> *And stealing still with love, and feare to Bed,*
> *Brings him not one, but many a Maiden-head.*[12]

The resumption of sexual relations could, if the woman were still young enough (and if she were not nursing her infant) lead to her beginning the process all over again within the next two years. The spacing of births tended to lengthen as a woman aged, and it was not uncommon for couples to attempt to space pregnancies relatively widely for various reasons. For the most part, however, women desired to become pregnant again relatively soon after giving birth or miscarrying. In other words, the rites, for most of a woman's reproductive life, had a more or less cyclical shape and logic, and many women were in that cycle more or less constantly throughout their reproductive years. This was especially so among upper-class women, many of whom did not nurse their own children and therefore were unaffected by the periods of lowered fertility caused by lactation.[13]

These rites of childbirth, in roughly this shape, were practiced, with minor variations, across class, cultural, religious, and geographical lines. The lying-in tended to be shorter, for example, for poorer women, who might also not have had access to a fully separate room, but almost all women observed some period of sequestration during and after the birth.[14] The practice of churching, as we will see, varied to some extent according to

[12] Robert Herrick, *The Poems of Robert Herrick*, ed. L. C. Martin (London: Oxford University Press, 1965), p. 269. See David Cressy's discussion in *Birth, Marriage, and Death: Ritual, Religion, and the Life-Cycle in Tudor and Stuart England* (Oxford University Press, 1997), pp. 222–4 and Gerald Hammond, *Fleeting Things: English Poets and Poems 1616–1660* (Cambridge, MA: Harvard University Press, 1990), pp. 263–4.

[13] See Dorothy McLaren, "Marital Fertility and Lactation 1570–1720," in *Women in English Society 1500–1800*, ed. Mary Prior (London: Methuen, 1986), pp. 22–53.

[14] Wilson, "Ceremony," in *Women as Mothers*, pp. 80–1 and Cressy, *Birth, Marriage, and Death*, p. 15. The experience of the poorest women – as well as prostitutes, prisoners, and those who gave birth out

the theological persuasion of the woman and her family (it was discouraged, for example, by many Puritan writers), but in the early seventeenth century it was practiced by the majority of women, even in the most Puritan parishes of London.[15] The work of Adrian Wilson, David Cressy, Sara Mendelson, Patricia Crawford, Linda Pollock, Audrey Eccles, Laura Gowing and others has shown, in various ways, how this complex series of practices gave an equally complex "social meaning" to the biological processes at its heart.[16] While to some extent the meanings of childbirth practices are so complex as to be overdetermined, and therefore difficult to analyze, certain matters of emphasis and purpose are noted in almost all of the historical studies. "The primary work of childbearing," as Cressy puts it, "... was not the production of a child but the deliverance of a woman."[17] As Adrian Wilson puts it, with a slightly different emphasis, the rites constituted "a coherent system for the management of childbirth, a system based on [the]...collective culture" of women and designed to satisfy "their own material needs."[18] The matters of primary importance for the shape of the rites were, in other words, the needs of the mother. As Wilson defines them, these needs were not only physical but psychological and social in the sense that they helped women to negotiate not only the pains and dangers they were subject to, but also the fears that such pains and dangers occasioned, the social uncertainties that came with taking on the role and responsibilities of motherhood, as well as the power dynamics peculiar to the institution of marriage in the cultural and legal context of the age.

of wedlock, of course – differed. See Laura Gowing, *Common Bodies: Women, Touch, and Power in Seventeenth-Century England* (New Haven, CT: Yale University Press, 2003), pp. 149–76, and Pollock, "Childbearing and Female Bonding," 301–4.

15 See Jeremy Boulton, *Neighborhood and Society: a London Suburb in the Seventeenth Century* (Cambridge University Press, 1987), pp. 276–9; Peter Rushton, "Purification or Social Control? Ideologies of Reproduction and the Churching of Women After Childbirth," in *The Public and the Private*, ed. Eve Garamarnikow (London: Heinemann, 1983), pp. 118–31; Wilson, "Participant or Patient," in *Patients and Practitioners*, pp. 139–40 and "Ceremony," in *Women as Mothers*, pp. 88–9; and Cressy, *Birth, Marriage, and Death*, pp. 197–229.

16 The phrase is Cressy's. See *Birth, Marriage, and Death*, p. 15. See also Sara Mendelson and Patricia Crawford, *Women in Early Modern England, 1550–1720* (Oxford: Clarendon Press, 1998), pp. 148–64; Angus McLaren, *Reproductive Rituals: the Perception of Fertility in England from the Sixteenth Century to the Nineteenth Century* (New York, NY: Methuen, 1984); Patricia Crawford, "The Construction and Experience of Maternity in Seventeenth-Century England" and Linda A. Pollock, "Embarking on a Rough Passage: the Experience of Pregnancy in Early-Modern Society," both in *Women as Mothers*. See also Pollock, "Childbearing and Female Bonding"; Gowing, *Common Bodies*, pp. 149–76; Howard, "Imagining the Pain and Peril"; R. V. Schnucker, "The English Puritans and Pregnancy, Delivery, and Breast Feeding," *History of Childhood Quarterly* 1 (1974), 637–58; Raymond A. Anselment, *Realms of Apollo: Literature and Healing in Seventeenth-Century England* (Newark, NY: University of Delaware Press, 1995), pp. 49–90; and Audrey Eccles, *Obstetrics and Gynaecology in Tudor and Stuart England* (Kent, OH: Kent State University Press, 1982).

17 Cressy, *Birth, Marriage, and Death*, p. 15.

18 Wilson, "Ceremony," in *Women as Mothers*, p. 70.

Some recent studies have tended to emphasize the socially regulative purposes of the rites, the ways in which they, for example, gave women a public opportunity for enforcing standards of morality and behavior within their own communities. Laura Gowing's recent work has suggested various ways in which the complex relationships among women at a birth could provide "an arena for the exercise of authority and deference" that echoed more general political, legal, and economic relationships. She also discusses how the birthing chamber could provide women of the middling and upper classes with public theaters for the conspicuous display of piety, class identity, and/or wealth, and how, especially in the case of illegitimate births or of possible infanticides, it could become an arena for the policing of general sexual mores.[19] Others have focused on the ways in which church authorities or individual male preachers and theologians sometimes attempted to reform the rites themselves or to use them to police or control women's behavior.[20] It is clear, however, that under normal circumstances the rites were primarily designed to serve rather than to control women, and that they were, above all, designed to help a woman make sense out of an experience that was likely to have terrified her. Stages were delineated so that she would know what was likely to happen next. Even experienced mothers would have needed markers of the various stages of the process, so that they would know how things were progressing.[21] Other aspects of the rites helped to designate the mother's special – and, if it was her first birth, rapidly changing – social role and status.[22] Still others made childbirth seem subject to the individual and collective wills of those involved, suggesting that the outcomes could be controlled, even when they could not. Of particular importance was the consoling presence of the other women themselves, many of whom would have successfully given birth and lived to raise children to adulthood.[23] Certainly an experienced midwife would

[19] See Gowing, *Common Bodies*, pp. 149–76. See also Pollock, "Childbearing and Female Bonding."

[20] Cressy, *Birth, Marriage, and Death*, pp. 16–28 and Jennifer Hellwarth, *The Reproductive Unconscious in Medieval and Early Modern England* (New York, NY: Routledge, 2002), pp. 1–24, 61–88.

[21] Howard notes the important role that time and duration played in many accounts of childbirth. See Howard, "Imagining the Pains and Perils," 377.

[22] Wilson argues that the rite marked a transition from one social role to another, although it was not necessarily a "rite of passage" in the classic anthropological sense. See Wilson, "Ceremony," in *Women as Mothers*, pp. 83–8.

[23] This is a central concern for Wilson, but even Pollock, who warns us not to overemphasize or romanticize the nurturing, sisterly aspects of the rites and shows how they could often have harsh, regulative purposes, admits that "pregnant women indisputably sought out and relied upon" the emotional and spiritual support of other women, both those who actually attended them and those who might offer advice before a birth or prayers during one. See Pollock, "Childbearing and Female Bonding," 290–3.

have been able to say that she had seen many women in similar circumstances and everything had come out well in the end for most.

This temporary and exclusively female ritual community, made up not only of friends and relations but possibly midwives in training, local aristocratic women with either a charitable or a political interest, and/or women brought by the midwife or by neighbors to help with various menial tasks,[24] was in several significant ways constructed along lines quite different from those of the community that normally surrounded the mother. As Wilson's earlier studies argued, it may have indeed been created in contrary reaction to the structure of the mother's normal life. The rites separated the pregnant, laboring, and recovering woman from her various other roles and responsibilities. Its enclosed space gave her a special status, making her the locus of household activities, the ordinary workings of which were taken out of her hands and given to her gossips and to some extent to her husband. She became the central concern of her temporary community of attendants for upwards of a month, and that community not only performed the various ritual activities of childbirth but also maintained her sequestration and guarded her special status. The female exclusivity of the rite may have actually created a carnivalesque inversion of the normal power dynamics of family and society, working in part as a hedge against, or as a temporary relief from, the pressures of the society's patriarchal structure.[25]

Even if we cannot be sure that childbirth practices did constitute a form of resistance or relief, it is clear that they were – unlike nearly everything else in early-modern English life – the almost unchallenged provenance of women. Men were of course involved in various ways, but usually at the periphery. They paid for things, often had a hand in choosing practitioners and inviting the gossips, but with the exception of surgeons brought in for emergencies and the occasional clergyman, few men actually entered the birthing chamber (or remained in it for very long). The rites themselves were therefore enacted within a space governed by its own female subcultural rules and customs. These, in addition, were handed down orally, and were largely unaffected by the dominant – and predominantly male – culture that surrounded them. As Wilson observes, although some men did complain in a resigned fashion, most men passively accepted the female domination of birth practices as natural and right (pervasive notions of female modesty, for example, demanded it).[26] A dynamic of grumbling

[24] See Pollock, "Childbearing and Female Bonding," 296.
[25] See, for example, Wilson, "Ceremony," in *Women as Mothers*, especially pp. 85–8.
[26] Wilson, "Ceremony," in *Women as Mothers*, pp. 81–3.

resignation in the context of wide acceptance is expressed throughout the surviving literature in many different ways: in plain descriptions and prescriptions, in satires warning prospective husbands and fathers about the expense and the disempowerment they could expect, and even in the uneasiness expressed by various authors of medical texts, midwifery handbooks, conduct books, and marriage sermons when they came to speak of what were over and again called "women's secrets."[27] It was also expressed, as Wilson has compellingly argued, in the reluctance of midwives and gossips to declare an obstructed birth impossible for them to remedy, necessitating the calling in of a male surgeon. Such a declaration was a tacit admission that the rites themselves and the female community that maintained them had failed. The extraction of an infant was, moreover, done only when it was concluded that the infant was dead, and it was accomplished by internal dismemberment and extraction through the vagina. Such surgical procedures, which Wilson identifies as a primary locus of obstetric anxiety, were nightmarish, and few women survived them, either because of the direct dangers of laceration and infection or because delays had already put them at risk by weakening their condition. Wilson argues that the reluctance itself, because it encouraged delays, may have led in many cases to the mother's needless death, but it is clear that the problem did not stem from ignorance or irresponsibility on the part of the birth attendants. It stemmed from their faith – seemingly vindicated in most cases – that the customs and dynamics of the female rites actually helped births to go easily.[28] In other words, much was at stake in female exclusivity, and women and midwives were loathe to give up the benefits of the woman's circle by rupturing it to allow a man to attend to a birth. Men, for their part, were reluctant to intrude. This only changed gradually toward the end of the seventeenth century, significantly altering only in the eighteenth with the rise of the male obstetric practitioner and eventually with the "medicalization" of what had been for ages almost completely a matter of social ritual.[29]

We know, from various accounts that have been preserved in the written records, that the oral subculture of the birthing chamber passed down

[27] See Audrey Eccles, "The Early Use of English for Midwiferies 1500–1700," *Neuphilologische Mitteilungen* 78 (1977), 377–85; Cressy, *Birth, Marriage, and Death*, pp. 39–41 and 55–9; Hellwarth, *The Reproductive Unconscious*, pp. 1–24; and Mendelson and Crawford, *Women in Early Modern England*, pp. 208–9.

[28] Wilson, "The Perils" and *The Making of Man-Midwifery*, pp. 33–8 and 49–53.

[29] See Wilson, *The Making of Man-Midwifery* for an extended account. See also Jean Donnison, *Midwives and Medical Men: a History of Inter-Professional Rivalries and Women's Rights* (New York, NY: Shocken, 1977).

various childbirth practices and beliefs that might be thought of as, if not subversive, then at least subaltern, suggesting that the rites were to some extent unaffected by some of the larger changes in the dominant culture. The rites of childbirth constituted what we might even call a sort of temporary (cyclically restored and dissolved) parallel church for the tending of the body and soul of the laboring woman. For example, as Cressy and others have observed, childbed rituals preserved a corpus of prayer with roots in Catholic practices and perhaps in even earlier non-Christian magical lore, well into the Protestant seventeenth century. The application of sympathetic magic in various forms was common, as was the application of saints' relics and the use of certain folk remedies based on various quasi-medical theories about the body and its behavior; such theories and magical practices often ran counter both to the emerging scientific culture of the age and to many of the central tenets of reformed Christianity. The customs of the birthing chamber even included the wholesale rewriting or adaptation of certain conventional prayers and biblical texts to the requirements of the mother's particular trials, suggesting energetic traditions of religious creativity that were sometimes in line and at other times at cross-purposes with prevailing theologies and ideologies.[30]

Commenting on this aspect of the rites, Cressy refers to the world of childbirth as constituting a distinctly "female subculture" that, as he puts it, "included intimate practices and beliefs that were barely suspected by husbands or priests, were long resistant to reform, and which remain virtually inaccessible to historians."[31] The final remark is an important warning that the record we are working from is incomplete. The practices that concern us were enacted as part of an oral culture that maintained a certain level of secrecy even in its own time, and it does not give up its mysteries very easily to the curious modern historian. As Cressy goes on to observe, most of what we must rely on in the written record was written from the "male point of view" and, therefore, "exploiting this evidence and seeing beyond its limits requires an unusual effort of empathy and imagination."[32] We will need to keep this warning in mind as we later attempt to expand that effort of empathy and imagination into the realm of literary practice, which was also, largely (but not exclusively) a matter of men coming to terms with what went on behind the veil of the lying-in chamber.

[30] One of the most striking examples of this is the adaptation of Psalm 22 printed in Bentley, *Monument*, pp. 109–12. See Carolyn Whitney-Brown, *Tudor and Stuart Birth Stories by Shakespeare and Others*, Doctoral Dissertation (Brown University, 1991), pp. 73–8; Otten, "Women's Prayers"; and the discussion below.

[31] Cressy, *Birth, Marriage, and Death*, p. 21. [32] Cressy, *Birth, Marriage, and Death*, p. 16.

CHAPTER 2

When things went wrong: maternal mortality and obstetric anxiety

Although in the majority of cases childbirth and its rites occurred predictably and with a positive outcome, the rate at which deadly or debilitating complications occured was relatively high, especially in London. The rites, in other words, were often maimed, and they were themselves designed to ward off thoughts of their own possible defeat. Fear of death in childbirth was a conscious part of peoples' lives, and it deeply affected both the ways in which they practiced the rites of the childbed and the ways in which they described and thought about those rites. This fear (for various reasons we will explore later) was, however, usually expressed in carefully managed terms.[1] We will therefore be less subject to the pitfalls of alarm, anachronism, or exaggeration for rhetorical effect if we search for indications, not of acute terror (although examples of that do exist, especially in crisis situations), but of managed anxiety, evidence of terror being kept at bay.[2]

Let us first look, however, at what historians have been able to tell us about maternal mortality itself and the ways in which it may have been perceived.

[1] Some recent research has suggested that we should abandon pessimistic or even alarmist interpretations of the evidence that survives (what Adrian Wilson calls the "fear thesis") and recognize that women did not go about their daily lives in constant terror of pregnancy and birth. He is clearly right in warning us against projecting our own shock and discomfort on people who lived day in and day out with particular conditions. In "The Perils of Early Modern Procreation: Childbirth With or Without Fear?," *British Journal for Eighteenth Century Studies* 16 (1993), 1–19, Wilson points out that the autobiographical literature we have from the period is more commonly full of expressions of religious equanimity in the face of suffering than it is of explicit expressions of fear. As we will see, however, such passages need to be read in light of the rhetorical decorum that governed their composition. See also Jennifer Hellwarth's argument that the rhetoric of fear found in handbooks and other texts may have been designed to create anxiety about birth in order to scare both mothers and their midwives into acquiescing to the authority of the men who composed such materials: Jennifer Hellwarth, *The Reproductive Unconscious in Medieval and Early Modern England* (New York, NY: Routledge, 2002), pp. 14–24. The approach may be correct in some instances, but it downplays the fact that women often did face circumstances that created acute anxiety as well as whatever genuine interest medical and religious writers may have had in alleviating suffering.

[2] The following general studies of fear in early modern Europe have been helpful: *Fear in Early Modern Society* eds. William G. Naphy and Penny Roberts (Manchester University Press, 1997); W. J. Bouwsma, "Anxiety and the Formation of Early Modern Culture," in *After the Reformation*,

Estimates have fluctuated over the past forty years or so, but the consensus among historians at this point is that in the course of the seventeenth century, even if rates for England as a whole were not quite as high as some earlier studies had suggested, rates in London were comparable with some of the highest rates recorded for any human community. In 1982, in *Obstetrics and Gynaecology in Tudor and Stuart England*, Audrey Eccles estimated that, according to pilot studies done in the 1970s, the rate of maternal mortality in early modern England might have reached as many as 25 deaths per 1,000 "birth events" (the term covers both live births and stillbirths). In other words, one woman died for every 40 births.[3] In 1971, Thomas Forbes had reported a rate of approximately 23.5 deaths per 1,000 baptisms for the years 1583–1599 in St. Bartolph's Parish, London.[4] Since this could only have included live births (stillborn infants were not baptized), it has made sense for historians to assume that the actual numbers were somewhat higher (stillbirths often brought with them fatal complications). In his D. Phil. thesis in 1982, Wilson, for example, trying to bring together early estimates of deaths in the case of live births with what he had gathered about stillbirths and other possibly fatal complications, arrived at a rate of as much as 30 per 1,000. That same year, B. M. Willmot Dobbie estimated from parish records in Somerset rates ranging from 24.4 to 29 per 1,000.[5] In 1986, however, Roger Schofield argued, in a widely influential essay entitled "Did the Mothers Really Die?," that the national rate was actually significantly lower. He based his study on statistics from 13 rural parishes and introduced a new and more accurate way of calculating the effect that the incidence of stillbirth may have had. Taking into account both his own findings and those of the previous studies, he concluded that:

> the "best" estimates suggest that the maternal mortality rate was just under 10 per 1,000 in the late sixteenth century, and just over that figure for the first half of the seventeenth century. The rate then jumps sharply upward to just under

ed. B. C. Malament (Manchester University Press, 1980); and Michael MacDonald, "*The Fearefull Estate of Francis Spira*: Narrative, Identity, and Emotion in Early Modern England," *Journal of British Studies* 31 (1992), 32–61.

[3] Audrey Eccles, *Obstetrics and Gynaecology in Tudor and Stuart England* (Kent, OH: Kent State University Press, 1982), p. 125. These early studies were based on examinations of contemporary Bills of Mortality. John Graunt's *Natural and Political Observations…Made upon the Bills of Mortality* (London, 1676), pp. 42–3, for example, provides an estimate of 15 maternal deaths per 1,000 births for the years 1631 and 1659. The numbers, however, refer only to women who actually died in labor, and Graunt points out that there were many reasons for a woman to die "within the Month." The number of women who died days or weeks after a birth from various complications would have been higher.

[4] Thomas Forbes, *Chronicle from Aldgate: Life and Death in Shakespeare's London* (New Haven, CT: Yale University Press, 1971), p. 106.

[5] Adrian Wilson, *Childbirth in Seventeenth and Eighteenth-Century England*, University of Sussex, D. Phil. Thesis (1982), p. 309; B. M. Willmott Dobbie, "An Attempt to Estimate the True Rate of Maternal Mortality, Sixteenth to the Eighteenth Centuries," *Medical History* 26 (1982), 79–90.

16 per 1,000 in the later seventeenth century, to fall back to just under 10 per 1,000 again in the first half of the eighteenth century.

The rates then dropped steadily to "between 5 and 6 per 1,000 in the early nineteenth century."[6] He notes, however, that the rates in London were some 30 to 50 percent higher than in the rural samples he worked with, reaching levels of over 20 per 1,000.[7] Wilson, drawing on Schofield and on some research of his own, later estimated that rates for different parts of England could fall anywhere between 10 and 20 per 1,000.[8] In his 1992 study of maternal mortality in Europe, the United States of America, and Australia, Irvine Loudon notes the same historical rise and fall of the rate as Schofield, estimating that, before the decline, maternal mortality in early modern England was about 15 to 16 per 1,000 in rural areas and about 21 in London.[9] More recently, David Cressy has concurred, noting both that rates increased in the course of the seventeenth century and that "conditions were always worse in London – sometimes twice the national rate."[10] These estimated rates are several hundred times higher than those typical today in the industrialized west, which average around 6 or 8 maternal deaths per *100,000* live births.[11] They are also some 2 to 5 times higher than is common in modern contexts where births regularly occur with no medical intervention, and a good deal higher than those regularly encountered in the developing world, even in nations experiencing considerable stress from economic deprivation, conflict, and/or natural disaster.[12]

6 "Did the Mothers Really Die? Three Centuries of Maternal Mortality in 'The World We Have Lost,'" in *The World We Have Gained: Histories of Population and Social Structure*, eds. Lloyd Bonfield, Richard Smith, and Keith Wrightson, (Oxford: Basil Blackwell, 1986), pp. 231–60, especially p. 250.

7 Schofield, "Did the Mothers Really Die?," in *The World We Have Gained*, p. 252.

8 See Wilson, "The Perils," 5, and *The Making of Man-Midwifery: Childbirth in England, 1600–1770* (Cambridge, MA: Harvard University Press, 1995), p. 19.

9 Irvine Loudon, *Death in Childbirth: an International Study of Maternal Care and Maternal Mortality, 1800–1950* (Oxford: Clarendon Press, 1992), p. 160. Loudon gives rates per 10,000. I have recalculated the rate to per 1,000 for easier comparison.

10 David Cressy, *Birth, Marriage, and Death: Ritual, Religion, and the Life-Cycle in Tudor and Stuart England* (Oxford University Press, 1997), pp. 30–1.

11 *United Nations Statistical Yearbook*, 38th edn. (New York, NY: United Nations, 1993), pp. 164, 167.

12 Loudon, *Death in Childbirth*, pp. 395–7. In a 1996 UNICEF study, only 27 out of the 144 countries surveyed showed rates of 900 per 100,000 or higher. The highest rates cited for that year were between 1,600 and 1,800 for Bhutan and parts of sub-Saharan Africa. An overview of the available statistics shows that, while modern rates can rise above 1,000 per 100,000, it is rare for rates to go much higher. The rate Loudon gives for London in the period under consideration, translated into the modern numbers, would be 2,100 per 100,000 births, but even Schofield's national rate of 1,000 per 100,000 is high given human historical experience. See UNICEF, *The Progress of Nations 1996*, "League Table of Maternal Death," at www.unicef.org/pon96/leag1wom.htm and the similar statistics in UNICEF, *Progress for Children: A Report Card on Maternal Mortality (No. 7)* (2008), pp. 44–7, at www.unicef.org/publications/files/Progress_for_Children-No._7_Lo-Res_082008.pdf [both last accessed March 10, 2009].

Historians are unsure just why rates rose in the seventeenth century and why they were worse in the city. It is clear, however, that most of the causes for high rates of maternal mortality that have been identified by modern social scientists were present in seventeenth-century London. According to the literature, there are, and always have been, three major *direct* causes of maternal death: (1) sepsis leading to puerperal fever; (2) toxemia, a condition in which the woman's body produces toxins that affect her nervous system and can result in the severe convulsions known as eclampsia; and (3) hemorrhaging.[13] All three of these conditions are treatable by modern medicine as long as the mother can get to a well-equipped hospital or clinic, and this is the primary reason that maternal mortality rates are so low in the developed world today. The literature also describes a set of *indirect* determinants, conditions that are likely to increase the rate of maternal mortality by either making the above conditions more common and/or by making them harder to treat: (1) maternal age (young women and older women are at higher risk, so the more women at either extreme who give birth in a given community, the higher the rate can be as a whole); (2) high parity (the more children a woman has already had at the time of a given birth, the higher her risk, so high fertility rates can contribute to higher mortality rates); (3) short birth intervals (the shorter the time between births, the higher the risk, so communities in which women tend to get pregnant again as soon as possible tend to have higher mortality rates); (4) lack of sufficient food for pregnant mothers (this creates situations in which women do not have the strength to cope with various complications, or in which pre-existing conditions create greater dangers); (5) cultural practices ranging from attitudes that keep women from seeking medical care to customs like female circumcision or infibulation that can expose women to additional risks; (6) lack of access to health care services (this could mean the absence of clinics or hospitals, or problems with transportation to such institutions); and (7) lack of trained obstetric practitioners (either because they are not well distributed geographically, because their training is substandard, or because there simply are none).[14] The presence of the first five of these determinants is likely to create more cases of the three direct causes. In the cases of the last two,

[13] Loudon notes that puerperal fever has historically been the most common cause. See London, *Death in Childbirth*, pp. 43, 77–9, 534–41 and *Childbed Fever: a Documentary History* (New York, NY: Garland, 1995).

[14] I have derived this list from several different studies: Bimal Kanti Paul, "Maternal Mortality in Africa: 1980–87," *Social Science & Medicine*, 37 (1993), 745–52; T. K. Sundari, "The Untold Story: How the Health Care Systems in Developing Countries Contribute to Maternal Mortality," *International Journal of Health Services*, 22 (1992), 513–28; Sereen Thaddeus and Deborah Maine, "Too Far to Walk: Maternal Mortality in Context," *Social Science & Medicine* 38 (1994), 1091–110.

preventable deaths are simply not prevented because of a number of systemic failures (bad roads, no medical schools, few hospitals, lack of funds, etc.).

As I said, most of these factors were present in seventeenth-century London, although some appreared in different forms. It should be obvious, for example, that the medicine of the day was unable to cope with severe infections, toxemia, or hemorrhaging. Women who experienced these conditions usually died, and little could be done to prevent their deaths. Some practitioners were, however, able to handle certain other complications – like those stemming from malpresentations – in ways that could have, and sometimes did, keep a woman from becoming infected or bleeding to death. Podalic version, for example, was known to be highly effective in cases of breech birth,[15] and since such a technique could help a woman avoid two of the most common causes of death, it is clear that the abilities of the practitioner could be a crucial factor when it came to some obstetric crises. But at this point, cultural factors took over. Certain aspects of the way most midwives practiced kept some of them from gaining knowledge of or expertise in such helpful techniques. Certain aspects of the childbirth rites themselves also militated against the bringing in of surgeons who might have been able to help. It was surgeons – practicing over a wider area than most midwives and only in emergency cases – who often knew and became expert in these techniques, but they were often brought in too late to remedy a situation. As Wilson has compellingly argued, such male surgeons were the objects of very acute fear since most women knew that their midwife was only likely to call upon one of them when she herself had given up on her, her infant, or both. Midwives and other female birth attendants were understandably loathe to give up on the women in their care and admit that they could not be saved by ordinary means. Wilson goes so far as to argue that the arrival of the male practitioner was "the real location of fear in early modern childbirth."[16]

Practitioners with experience in complications railed against such delays and against some of the actual practices of ordinary midwives. As we saw, some practitioners (e.g. Willughby), attacked practices that, as Eccles observes, may have derived from the recommendations of the single most influential midwifery handbook for the earlier part of the period, *The Birth of Man-kinde*, which for a long time was one of the few texts available to a literate midwife or surgeon.[17] Given the danger of infection, even more

[15] Eccles, *Obstetrics and Gynaecology*, pp. 115–17.

[16] Wilson, "The Perils," 14 and *The Making of Man-Midwifery*, pp. 33–8 and 49–53.

[17] Eccles, *Obstetrics and Gynaecology*, pp. 11–12, 86–8 and "The Early Use of English for Midwiferies 1500–1700," *Neuphilologische Mitteilungen* 78 (1977), 377–85.

troubling than the "hailings" and "pullings" recommended in the book is the fact that it recommends over and over again ointments made out of animal fats, especially "Hens...Ducks...[and] Goose greace" for "annointing" the "private" or "secret" parts, and even for insertion into the uterus through the vagina on a sponge.[18] Eccles notes, ironically, that because the practices were recommended in the book, it might have been, at least in the earlier period, "the better educated and more consciously professional midwife who learned them."[19]

In any case, the pains that may have been caused by practitioners were not always considered preventable. Many women may have even lacked an incentive to demand that midwives change their situations. Eccles argues, for example, that the use of such practices as those recommended in *The Birth of Man-kinde* may have been sustained by a sort of "cult of difficulty" among middle-class women who believed that difficult birth was a sign of greater cultural and spiritual refinement.[20] Many otherwise normal births may have been, as a result, more torturous and disfiguring than they had to be for some middle class women precisely because they saw themselves as belonging to a virtuous social class, and simply expected their births to be that way. The following quotation from Jane Sharp's *The Midwives Book* articulates some of the beliefs that underlay this index of pain and virtue:

> Child-bearing is so dangerous that the pain must needs be great, and if any feel but a little pain it is commonly harlots who are so used to it that they make little reckoning of it, and are wont to fare better at present than vertuous persons do, but they will one day give an account for it if they continue impenitent, and be condemned to a torment of hell which far surpasses all pains in Child birth, yet these doubtless are the greatest of all pains women usually undergo upon Earth.[21]

[18] See, Thomas Raynalde, *The Birth of Man-kinde* (London, 1626), pp. 98–9.

[19] Eccles, *Obstetrics and Gynaecology*, p. 88.

[20] See Eccles, *Obstetrics and Gynaecology*, pp. 88–90.

[21] Jane Sharp, *The Midwives Book* (London, 1671), p. 170. Sharp's handbook was the first published in English by a practicing female midwife (she claims to have been practicing for thirty years). Some other texts explained the discrepancy between upper-and lower-class women in more strictly physical terms. Thomas Willis, for example, did note that "poor Women, Hirelings, Rusticks...also Viragoes, and Whores...bring forth without great difficulty," while wealthier women "as tho they partak'd of the Divine Curse after a more severe manner, *bring forth in Pain*." However, he then goes on to explain that the difference had more to do with the fact that lower-class women got more exercise: see Thomas Willis, *The London Practice of Physick* (London, 1685), pp. 631–2. This passage is from the 1685 translation of a chapter on childbed fevers that Willis added to the second edition of his Latin treatise, *De Febribus*. See *Diatribae duae Medico-philosophicae, Quarum prior agit de Fermentatione sive De motu intestino particularum in quovis corpore. Altera De Febribus...* (London, 1660), pp. 277–8. Eccles quotes the English passage, but misses the force of Willis' "as tho" (Eccles, *Obstetrics and Gynaecology*, p. 90).

So it is possible that middle- and upper-class women had, to some extent, if not an incentive to undergo pain then at least an explanation for why they underwent it, one that flattered their sense of class identity. This may have kept them from demanding midwives who could promise a reduction in pain. An unintended result may have been an increase in the number of infections and hemorrhages.

Birth was, in addition, experienced under highly septic conditions, the densely populated city providing a breeding ground for highly infectious diseases such as influenza, smallpox, tuberculosis, and plague. This made London a particularly hostile environment in which to be pregnant. As modern researchers have established, pregnant women undergo a period of depressed immunity in the third trimester called PAID ("pregnancy-associated immune deficiency syndrome"). The depression is not very great, but is possibly just significant enough to have raised the mortality rate in London.[22] It might be best, in fact, to think of London itself as a primary indirect cause of its own higher rates of maternal mortality, although it is difficult to say to what extent people were aware of this at the time.[23] The city was experiencing phenomenal population growth, mostly a result of migration rather than a high birth rate, and this caused a disruption of many basic economic, social, and religious relations, as well as a great strain on whatever public infrastructure could be held in place. The very bad septic conditions, the overcrowding, and the attendant massive outbreaks of plague and other infectious diseases clearly must have created a backdrop of greater risk.[24]

In addition, high parity rates and short birth intervals were commonplace, especially among upper-class women who did not usually nurse their own children. These women also tended to marry young and continue giving birth as long as they could into middle age, and this put them at risk both early and late in their procreative careers. It is hard to say, however,

[22] Schofield, "Did the Mothers Really Die?," in *The World We Have Gained*, p. 254. Andrew Wear, *Knowledge and Practice in Early Modern English Medicine, 1550–1680* (Cambridge University Press, 2000), p. 280 notes that at the time many believed pregnancy predisposed a women to contracting the plague.

[23] Wear notes, however, that people were aware that the city offered a far less healthy environment than the countryside: see Andrew Wear, "Making Sense of Health and the Environment in Early Modern England," in *Medicine in Society: Historical Essays* (Cambridge University Press, 1992), pp. 130–7.

[24] Some historians have suggested that a vitamin D deficiency may have led to a higher than average rate of childhood rickets among both urban and upper-class women, and therefore to a higher rate of obstructed labors due to pelvic malformations in the mother. See Eccles, *Obstetrics and Gynaecology*, pp. 126–7. Wilson, however, notes that this was probably not a big factor in the *different* rates of upper-and lower-class women (*Childbirth*, pp. 21–2). Loudon is uncertain about how much rickets affected maternal mortality, but notes that it may have had some effect (*Death in Childbirth*, pp. 143, 445–58).

how large and how visible this difference was. Roger Finlay's figures show, in any case, that marital fertility was relatively high across class lines, even if the rates for upper-class women were somewhat higher.[25]

Of the determining factors I have mentioned as probable causes for the high rates of maternal mortality in the seventeenth century, high fertility rates, relatively short birth intervals, continuous births throughout the fertile years, and the practices and technical competence of birth attendants and practitioners seem to have been the ones of particularly acute importance across class and geographical lines. They were merely exacerbated in the city, and perhaps also among upper-class women. Loudon's suggestion that the "significant rise in the number, status, skill, and efficiency" of English midwives in the latter part of the period was the most important reason for the rapid *decline* in the maternal mortality rate after the late seventeenth century supports this general conclusion.[26] In the late sixteenth and early seventeenth centuries, the rites of childbirth worked in a way that allowed mortality rates to remain at a reasonably high, but not extraordinarily high, level. In the city, however, and to a lesser extent all across England from the mid seventeenth century until early in the eighteenth century, certain disrupting conditions came into play that significantly increased the rate. At the same time, however, other factors began to have the opposite effect. Reorganization, dissemination of printed knowledge, and increased literacy worked to reduce the rates as midwives came to understand better how to handle dangerous complications. All of this began to happen well before the medicalization and masculinization of obstetrics had any profound effect on maternal mortality. Most historians agree that by the time childbirth ceased to be a social ritual and became a medical procedure, it was already well on the way to becoming much safer than it had been. The positive effects of medicalization itself were not felt until much later.

[25] The mean fertility rate for married London women of the wealthier classes was approximately 1 birth per interval of just under 2 years (23 months) from the date of marriage to the end of a woman's period of fertility, with some sets of statistics yielding mean intervals as short as 20.5 months. Finlay notes that the rate was only slightly lower for lower-class women (27 months) because they nursed their own children. See Roger Finlay, *Population and Metropolis: the Demography of London 1580–1650* (Cambridge University Press, 1981), pp. 133–50. See also Dorothy McLaren, "Marital Fertility and Lactation 1570–1720," in *Women in English Society 1500–1800*, ed. Mary Prior (London: Methuen, 1986), pp. 22–53. McLaren was uncertain about how much high fertility affected maternal mortality, and she doubted Dobbie's calculations. The rates do, however, figure in Schofield's calculations.

[26] Loudon, *Death in Childbirth*, p. 161. See also Cressy, *Birth, Marriage, and Death*, pp. 35–41.

THE PERCEPTION OF OBSTETRIC RISK

The most important questions for our purposes, however, are what all of this meant for the experience and perceptions of particular women in the period, and how such experiences and perceptions were reflected in the texts, especially the literary texts, that have survived. In answering such questions, we should first note that because more women died in the city, and because the literate and literary culture of the period was largely an urban culture centered in London, we may expect that to whatever extent this culture responded to death in childbed, it was responding to the highest levels experienced in the period, especially as the seventeenth century wore on. Milton's career, for example, was spent almost entirely in and around London, and the years with which we are concerned (between the early 1630s to the later 1660s) are the years in which the rates rose sharply.

Schofield offers a few other useful statistics that may be applied more widely to England as a whole, as well as to London, and they can help us to fix our attention on the factors that would have affected the perception and ultimately the representation of childbed risks. Schofield estimates that, given what we know about marital fertility rates, and given a maternal mortality rate of 10 per 1,000, a woman in early modern England "on average would have run about a 6 to 7 percent risk of dying in childbed at some point in her procreative career."[27] Assuming a rate of about 20 for London in the later seventeenth century, this means that the lifetime risk a woman might have run in the city would have been somewhat higher, about 12 to 14 percent.

But how would women have perceived such risks? Would they have even been aware of them? They obviously would not have had access to statistical calculations, and as Schofield notes, they would not have been likely to think in terms of something as abstract as lifetime risk. He suggests that it is more likely that they evaluated their risks "afresh toward the end of each pregnancy."[28] As Wilson's work has shown, several factors, as we might reasonably assume, would have greatly affected a woman's state of mind about a coming birth. Most important among these would have been her present state of health. For a reasonably healthy woman, however, a particularly important factor as the time of a birth actually neared would

[27] Schofield, "Did the Mothers Really Die?," in *The World We Have Gained*, pp. 258–9. This is assuming that a woman experienced about 6 to 7 full-term pregnancies in her life time. In individual cases, of course, women could have had more children, or less, and this would have affected their lifetime risks. How that affected their *perceptions* of risk is hard to say.

[28] Schofield, "Did the Mothers Really Die?," in *The World We Have Gained*, pp. 259–60.

have been the possibility that particular complications might emerge. The thing women feared more than anything else in the early stages of a pregnancy was miscarriage. In the later stages, they feared obstructions, malpresentations, and stillbirths. The first two of these late-stage complications were known to make very likely one of two related results: (1) the death of the infant and (2) the need for a surgical procedure to remove that infant. The third also often required a surgical removal. Most women knew that all three involved not only the death of the child, but probably their own as well.[29]

A woman's perceptions of risk would also have been affected by how often she saw other women die. Schofield, for example, notes that in his data set, "averaged over all age groups there were 1.3 deaths per year per 1,000 women of reproductive age." In a hypothetical village of 1,000 *inhabitants*, containing about 250 women between the ages of 15 and 49, "the death of a fellow villager in childbed would" have occurred on average once every three years. Another thing that might have affected women's perceptions of obstetric risk as they went from birth to birth was their age. They might very well have been aware that risk of death changed with age, although they might not have gathered from their experience a wholly accurate picture of how that risk was really distributed. For example, young women (under 20) and older women (over 40) ran the greatest risks of dying in childbed, but it may not have seemed so to women at the time. It was among women between the ages of 25–34 – years that were actually less risky individually – that maternal mortality would have been most visible. Since more women gave birth during those years, there were more actual deaths to be witnessed among them, and it may have seemed that most women died in childbed in the middle of their reproductive years, rather than at the beginning or the end. For example, given what we know about the average age at which most women married, and about marital fertility over the course of women's lives as a whole, in a hypothetical group of 1,000 *women* of various ages giving birth each year, a woman in her teens would have died only once every ten years, a woman in her forties once every three. On the other hand, about three women between the ages of 25 and 34 might have died *each* year. Schofield notes that because of this distribution, women may have had a somewhat distorted sense of how their risks might have changed as they aged,[30] but

[29] See Wilson's argument in "The Perils." See also Raymond A. Anselment, *Realms of Apollo: Literature and Healing in Seventeenth-Century England* (Newark, NJ: University of Delaware Press, 1995), pp. 49–68.

[30] Schofield, "Did the Mothers Really Die?," in *The World We Have Gained*, pp. 257–9. It was known that the risk was greater for *very* young women. See, for example, the warning in *The Birth of Mankinde* about women younger than "twelve or fifteen years of age" (Raynalde, *The Birth*, p. 91).

it is clear enough that since most women had most of their children in the years between 25 and 34, their sense of risk, though slightly skewed from a statistical perspective, would have matched their experience reasonably well, rising when they were most fully engaged in reproductive life and falling as they disengaged from it in their later years. This would have been so even if, strictly speaking, they were at greater risk of dying in each birth as they aged.[31]

Schofield also suggests that we try to imagine how a woman might have thought about her possible death in childbirth against the backdrop of the risks she ran of dying from other causes. A woman's chances of dying from any number of other causes unrelated to childbirth, especially from infectious diseases, was, according to Schofield, "between 7 and 16 per 1,000, depending on her age."[32] This was no greater in any given year between births than the risk most pregnant women ran of dying when they came to term. Schofield therefore suggests cautiously that against the background of general mortality, death in childbirth may not have stood out enough to be the cause of any very specific or high level of anxiety.[33] However, beyond pointing out that childbirth was probably less risky on the whole than many historians had up to that time suggested, Schofield does not make any conclusive claims about how the risk was perceived. He himself notes, as I said before, that "it is doubtful whether people in the past thought in terms of probabilities cumulated over a span of years." Therefore, his suggestion that a woman might think about her possible death against the backdrop of general mortality seems just as unlikely, given that it too would have depended on a knowledge of statistical probabilities rather than on the raw confrontation with a possible death.

As Mendelson and Crawford have rightly observed, despite what might have been only a 6 to 7 percent lifetime risk, or as low as a 1 percent risk, in any given birth (although perhaps twice these figures in London), women clearly calculated their sense of risk in simpler and more immediate terms.[34]

[31] Wear points out that maternal mortality would have accounted for up to 20 percent of all female deaths between the ages of 25 and 34 (about 11 to 14 percent of women of reproductive ages older than that and younger) (*Knowledge and Practice*, p. 13). These were the ages in which women's general mortality rate was at its lowest (most women – and men for that matter – died at earlier and later ages). There were fewer deaths overall among these women, and for 20 percent of those to have been from a specific and highly distinctive cause is significant.

[32] Schofield, "Did the Mothers Really Die?," in *The World We Have Gained*, p. 260. As Cressy notes, general mortality rates tended to hover around 25 per 1,000, with rates reaching 35 per 1,000 in particularly bad seasons (*Birth, Marriage, and Death*, p. 380).

[33] Schofield, "Did the Mothers Really Die?," in *The World We Have Gained*, pp. 259–60.

[34] Sara Mendelson and Patricia Crawford, *Women in Early Modern England 1550–1720* (Oxford: Clarendon Press, 1998), p. 152.

Many found themselves having to manage very acute anxieties; some expressed them in muted terms, others more directly. Even Schofield's estimate of 10 deaths per 1,000 births (a death every three years in his hypothetical village) would have meant that most people approaching a childbirth of their own or within their immediate family would have known someone who had died in childbirth within very recent memory. A young woman in her early twenties facing her first birth might have known as many as three women who died in her village or her neighborhood since she was about twelve. We cannot so easily discount, on the basis of real statistical risk, the sort of effect that kind of experience would have had on a young woman's consciousness, especially given that she might have been quite closely associated with one or more of the events. Her mother might have been one of the gossips, for example, or the deceased might have been a relative. She might have heard eyewitness accounts of what must have seemed horrifying to those who participated, given that the death might have involved a prolonged, obstructed labor, hemorrhaging, fever, or some terrible surgical procedure.[35] The risk of dying in childbirth was also, we must remember, an added risk, laid on top of the general risk, a risk specific to women and therefore a part of their self-conception as distinct from men. It was also a risk that always shadowed a family's highest hopes and greatest joys. It might seem to a modern demographer from the numbers alone that maternal mortality would disappear into the backdrop of a high general rate of mortality (one that is already hard for modern readers to imagine living with), but as Loudon reminds us:

> deaths in childbirths were always different from other deaths. Childbirth was the only major cause of mortality that was not a disease, and in that way it stood apart. It was always a tragedy…a sudden and brutal disruption of a family.[36]

One example should suffice to illustrate what Loudon means. In the memoir he composed while in exile during the 1650s, Gervase Holles describes his state of mind before and after the death of his first wife, Dorothy, in 1635. After briefy recounting the presumably uneventful births of his first and second children, he goes on for several pages about the painful shock that attended Dorothy's death while giving birth to their third. He claims to have dreamed the night before that his wife would give birth to a daughter and that both would die. The dream connects what

[35] See, for example, Alice Thornton's account of the death of her sister, who died giving birth to her sixteenth child when Alice was nineteen. Alice Thornton, *The Autobiography of Mrs. Alice Thornton*, ed. Charles Jackson, Surtees Society (Durham: Andrews and Co., 1875), vol. LXII, pp. 49–53. See below.

[36] Loudon, *Death in Childbirth*, p. 164.

would happen the next day with Gervase's memory of his own mother, who, like his wife, died giving birth to *her* third child when he himself was about one year old (in both cases, the children, both of them also daughters, died as well). This suggests that the "surprise" of his wife's death was a matter of its shock to his hopes, as well as the sheer shock of the loss itself, rather than a response to its rarity. Holles fills several pages with an account of the dream, the birth and death, and with remembrances of his wife, including a set of elegies written for her by others. He then goes on to explain how this loss, which he says was "not courted from [him] by any ling'ring sicknes but ravished away before [he] could suspect [he] should have been so miserable" afflicted him "strangely." He reports that he was "scarse able to move out of dores" for nearly three months.[37]

In her fascinating study of late sixteenth and early seventeenth-century tomb sculptures for women who died in childbirth, Judith Hurtig noted that such specific funereal sculptures appeared on English tombs for the first time during this period. She shows how a particular iconography was developed for the depiction of the deaths of a wide range of middle- and upper-class women, suggesting that the sudden appearance of such tomb sculptures and their apparent popularity indicates "a time when childbirth and its perils appear to have been the subject of particular concern and anxiety."[38] Hurtig also briefly notes, and I will explore this material in some depth in the next section, that it is in this period that private devotional texts and prayer collections like Bentley's first began to include prayers specifically designed for women in childbirth, as well as for birth attendants and for family and friends who watched and waited anxiously.[39]

As Linda Pollock has argued, we must also remember that women had "several long months" in which to contemplate what was to come, and that they were, as I said before, quite aware that, should anything go seriously wrong, their chances of survival were slim.[40] As a result, Mendelson and

[37] Gervase Holles, *Memorials of the Holles Family 1493–1656*, eds. A. C. Wood and B. Litt (London: Offices of the Royal Historical Society, 1937), pp. 230–5. For further details, see A. C. Wood, "The Holles Family," *Transactions of the Royal Historical Society*, (London: Offices of the Society, 1936) 4th series, vol. XIX, pp. 145–65. I am grateful to Stuart Clark for suggesting this reference.

[38] Judith W. Hurtig, "Death in Childbirth: Seventeenth-Century English Tombs and Their Place in Contemporary Thought," *The Art Bulletin*, 65 (1983), 603–15. Hurtig's article is the first that I am aware of that mentions Milton's epitaph in connection with the general culture of childbed suffering. Anselment also discusses tomb sculptures and paintings of deceased mothers and newborns (*Realms of Apollo*, pp. 49–50).

[39] Hurtig, "Seventeenth-Century English Tombs," 613–14.

[40] Linda A. Pollock, "Embarking on a Rough Passage: the Experience of Pregnancy in Early-Modern Society," in *Women as Mothers in Pre-Industrial England: Essays in Memory of Dorothy McLaren*, ed. Valerie Fildes (London: Routledge, 1990), pp. 47–8.

Crawford conclude, perhaps a bit too bluntly but I think accurately enough, that "during every pregnancy, each woman feared her own death."[41] The fact that most of the childbed prayers collected in Bentley's *Monument of Matrones* – to take one particularly large set of examples – paraphrase Genesis 3:16 with some added intensity clearly demonstrates the point that *mortality*, not simply sorrow or pain, was always understood as part and parcel of the women's childbed condition. The surviving texts (diaries, letters, prayers, sermons, handbooks, etc.) are, in addition, full of stark statements like the following, quoted in Mendelson and Crawford's study from Mary Carey's correspondence with her husband: "I am now near the time of my travail and am very weak, faint, sickly, fearful, pained, apprehending much suffering before me, if not death itself, the King of Terrors."[42]

Even more common are the less direct and more carefully managed terms one finds in many religious texts. Here, for example, is a passage from one of the set prayers in Bentley's collection, where a woman is directed quite explicitly to pray for the strength *not* to feel fear. After acknowledging that the pains she is about to experience are richly deserved, given her sinfulness, she also reminds herself of God's great love and mercy:

> Wherefore, oh most merciful father, I am bold to run presentlie vnto thee with all my trust, hope and confidence, that thou hast giuen me, praieng and beseeching thee, for thy great mercies sake, for thine infallible promise and truth sake, which neuer faile anie that put their trust in thee…that thy clemency may refresh and restore in me, that which my sins haue hindered and corrupted; and either take from me the great labour and dangerous trauell that my sins have deserued, & the feare that it hath brought me into for the same, so that I shall not need such power and strength, such care and industrie as my corruption now seeketh and requireth; or else to qualifie, mitigate and order all my throwes, paines, pangs, and pinches of this my child-birth, that the trauell thereof doo not surmount, nor ouercome my strength, further than thou, oh father wilt make mee able to beare, & endure the same, or else encrease my strength, encourage my mind, and fortifie my senses so, that I may without mistrust, despaire, or grudging against thy maiestie, beare the labour to the end.[43]

The woman figured as the speaker of this prayer (the prayer represents and offers this speaker as a religious subject position to any woman preparing

[41] Mendelson and Crawford, *Women in Early Modern England*, p. 152.

[42] Mendelson and Crawford, *Women in Early Modern England*, p. 152, and Mendelson's "Stuart Women's Diaries and Occasional Memoirs," in *Women in English Society*, pp. 196–7. Anselment, *Realms of Apollo*, pp. 57–8, notes how often a mother's fear of her own death combined with fear that her infant might die.

[43] Thomas Bentley, *The Monument of Matrones: Conteining Seuen Seuerall Lamps of Virginity* (London, 1582), p. 103.

herself for childbirth) is worried that the pain and the danger will be so bad that she will lose sight of God's love and mercy, and that this will confirm her sinfulness and make her more deserving of punishment than of a vindicating trial. She does not ask that the pain and danger be removed or mitigated because she is simply scared of them directly. She is primarily worried about what they might make her feel or say or do in relation to God. She is worried that the trial will be beyond the capacity of her faith in His goodness, and that her reaction will be despair or rebellion. As another prayer in the volume puts it, she fears being "swallowed vp of greefe and sorrowe,"[44] states of mind and spirit that might lead to her being swallowed up in death and damnation. She asks to have less to fear, or, barring that, for the strength to face a painful death as just, fitting, and good. The state a woman wished to achieve was one of poised acceptance and confidence in a coming salvation:

> Thus O Lord I me in thy will
> doo put, eke wholie in thy hand,
> I will not once swarue from thy skill,
> to die, or liue, to fall, or stand, Amen.[45]

A woman confident in God could free herself from worry, but achieving such confidence was not an easy matter. Expressions of calm, confident acceptance were themselves often evidence of significant anxiety, signs of a struggle to overcome what was recognized not simply as a physical peril but as a great *spiritual* peril.

Anxiety was also expressed in the interest people took in stories about spiritually heroic women who died with their faith intact. Such interest is amply attested to by the popularity of such public expressions of fortitude as those found in "maternal deathbed" books like Elizabeth Jocelin's *The Mother's Legacie to Her Unborne Childe*, which tells of how Elizabeth, feeling early in her pregnancy that she was going to die, calmly bought herself a winding sheet and prepared a book of religious teaching for the child she was about to bear. As she believed she would, she did die of "a violent fever" about nine days after giving birth to a daughter.[46] We can also see this interest expressed in such memorial volumes as those published by Phillip Stubbes and William Crashawe in honor of their wives. Both spend a great deal of time

[44] Bentley, *Monument*, p. 107. [45] Bentley, *Monument*, p. 106.

[46] Elizabeth Jocelin, *The Mother's Legacie to Her Unborne Childe* (London, 1624). This and other books like it were highly popular. Jocelin's book went into eight editions between 1624 and 1684. See Betty S. Travitsky's introduction to the volume of *Mother's Advice Books* in *The Early Modern Englishwoman: Printed writings, 1500–1640*, (Burlington, VT: Ashgate, 2000) Series 1, Part 2, vol. VIII and Sylvia Monica Brown's *Women's Writing in Stuart England: the Mother's Legacies of Dorothy Leigh, Elizabeth Joscelin, and Elizabeth Richardson* (Thrupp: Sutton Publishing, 1999).

recounting the perfect faith these women manifested as they neared death, and both volumes were published to provide other women with spiritually heroic exemplars.[47] To provide a more private example, Alice Thornton, in her memoir, spends a good deal of time recounting the poise and religious equanimity with which her older sister Catherine faced her death in childbed. She spends more time on that, in fact, than she does on the circumstances of the death itself. Her sister died in 1645 while giving birth to her sixteenth child (she lost six of them in mid-term miscarriages brought on, Alice thought, by falls). Catherine's behavior made a strong impression on her younger sister, who was about nineteen years old at the time and as yet unmarried, and Alice clearly modeled her own reactions to her later childbed sufferings on what she took to be her sister's edifying example:

> Affter exceeding sore travill she was delivered of a goodly son about August 3d, by one dame Sworre...This childe came double into the world, with such extreamity that she was exceedingly tormented with paines, so that she was deprived of the benefitt of sleepe for fourteen daies, except a few frightfull slumbers; neither could she eate any thing for her nourishment as usuall. Yett still did she spend her time in discourse of goodnesse excelently pieous, godly, and religeous, instructing her children and servants, and prepairing her soule for her deere Redeemer, as it was her saing she should not be long for Him.[48]

Alice goes on for another three pages describing Catherine's piety, including an account of how her own "grief and sorrow" brought her "into a very weak condition," making it necessary for her mother and a serving woman to come and relieve Alice of caring for her sister, sending her home. Alice even tells us that Catherine was inspired by the intensity of her religious feeling to utter, "in a manner," prophecies about the future of the kingdom, even going so far as to pray for "our enimies" (the Thorntons were Royalists), "for they stood in need of our praiers for the forgivenesse of all their evills."[49]

A close association of childbirth with death shows up in the culture in any number of other ways as well. For example, William Perkins' widely read

[47] Phillip Stubbes, *A Chrystall Glasse, for Christian Women* (London, 1591); William Crashawe, *The Honovr of Vertve or the Monument erected by the sorowfull Husband* (London, 1620). Crashawe contains one of the most extensive collections of elegies we have on the occasion of a maternal death.

[48] Thornton, *Autobiography*, pp. 49–53. See also Sharon Howard, "Imagining the Pain and Peril of Seventeenth Century Childbirth: Travail and Deliverance in the Making of an Early Modern World," *Social History of Medicine* 16 (2003), 367–82, especially 370–2 and Lucinda McCray Beier, *Sufferers and Healers: the Experience of Illness in Seventeenth-Century England* (London: Routledge and Kegan Paul, 1987), pp. 234–5.

[49] Thornton, *Autobiography*, p. 51. The twelfth of the meditations that John Oliver offers for women nearing a birth similarly suggests that a woman's suffering could confer a powerful spiritual and moral authority: John Oliver, *A Present for Teeming Women* (London, 1663), p. 57.

spiritual handbook for the dying, *A Salve for a Sicke Man*, has the following subtitle: "*A treatise containing the nature, differences, and kindes of death; as also the right manner of dying well. And It may serue for spirituall instruction to 1. Mariners when they goe to sea. 2. Souldiers when they goe to battell. 3. Women when they travell of child.*"[50] It is also, surely, no coincidence, as Heather Dubrow has pointedly noted, that the "Form of Solemnization of Matrimony" in the *Book of Common Prayer* should contain a prayer for fertility that, without pause, becomes in the end a prayer for long life:

> O MERCIFUL Lord and Heavenly Father, by whose gracious gift mankind is increased: We beseech thee assist with thy blessing these two persons, that they may both be fruitful in procreation of children, and also live together so long in godly love and honesty, that they may see their children's children, unto the third and fourth generation, unto thy praise and honor; through Jesus Christ our Lord. Amen.[51]

MORBIDITY AND MENTAL ILLNESS

Factors other than death must also be taken into account if we are to understand fully the ways in which women confronted the pain and danger of childbirth. For example, the frequency and difficulty of birth in early modern England caused a great deal of sickness among women, who were far more often sick than men, and often chronically so. Ralph Josselin's diary contains a fascinating account of his wife's various illnesses over the course of their long and fertile marriage. Jane lived to a ripe old age having experienced at least 15 pregnancies.[52] Ralph, who paid a great deal of attention to his own health and to that of his family members, recorded 131 instances in which Jane was ill during the first 22 years of their marriage (her child-bearing years). At least 73 of these were directly the results of pregnancy or childbirth, and many others were probably indirectly related. In her final 20 years, however, after she stopped giving birth, he recorded only 17.[53]

Obstetrical practices that led to permanent disfiguration were also very common in the period. A certain amount of tearing of the perineal tissues is

[50] William Perkins, *A Salve for a Sicke Man* (Cambridge, 1595).

[51] *The Book of Common Prayer, 1559: the Elizabethan Prayer Book* ed. John E. Booty (Charlottesville, VA: University Press of Virginia for the Folger Shakespeare Library, 1976), p. 296. The conjunction is preserved in later versions. Heather Dubrow notes this conflation in *A Happier Eden: The Politics of Marriage in the Stuart Epithalamium* (Ithaca, NY: Cornell University Press, 1990), p. 120.

[52] *The Diary of Ralph Josselin: 1616–1683* ed., Alan Macfarlane (London: For the British Academy by Oxford University Press, 1976). See Beier's discussion in *Sufferers and Healers*, pp. 182–210.

[53] See Alan Macfarlane, *The Family Life of Ralph Josselin, a Seventeenth-Century Clergyman: an Essay on Historical Anthropology* (Cambridge University Press, 1970), pp. 81–9. See also Alice Thornton's account of her own experiences (*Autobiography*, pp. 49–53, 84–98, 123–7, 139–67) and Beier's discussion in *Sufferers and Healers*, pp. 231–5.

common in normal childbirth, but little could be done at the time to help such tears to heal smoothly, and the sorts of strains that accompanied abnormal births as well as the techniques some midwives used to hasten or "ease" a birth could turn an otherwise normal situation into a nightmare. Willughby, for example, gives some terrifying accounts of cases in which he and his sister (his partner in the practice and later a midwife on her own) were called in to aid women who were harmed by what he thought were disturbingly common practices:

> Let all cruelties, as cutting of children in pieces in the mother's womb, with all violent wayes in every difficult labour, bee forborn. For it retardeth the births, and, oft lacerating the body of the woman, maketh her paines intolerable, which renders her so weake, and heartles, that shee hath no strength left to endure her throws, and the child's enforcements. Whosoever useth such harshnes, may well be branded with cruelty, and ignorance in midwifery.
>
> A London midwife, very officious, endeavouring to have a speedy delivery, through haling, and stretching those tender parts, made a labour of long continuance, and, with her halings, a breach about an inch long into the fundament. With this affliction the woman was much disquieted. For ever afterward her excrements came forth by the birth place; yet this woman did much commend her laborious midwife, and said that shee took great paines to deliver her, to save her life.
>
> This fact was done in Fleet-street. The woman came to mee for help, and shewed me her torn body.

The injuries suffered in a difficult birth could follow a woman for years as a permanent disfiguration, one that could make her subsequent births even more frightening and painful. Willughby goes on to recommend, for this reason, that if a woman can endure the kind of problem he describes, it is better to leave it than to cure it:

> Where this grief can, without trouble bee suffered, it will bee much better not to meddle with it, then to endeavour to cure it. For it will cause the next labour to bee more dolorous, and difficult, by making new laceration, or incision.

He argues that the woman's physical state should be left in the condition most conducive to further child-bearing:

> [This condition]...not being cured, the ensuing births will bee more easy, by reason of the spaciousnes of the breach, the vulva and intestinum rectum being laid together, and making but one passage.[54]

[54] He goes on to relate and cite several more cases. Percival Willughby, *Observations in Midwifery*, ed. Henry Blenkinsop (Warwick: Printed by H. T. Cooke, 1863; rpt. Wakefield: S. R. Publishers, 1972), pp. 54, 159, 252.

Eccles notes that this practice was common: "It seems likely," she states, "that unless the tear was too extensive to live with it was more usual to leave the cure to nature, or to use medicines only."[55] The rigidity of the scar would, it was believed, make another breech unavoidable, and this was thought undesirable despite the fact that some writers recommended stitching for reasons related as much to sexual pleasure as to procreation: "the Excrements coming that way disgust the Husband," noted one French surgeon, "and the Woman is by no means fit for his Caresses."[56]

As one can imagine, the physical alteration of a woman's body was the source of some anxiety. In *The Body Embarrassed*, Gail Kern Paster notes, for example, a fascinating passage from Guillemeau's *Child-Birth or, the Happy Delivery of Women* (translated into English in 1612). In Jacques Guillemeau's discussion of restoration of the parts of a woman's body that "have beene strayned, and as it were quite changed, through a long and painefull travaile," he, as Paster puts it, "wistfully" fantasizes about antipodean women of whom he has heard:

> There are women…that dwell beyond the Antartique Pole, whose bodies are entire and Virgin-like, euen after often child-bearing, and in whom there is perceiued no difference from them that are Virgins, as they that haue opened them, hauing made diligent search, doe testifie: But since there bee no such women found in our quarters, (though I dare boldly say, there be some, not much different) therefore will it be very necessary to have a care what is to be done, to their belly, breasts, and nether parts.

He goes on to prescribe bandages and ointments for most cases, with stitching to be done only when the tears were particularly severe.[57]

There is also evidence that anxieties about mortality, morbidity, and disfiguration were the cause of a significant amount of mental illness among women. For example, Michael MacDonald's study of the medical practice

[55] Eccles, *Obstetrics and Gynaecology*, pp. 106–7.

[56] M. de La Vauguion, *A Compleat Body of Chirurgical Operations* (London, 1699), p. 239. La Vauguion's text is late and reflects French practices and attitudes, but some of these may have come to England much earlier. Jacques Guillemeau, whose text was translated into English in 1612, also recommended stitching in cases where the tear reached into the fundament, although he seems less concerned about cosmetic matters: see Jacques Guillemeau, *Child-Birth or, the Happy Delivery of Women* (London, 1612), pp. 194–9, 211–15. Ambrose Paré recommends stitching, but thinks it is an unfortunate necessity, making a woman's tissues too rigid to stretch for the next birth and requiring a surgeon to later cut through the scar. See Ambroise Paré, *The Workes of that Famous Chirurgion Ambrose Parey*, trans. Thomas Johnson (London, 1634), pp. 917–18. See also Eccles, *Obstetrics and Gynaecology*, p. 107.

[57] Guillemeau, *Child-Birth*, p. 195. See Gail Kern Paster, *The Body Embarrassed: Drama and the Disciplines of Shame in Early Modern England* (Ithaca, NY: Cornell University Press, 1993), p. 196. The women he speaks of as "not much different" are probably prostitutes.

notes of Richard Napier, an astrological physician and Anglican divine active in Oxford and Buckinghamshire from 1580 to 1634, cites the tribulations of childbirth as an important factor in mental disorders:

> Women who survived were sometimes irreparably mangled. The suffering childbirth caused cannot be estimated accurately, but the fear, stress, and illnesses induced by difficult births contributed to the mental disorders of 81 of Napier's patients, including one man who was so frightened by his wife's awful pain that he went mad.[58]

Napier's patients came from all social strata and from both rural and urban populations, and his notes are an invaluable resource for understanding the nature of medical practice in the period. All told, he recorded 2,039 cases of mental illness in his years of practice. Of those cases, 1,267 were women over the age of 14 (19 were younger than that and unlikely to have had obstetric or gynecological problems), 748 were men, and in 5 cases the patients had ambiguous names and the details of Napier's accounts do not clearly indicate their gender.[59] In addition to the 80 cases in which mental disturbance in women was caused by difficult birth, another 204 women – or all together 22.4 percent of all the women over 14 who complained to Napier of mental or emotional disturbance – also suffered from some form of obstetric or gynecological illness.[60] In her memoir, Lucy Hutchinson, who included a complementary account of childbed woes in her biblical epic, *Order and Disorder*, tells the story of her mother-in-law's mother, who went insane after giving birth to triplets (three daughters, one of whom was stillborn). We can only speculate as to what it was like to give birth to triplets in the seventeenth century, but as far as Lucy was concerned it was evidently difficult enough to cause some form of mental imbalance. As she puts it, "after that, all the art of the best physicians in England could never restore her [sister's] understanding."[61]

[58] Michael MacDonald, *Mystical Bedlam: Madness, Anxiety and Healing in Seventeenth Century England* (Cambridge University Press, 1981), pp. 108–9; see also pp. 19–20.

[59] MacDonald, *Mystical Bedlam*, p. 38.

[60] MacDonald, *Mystical Bedlam*, p. 259, n. 87.

[61] Lucy Hutchinson, *Memoirs of the Life of Colonel Hutchinson Written by His Widow Lucy* (London: J. M. Dent, 1908; rpt. 1913), pp. 33–6. For the remarkable lament over Eve's curse in the epic, see *Order and Disorder*, Book 5, lines 127–80, 221–36: Lucy Hutchinson, *Order and Disorder*, ed. David Norbrook (Malden, MA: Blackwell, 2001), pp. 69–72.

CHAPTER 3

Religious frameworks

As much of what I have already said makes clear, in Milton's world, religious beliefs and practices were central to the ways in which people accommodated themselves to the difficulty of their obstetric experiences, providing what David Cressy calls the era's "master-narrative for understanding the mystery of childbirth."[1] While the religious practices of the birthing chamber sometimes edged over into the manipulation of charms, magical incantations, and sacred relics of various kinds (the last being the most common hold-over from earlier Catholic practices),[2] the central rites of childbirth were, along with the churching ceremony, a series of individual and group prayers and meditations performed by the mother, her attendants, her family members, and other interested members of her community in preparation for her coming labor. These were, for the most part, conducted in the birthing chamber itself and in the domestic and social circles that surrounded it, and they drew on a particular set of theological concepts, devotional traditions, and biblical passages and images. The purpose of these practices, along with the various social and practical aspects of the childbirth rites as a whole, was to help women and others involved with the birth cope with their fears about what might happen, and they worked by turning what could inspire despair into an opportunity for the

[1] David Cressy, *Birth, Marriage, and Death: Ritual, Religion, and the Life-Cycle in Tudor and Stuart England* (Oxford University Press, 1997), p. 16.

[2] The use of charms like "eagle stones" was more usually thought of as a "medical" application. See Jane Sharp, *The Midwives Book* (London, 1671), pp. 182–4, 198. Some thought belief in them was superstitious. Richard Adams' sermon on 1 Timothy 2:15, for example, distinguishes between such semi-magical practices and the effectiveness of a truly religious sensibility. For him, a woman's sense of holiness was "the true Eagle-stone to be constantly worn for the prevention of miscarrying." See Samuel Annesley, *A Continuation of Morning-Exercise Questions* (London, 1683), p. 655. It was common among Catholics for women to make a point of confessing and taking communion in preparation for the day of delivery. Sometimes masses were said on behalf of a woman in travail. Some of these practices remained common among Protestants as well. Many took communion, and some non-conformists organized prayer vigils for particular women. See Cressy, *Birth, Marriage, and Death*, pp. 22–7.

demonstration of a confident faith. Prayers and meditations were, of course, also thought of as practically efficacious. God might very well, it was thought, intervene in response to earnest prayer and make the travail mild or at least preserve the lives of the mother and child. It was the *spiritual* state of the mother, however, that took center stage, and concern for salvation often pushed the hope women had of simply surviving their ordeals to the wings.

Within this general framework of trial and petition, the facts of maternal mortality, the fears that came with them, and their spiritual significance could be thought of in several different ways. A death in childbirth could be thought of, for example, as part of a divine punishment visited upon England (or urban England or some particular part of England) by a God angry at the excesses of city life, a falling off of sincere worship, or any number of collective sins of which the nation or some part of it might be thought guilty. It was more common, however, for people to frame their religious thinking in more specifically personal terms. They might, for example, blame a particular death on the woman's or her family's particular sins.[3] However, since most texts that recounted the deaths of particular women were primarily concerned with consoling mourners and/or with the representation of the deceased as a model for emulation, they tended to blame the death on the transhistorical and universal condition of original sin, rather than on any conditions, spiritual or otherwise, particular to a given woman. This allowed writers, especially in the texts written by Protestant divines, to focus on the ways in which each woman, her attendants, and the members of her family or community faced the death as a manifestation of God's universal will, revealing each believer's true spiritual nature and investments.

The set prayer texts would have provided Milton with his most accessible source for a theologically informed childbirth discourse. He would have come across many of them in published devotional books, collections of sermons, and conduct books, and the concepts underpinning such prayers find expression – often quite systematic expression – in these texts, as well as in some books of biblical exegeses and theology, all of which Milton read

[3] People were more likely to imagine before a birth that death might come as a possible punishment for particular sins than they were after the death to claim that a woman had died because of her own sins. The nature of such evaluations depended a great deal, however, on who was doing the evaluating and on whether they were discussing a particular individual or an abstractly conceived class of women. For some discussion of the way preachers urged people not to "judge others on the basis of their afflictions," see David Harley, "Spiritual Physic, Providence and English Medicine, 1500–1640," in *Medicine and the Reformation*, eds. O. P. Grell and A. Cunningham, (London: Routledge, 1993), pp. 101–17, especially p. 103.

voraciously. A fairly large number are preserved in the autobiographical and personal literature, some of which found its way into publication and might have been available to Milton. What was not available to him, of course, can still be an important source for us as we try to reconstruct the larger context in which he operated. As I have already said, many of the prayers actually used by women in the birthing chamber were handed down as part of an oral tradition that was essentially the possession of women, but that does not mean that an interested man could not have observed women praying or overheard the prayers they uttered. It is useful, of course, to distinguish between what Milton might have overheard or witnessed, the materials preserved in surviving letters and diaries, and those preserved in the published works. The latter were, for the most part, the products of a more "official" – and certainly male – religious and intellectual culture. Still, all of the surviving materials and indications of oral practice must be dealt with together if we are to get as complete a picture as is possible, not only of what happened in the birthing chamber, but of how such activities might have been perceived. I will therefore treat these materials together, making whatever distinctions seem relevant as I go along.

CENTRAL BIBLICAL TOUCHSTONES

The religious rhetoric of childbed suffering was deeply informed in all of the surviving materials by reference to and adaptation of a particular set of biblical touchstones. Three, in particular, stand out as of special importance: Genesis 3:16, 1 Timothy 2:14–15, and John 16:20 (all three, along with a few others I will discuss below, were alluded to directly by Milton).[4] The first of these is, of course, the most universal. All childbed prayers or sermons, and many passages on childbirth in the autobiographical writings of the period, contain at some point a direct proclamation regarding the need for a woman to accept her suffering and possible death in terms of Eve's curse:

> I will greatly multiply thy sorrow and thy conception; in sorrow thou shalt bring forth children; and thy desire shall be to thy husband, and he shall rule over thee. (*KJV*)

[4] Carolyn Whitney-Brown singles out the same three passages for specific discussion (see *Tudor and Stuart Birth Stories by Shakespeare and Others*, Brown University, Doctoral Dissertation [1991], pp. 63–8). Raymond A. Anselment notes the importance of the passage from 1 Timothy in *Realms of Apollo: Literature and Healing in Seventeenth-Century England* (Newark, NJ: University of Delaware Press, 1995), p. 53. See also Cressy, *Birth, Marriage, and Death*, p. 17.

The curse was thought of, most obviously, as a punishment laid on women for Eve's sin, but it was also, and again almost invariably, seen as part of a scheme specifically designed for the redemption of women. Very few surviving texts indicate that anyone expected that the conditions of the curse could be altered, avoided, or even ameliorated.[5] The only way out of suffering, we might say, was through it. But a woman's passage through her pangs was thought of less as an experience simply to be endured than as a proving ordeal, a spiritual trial that perfectly mixed divine judgment *and* mercy. Women were exhorted – and exhorted themselves – to accept their pain and danger as both a just punishment for sin (a sign of their spiritual depravity) and as a gift that provided them the opportunity to transcend that sinfulness (a sign of their God-given capacity for the utmost spiritual dignity and even heroism).

All prayers for women in childbirth – and almost all early modern sermons or theological references to the childbed of any sort – understood the danger of death to be part and parcel of women's condition under the curse, and framed their petitions, prescriptions, proscriptions, and arguments in ways that emphasized the urgency of the birthing woman's physical and spiritual situation. Most paraphrases tended, for example, to ratchet-up the fearfulness of the curse in ways appropriate to the common perception that childbearing women ran risks greater than were captured by the word "sorrow," chosen by the *KJV* translators for the Hebrew words, עצבונך (*itz'vonekh* – "your sorrow" or "your pain") and בעצב (*b'ehtzehv* – " in sorrow" or "in pain").[6] In most of the prayers in Bentley's collection, to take just one particularly large set of examples, phrases like the following either replace or get added to the bare translation of the Hebrew when allusions are made to the verse: "that we should conceiue in sorrowe, *and beare in perill*"

[5] The passage from Willughby I quoted earlier (see pp. 19–20) is one of the rare partial exceptions. Even there, however, he still expects childbirth to be painful, just not necessarily deadly. See Percival Willughby, *Observations in Midwifery*, ed. Henry Blenkinsop (Warwick: Printed by H. T. Cooke, 1863; rpt. Wakefield: S. R. Publishers, 1972), p. 13. Some preachers hoped that the curse might not fall too hard, even in a sense that it might be lifted in particular cases, but these are usually somewhat hyperbolic expressions of hope that temporal salvation from peril will be the most common judgment of God in any given case. See, for example, the strange passage on pp. 657–8 of Adams' sermon, which seems to contradict much of the rest of what the sermon argues (Annesley, *A Continuation*, pp. 657–8).

[6] The root, עצב, could have both physical and emotional denotations, but did not necessarily imply mortal danger. The word used in verse 3:17 for what Adam will suffer in working the earth ("in sorrow shall you eat of it" [*KJV*]) is from the same root: בעצבון תאכלנה (*b'itzahvon tokhalehnah*). The root appears again at 6:6 in the description of the "grief" felt by God at having created creatures who had become so wicked: ויתעצב אל־לבו (*vayit'atsev el-libo*), "and it grieved him at his heart" (*KJV*). Milton's paraphrase of the curse in *Paradise Lost* 10.193–6 sticks close to the Hebrew, but he intensifies our sense of what "sorrow" entails by presenting the arrival of Sin and Death in Eden just thirty-three lines later. See Chapter 8.

(my italics), "perils both of soule and bodie," "and with great danger," "the vnspeakable pangs, intollerable paines, and most bitter agonie of death." The following example puts it particularly starkly:

> O most righteous Lord God, which for the offence of the first woman, hast threatened vnto all women high and lowe, a common, sharpe, and ineuitable malediction, and hast enioined them, that they should conceiue in sin, and being conceiued, should be subiect to manie & greevous throws and torments, and finallie, be deliuered with the danger and ieoperdie of their life.[7]

Over and over again, the prayers state not only that birth was originally ordained as a painless matter and sin had made it sorrowful, but also that sin had made it painful *and* deadly. Such a characterization was used by the authors of these prayers to concentrate the minds of childbearing women on the states of their souls by making it clear to them that they were quite possibly about to meet their maker and had to prepare themselves to die well.

Genesis 3:16 was also used to etch in stone a close relationship in people's minds between the conditions of female physical suffering and the everywhere-obvious social condition of female submission to male authority. Women were doomed not only to suffer physically and emotionally, but also to suffer the ascendancy of the male will, and this too was seen as central to God's scheme for both women's punishment and their salvation, tying a woman's hopes for redemption to her patient acceptance of both her pain and her social position. The two forms of suffering dovetailed in the way some divines conflated a woman's acceptance of her husband's sexual and reproductive desires with her acceptance of God's will for her, a will that pinioned her between the first commandment ("be fruitful and multiply" [Genesis 1:28]), and the conditions of punishment and trial she had to face in order to fulfill it.[8] Women themselves, of course, as we shall see a little later, tended to think in terms of *their own* sexual and reproductive desires, and worked to align those with what they believed was God's will for them. Some of the texts authored by men, however, betrayed a clear anxiety about how fear of childbirth might persuade women to put their own physical well-being ahead of whatever reasons God or their husbands (or, especially for

[7] Thomas Bentley, *The Monument of Matrones: Conteining Seuen Seuerall Lamps of Virginity* (London, 1582), pp. 95, 100, 103, 129, 145. Further expressions of fear of death can be found in the pair of long prayers recommended for women in the midst of a long travail (pp. 112–19) and the prayers of thanksgiving that follow. See also pp. 146–9.

[8] For more on this dynamic, see Jennifer Hellwarth, *The Reproductive Unconscious in Medieval and Early Modern England* (New York, NY: Routledge, 2002), pp. 14–24.

upper-class women, their families) had for asking them to bear children.[9] Such anxiety was usually expressed in the form of exhortations to women to do what the prevailing ideology identified as their duty.

The second most often quoted passage from the Bible in childbed contexts, 1 Timothy 2.14–15, is actually a centrally important New Testament comment on Genesis 3:16 itself, one that, according to the readings commonly applied to it, reinforced the schema of trial and redemption suggested by conventional understandings of Genesis. The passage tied both punishment and submission (social and religious) to the action of saving grace, while adding a set of resonances of its own. The key verse is the final one:

> Adam was not deceived, but the woman being deceived was in the transgression. Notwithstanding she shall be saved in childbearing, if they continue in faith and charity and holiness with sobriety. (*KJV*)

The passage is, perhaps, the most direct statement in the Christian scriptures regarding the religious dimensions of childbirth. It is also part of one of its most explicit and important discussions of how women were supposed to live and behave within the larger Christian community. It has therefore been at the heart of most debates since the earliest periods on such matters as whether or not women should be ordained as priests, whether they should be allowed to teach or preach in public, and whether they should even be allowed to speak in public. It also figures in discussions about the place of asceticism in Christian practice (the passage suggests that it should be rejected by women, but also by implication, by most men, in favor of married life). Finally, and most importantly for our purposes, it has always been central to discussions about the meaning of Genesis 3:16 itself, the particular burdens of sin that women carried because of Eve's role in the Fall, and the particular avenues by which they would therefore have to seek salvation or have it granted.

The passage presents a set of vexing interpretive problems that have given exegetes trouble from the time of the very earliest commentaries. There was, in particular, a fair amount of debate concerning the passage in the early modern period because of the way it seemed to some to imply that childbirth had a sacramental status. It therefore figured prominently in some of the founding arguments of the Reformation. It also proved unavoidable in

[9] Many such texts expressed anxiety that women might see their sufferings as something they could avoid either by abstinence, contraception, or abortion. See, for example, John Oliver's *A Present for Teeming Women* (London, 1663); Adams' sermon on 1 Timothy (Annesley, *A Continuation*); and Christopher Hooke, *The Child-birth or Womans Lecture* (London, 1590).

debates concerning the changing place of women in social and religious institutions. The passage continues to be of some controversy today, especially in modern discussions of gender relations in Christian religious and communal practice, in part because of the issues it raises and in part because of its exegetical difficulties.[10] Its problems have largely to do with the meaning of what the *KJV* renders as "saved" (*sōthēsetai*) (is it spiritual salvation or physical salvation?) and "childbearing" (*teknogonia*) (is it perhaps "child*rearing*?"), and with the ambiguous shift to plural at the end. Despite some evidence that the original author may very well have meant exactly what the plain sense of the text seems to say (that childbirth is a sacrament), the shift to the plural and the possibility of reading *teknogonia* as referring to "child*rearing*" led most early commentaries to associate women's salvation with the *raising* and *education* of children, rather than with trials encountered in their birth.[11] Such an association yields the following paraphrase: "the woman [Eve], being deceived, was in the transgression. Nevertheless, she [all womankind, descended from her] shall be saved by childrearing, if they [their children] continue in faith, etc." This, however, still suggests that women's salvation depends upon the good work of raising children (and this would, indeed, later be hard for Reformation commentators to square with a covenant of faith). It also seemed to make a woman's salvation precariously dependant upon the spiritual choices her children might go on to make after they had grown and left the circle of her influence and discipline. Some commentators avoided these problems by taking the shift to the plural ("they") as simply making explicit the shift already suggested earlier in the passage to the collective made up of all individual women across the span of sacred history (this is clearly implied by the fact that "she" is introduced in the future tense, which makes no sense in relation to Eve, and instead implies her future descendants).[12] This yielded a paraphrase that could refer either to childbearing or rearing, but focused only on the woman's own behavior in the course of her experiences: "Eve sinned. Nevertheless, womankind [each individual "she"] shall be saved in

[10] See the useful survey of the exegetical debates in Luke Timothy Johnson, *The First and Second Letters to Timothy: a New Translation with Introduction and Commentary*, *The Anchor Bible* (New York, NY: Doubleday, 2001), vol. XXXVA, pp. 20–54 and Stanley E. Porter, "What Does it Mean to be 'Saved by Childbirth' (1 Timothy 2.15)?," *Journal for the Study of the New Testament* 49 (1993), 87–102.

[11] See Johnson, *The First and Second Letters*, pp. 26–35. It is also possible that the idea of childbirth's sacramental status might be an expression of early Christian anti-asceticism. See Krijn van der Jagt, "Women are Saved through Bearing Children: a Sociological Approach to the Interpretation of 1 Timothy 2.15," in *Issues in Bible Translation*, ed. Philip C. Stine, UBS Monograph Series No. 3 (London: United Bible Societies, 1988), pp. 287–95.

[12] See Johnson, *The First and Second Letters*, pp. 202–3 and Porter, "What Does it Mean."

childbearing or rearing as long as they continue [that is, as long as each woman individually continues] in faith, etc." This reading, as we will see in a moment, is of fundamental importance to later Reformation readings of the verse because it suggests a way around the sacramental status of birth itself without recourse to the still problematic idea of child*rearing* as a good work.

Beginning around the ninth century, other interpretations began to be offered. For example, it was suggested by some that the verse concerned a woman's own baptism, and later that it referred to the Incarnation (she shall be saved, we might say, by "The Childbirth," the miraculous birth of Jesus through Mary, either because of the saving power of Christ himself or because of the dignity that Mary's pregnancy and birth conferred on all human births).[13] Until the Reformation, the tradition, however, is strongly weighted toward the idea of child*rearing*, largely, perhaps, because the grammar of the passage seemed most plainly to refer to some action or experience of women in relation to children, and child*rearing* was seen as a deliberate choice on a woman's part (she could choose to raise her children as good Christians or she could neglect them), while childbirth itself was seen as a physical process over which she had little control and about which she had little choice once she had accepted marriage. She was either fertile or barren, and in submitting either to her husband's will or to her own desires she had to take what came or did not come as a result of her sexual life.

With the Reformation, however, new concerns developed. Luther spent a good deal of time explaining how the passage, whether it refers to childbirth or rearing, "does not clash with the doctrine of salvation by faith."[14] Such an argument entailed showing how the passage had to refer not to some action chosen by women but to some way in which they exhibited the quality of their faith in response to particular circumstances. It therefore became less important for writers to avoid sacramental child*birth* by focusing instead on child*rearing*. It no longer mattered, in some sense, which action was being discussed, and attention moved away from the textual problems of the first part of the verse and toward the significance of its final words, which named the qualities a woman had to exhibit in whatever she did in order to show herself worthy of salvation.

Most of the sixteenth- and seventeenth-century English references to the passage I have come across in contexts directly related to childbirth clearly

[13] See Johnson, *The First and Second Letters*, p. 33.

[14] Quoted from Johnson, *The First and Second Letters*, p. 37. See also Calvin's sermons on Timothy, which were published in English as early as 1579 (*Sermons of M. John Calvin, on the Epistles of S. Paule to Timothie and Titus* [London, 1579], pp. 212–30).

understand the text as referring to the process of birth itself. Some of these references understand it in terms of physical salvation (if a woman is faithful, charitable, holy, and sober in her life and in the course of her labor, she need not fear dying, but God will allow her to give birth to healthy children and live to raise them). The vast majority, however, clearly concentrate on the woman's spiritual salvation, which they make dependant upon how the ordeal of labor reveals the quality and intensity of her faith.[15] Having made her choice to marry and procreate, the birth would serve as the climactic outcome of the woman's choice (should she by God's grace also prove fertile). As long as a woman could face the event properly, she could guarantee herself the only positive result that in the end really mattered: she would prove herself worthy of salvation. In addition, she would do so not because there was anything saving in the pains of birth itself, not even because the choice to marry and procreate was a fulfillment of a divine command, but simply because she had proved herself faithful under extreme duress. This, as we shall see, had the effect of putting a premium on a woman's ability to control herself spiritually and emotionally in her labor.

The passage also, however, lent travail a shapely figurative power in the minds of many women and commentators, suggesting, as some of the earlier commentaries would have it, a close typological relationship between Eve and Mary, as well as a figurative relationship between suffering and death in childbirth and Christ's suffering and death on the cross. It also lent weight to the connection commonly drawn between a woman's successful rising from her childbed (or her successful rising up to heaven should she die) with Christ's resurrection.

I will discuss the significance of such figurative thinking in more detail below. There is, however, one more biblical passage we should single out for discussion first, one that also tended to reinforce such Christological understandings. In the Gospel of John, Jesus comforts his disciples with an elaborate metaphor suggesting that the sorrow they will feel at his death will be like the sorrow of a woman in childbirth:

> A woman when she is in travail hath sorrow, because her hour is come: but as soon as she is delivered of the child, she remembereth no more the anguish, for joy that a man is born into the world. And ye now therefore have sorrow: but I will see you again, and your heart shall rejoice, and your joy no man taketh from you. (John 16:21–2, *KJV*)

[15] The most elaborate treatment is Adams'. The importance of the passage in the context of childbirth has not been much discussed. However, see Margaret Thickstun, "Mothers in Israel: the Puritan Rhetoric of Child-bearing," in *Praise Disjoined: Changing Patterns of Salvation in 17th-Century English Literature*, ed. William P. Shaw (New York, NY: Peter Lang, 1991), pp. 73–87 and Whitney-Brown, *Tudor and Stuart Birth Stories*, pp. 61–6.

The passage had wide application in the context of birth, and few writers on the subject could resist alluding to it or quoting it directly.[16] It was often used simply as a way of expressing the wish a woman had that her labor would be easy and her child born alive and healthy.[17] It also, however, allowed women to see their own suffering as like that of a sinful world, or a small group of the faithful awaiting and finally gaining salvation through God's self-sacrifice. Just as Christ suffered in the Passion, died, and returned to bring redemption, a woman could face with confidence her own Passion, knowing that a merciful God would watch over her and redeem her. The fact that Jesus thought to use this metaphor (one he may have derived from Micah 5:2–3, a passage quoted in Matthew as pertaining to His own birth), gave the pains of labor, in addition, a powerful dignity.[18] Because Christ thought of himself in terms of her experiences, a woman could think of herself as suffering as he did. She could think of herself as undergoing an ordeal caused not (or not only) by her own sins, but by those of mankind as a whole. Should she live, her sitting-up and eventual return to normal life was a resurrection that vindicated God's mercy, figuring the reward awaiting all the faithful. If she died maintaining her faith, facing death with the proper religious acceptance, with the humility of a creature facing a loving but just and exacting God, she would be thought freed from her sinful body by Christ's similar suffering in a way that provided a model for imitation by others. In less theologically correct contexts, and as we will see in both Milton's early "An Epitaph on the Marchioness of Winchester" (hereafter "An Epitaph") and in *Paradise Lost*, such logic could powerfully reinforce the typological relationship between Eve and Mary, allowing women to identify not only with the weakness that brought the Fall and the suffering that reversed it, but also the blessedness that prepared the way for this reversal: Mary's giving the Incarnation its local habitation. Such thinking tended to make women's submission to their childbed sufferings a central guarantor of the ultimate salvation of all of mankind. Had Eve not submitted, and all her daughters following, Mary would never have been born to bear Jesus. Such a schema made particular sense in Protestant contexts

[16] Successive versions of the *Book of Common Prayer* (1549, 1552, 1559, and 1662) all specified this passage (actually, verses 16–22) as a reading for the third Sunday after Easter. See also Anselment, *Realms of Apollo*, p. 53 on its range of meanings in the context of birth.

[17] See, for example, Bentley, *Monument*, p. 120.

[18] The first of the two verses from Micah, according to Matthew 2:5–6, predicts the birth of Jesus in Bethlehem; the second uses the metaphor of a woman's temporary childbed suffering as a figure for Israelite suffering in exile. The Geneva Bible's comment on these verses cites the passage from John as an analog. See *The Geneva Bible: A Facsimile of the 1560 Edition*, ed. Lloyd E. Berry (Madison, WI: University of Wisconsin Press, 1969), p. 375.

that sought to humanize Mary, denying the doctrine of the Immaculate Conception and treating her as simply an ordinary woman of the line of Eve chosen for an extraordinary role in reversing the effects of her foremother's sin. This is a reversal in which ordinary women could, in their small ways, participate.

SUBMISSION, DIVINE WILL, AND THE FEMALE BODY

The three passages from Genesis, Timothy, and John provided those involved in a birth with a range of possible responses within a complex schema of punishment and redemption, submission and transcendence, degradation and dignity, and all responses tended to hover suspended between the poles suggested by these dichotomies. They also tended to hover between temporal and eternal notions of reward and punishment. Their final logic, however, as I said before, tended to emphasize the hereafter at the expense of the here and now. This emphasis may have been simply an expression of the authors' piety (whether deeply felt or a matter of conventional expectation, whether as an expression of an individual's own beliefs or an ideal set forth for emulation by a preacher). It may also have been a reaction to the helplessness women felt in the face of what might happen to them physically. A concentration on spiritual preparedness allowed women to exert their wills toward activities that, if they could not necessarily save them from death, might help them to die well and achieve salvation. In any case, in the religious discourses, women are presented, and presented themselves, as radically dependent on God for any possibly happy end. This sense of helplessness and dependency is also echoed, as we have seen, in the characterizations and self-characterizations of midwives, gossips, surgeons, and physicians. It is said over and over again, for example, in the prayer texts and sermons that without God's aid, "all womens helpe, and all physicke" would be in vain.[19] Midwives themselves were exhorted to pray for God to allow them to do whatever *could* be done by human hands, given God's judgment on the spiritual state of the mother. This sense of ultimate dependency on divine will, the sense that no human action could be efficacious on its own, is pervasive in the surviving religious texts and central to their governing logic. With the Fall, childbirth became a sign not only of

[19] Bentley, *Monument*, p. 98. Note that "womens helpe" refers to all that the midwife and gossips might do, "physicke" to medical treatments prescribed by a physician. No mention is made in the prayer – and seldom in the prayers at all – of surgical practice. This may have much to do with what Wilson argues about fear of surgeons. See discussions in Chapters 1 and 2 (see pp. 27 and 33).

sin but of human weakness, one that mirrored, I would argue, the helplessness of the human will given classic Christian expression in the Epistle to the Romans, and of course made central to Reformation theology. Childbed suffering was thought to work, we might say, like the Law of the old dispensation in Paul's formulation. It forced women to see how much they needed God to save them both physically and spiritually, providing what Puritan thinkers especially considered a particularly acute lesson in the bondage of the will.

The question of whether redemption would come in the shape of physical survival or salvation after death hardly seemed to matter according to the hard logic of this theology.[20] In any case, a woman's best chance of having a safe physical delivery was over and again attached to her preparedness to die. As Richard Adams put it in his sermon on 1 Timothy 2:15:

> None ever repented of making ready to die. And every Christian is ready, who can entirely submit to God's disposal in Life and Death. Yea, and then a good woman is likest to have her will in a safe *temporal deliverance*, when she is most sincerely willing that God should have his in dealing with her as seemest best to himself.[21]

Eternal deliverance mattered most, especially in the works of male divines who were interested in trying to explain to suffering women the religious significance of their experiences in what Margaret Thickstun has called "theologically acceptable terms."[22] The danger of death is of central importance to such writers because it allowed them, as I said before, to emphasize the spiritual urgency of the event. Some scholars have gone so far as to suggest that some authors deliberately exaggerated the danger in their accounts of birth in order to frighten women into pious, controlled behavior.[23] However, given that small complications could quickly become emergencies for which there were no remedies, and because it was plain to everyone involved that a proper submissiveness to divine will did not in

[20] Adams provides a particularly emphatic sermonic example (Annesley, *A Continuation*, p. 659). In the prayer texts that survive, however, the possible outcomes (continued temporal life on the one hand and eternal life on the other) were often conflated, as if the authors or recorders of such prayers could not bear to let go of the possibility that no matter how bad things were getting in a particular birth, God might choose to save the mother and child *in life* rather than only in the *after-life*. See, for example, Bentley, *A Monument*, pp. 141–2. For comparison, the prayer recorded by Bentley on pp. 146–8 makes a distinction between physical and spiritual salvation that is closer to Adams'.

[21] Annesley, *A Continuation*, p. 654.

[22] See Thickstun, "Mothers in Israel," in *Praise Disjoined*, p. 74 and *Fictions of the Feminine: Puritan Doctrine and the Representation of Women* (Ithaca, NY: Cornell University Press, 1988), pp. 11–15.

[23] See Hellwarth, *The Reproductive Unconscious*, pp. 14–24. Kathryn McPherson's manuscript in progress, *Refiguring Maternity*, promises to extend this analysis. I am grateful to Professor McPherson for allowing me to see a copy of her manuscript.

any sense guarantee a safe or easy birth, women themselves may have been more powerfully comforted by the promise of eternal rather than temporal salvation as a difficult birth progressed. They may not have wished to contemplate a temporal reward that they had all too often seen go ungranted. A strategy based on patient submission to a physical condition that little could be done to alter, on the other hand, had obvious advantages. The assigning of such a condition to divine will had the effect, for example, of warding off despair no matter what outcome gradually or suddenly revealed itself, and this, in turn, to some extent restored agency to the woman by tying her will to God's. There was no human power that could alter her physical condition appreciably, but a belief that God's will was being done no matter what the outcome allowed women to imagine they participated in divine power, and that they were at the center of an event that had not only personal and social but also cosmic importance. Some of the prayer texts even praise God for giving women the special "aptnes and power" to conceive children, glorying in the role women had as the "shop and receptacle" of His "most excellent worke," although they stop short of calling her his partner.[24]

However, even in the event of a happy birth, it was salvation that was considered a woman's great reward, not her continued life, which would, in any case, have to be led in continued faith, charity, holiness, and sobriety if salvation were to be granted to her in the end. In most of the texts I have examined, celebrations of women's creative powers quickly give way to expressions of acceptance of God's will should He decide to close her womb, cause it to miscarry, or through long and difficult labor bring her life to an end.[25] Some writers even went so far as to warn that a successful birth should not be mistaken for a sign of God's favor. A woman might be saved, as Adams puts it, "temporally" and yet not receive salvation.[26] John Oliver, in his *A Present for Teeming Women*, asserts that women, "*if they be delivered* while yet they retain...[an] unwillingnesse of mind to prepare for

[24] Bentley, *Monument*, p. 102. Although I am as yet unaware of any direct allusions to the passage, I suspect that such praises would have suggested – in a controversial way – Eve's declaration in Genesis 4:1 about the birth of Cain. The *KJV* renders the verse "I have gotten a man from the Lord," but the Hebrew verb קניתי ("*kaniti*") can mean both "I have acquired" and "I have created." Also the propositional phrase את־יהוה can be rendered not only as "from the Lord" but as "with the Lord," implying a partnership, although the exegetical traditions tend to see this as a boastful claim on Eve's part and to tie the pride it suggests to the subsequent experience of the child she bore. Cain's name, in any case, is a pun on "*kaniti*," and his descendants were creators, makers of technologies and founders of cities.

[25] Bentley, *Monument*, pp. 101–4 is a good example.

[26] Annesley, *A Continuation*, pp. 636, 639, 654, 655, 661–2.

death, ...are delivered in *anger not in favour, with Gods curse not his blessing*, and are (in all likelihood) reserved to the greater condemnation, when their sin is repined [ripened]."[27] It was important, therefore, that women arise from their beds with a renewed commitment to God, taking their survival as a merciful second chance. It was hoped that such mercy would melt the heart of even the hardest sinner.

Many texts, especially those written by women themselves, often also expressed a desire that women be allowed to live for the purpose of raising children to be good Christians, a desire in line with some of the traditional readings of 1 Timothy 2:15. Such desires, however, were not really an exception to the rule of concentration on the hereafter. If a woman lived, she could obviously live her life as a guide and spiritual example to her children, but even dead (or perhaps especially if she died), her behavior in extremity could offer a proper and edifying model for emulation. Elizabeth Jocelin and the other women who wrote death-bed books famously took pains to make sure their children would be properly instructed in the event of their own deaths. Such books prominently displayed death in childbirth as an instance of a good and exemplary death. They were more concerned with that death than with the ongoing life of a good mother, and they were often cited.[28]

Childbirth was itself often seen by preachers, composers of devotional handbooks, and by individual women as a kind of *momento mori*, and as sign of a collective human immersion in a sinful, physical condition.[29] In preparation for their proper deaths, women were invited to contemplate the physical processes of birth as synecdoches for the mutable grossness of physical life as a whole.[30] The rhetoric such exhortations inspired was often grotesque in its contempt for the material world as figured in the body of a travailing woman. This could, of course, make women behold themselves with loathing, but it could also help make a kind of sense out of the physical horror of a birth that was proceeding badly. All of the blood and sweat and even the excrement of a suffering woman were not evoked gratuitously, nor were they simply signs of a misogynistic horror at the

[27] See the prefatory epistle, "To The *Christian Reader*," (Oliver, *A Present for Teeming Women*, a5). The 1663 edition reads "repined," but later editions correct the spelling. See also Thickstun, "Mothers in Israel," in *Praise Disjoined*, pp. 81–2.

[28] Adams, for example, cites Joceline's case several times. The first is on p. 652, and he cites her again at least four more times (Annesley, *A Continuation*). The relationship of maternal mortality to the larger traditions and conventions of the *ars moriendi* are discussed at length in Lucinda M. Becker, *Death and the Early Modern Englishwoman* (Aldershot: Ashgate, 2003), pp. 34–40, 103–28.

[29] Thickstun, "Mothers in Israel," in *Praise Disjoined*, pp. 79–82.

[30] Thickstun, "Mothers in Israel," in *Praise Disjoined*, p. 81.

female body. I would not argue that such evocations were untainted with misogyny, but it is also true that they helped all concerned to see birth as part of the human condition of physical mutability and frailty, a condition that everyone faced, male or female. John Donne, for example, in a sermon he preached in 1618 on the churching of Lady Doncaster, described the sin-worn physicality of human conception and birth in vivid terms, comparing birth within marriage to a flower bed fertilized with dung, and birth itself to a bloody cataclysm (but one created by God for a purpose). The passage continues: "we come into this world, as the Egyptians went out of it, swallowed, and smothered in a red sea, *Pueri sanguinum, & infirmi*, weake, and bloudy infants at our birth."[31] His address is clearly to both men and women, and the sinfulness Donne is concerned with (part of an argument for our need of baptism) is general.[32]

Preachers and women themselves did, however, have special ways of applying such general meditative figures to women's own physical experiences, and in the process, some authors developed a startlingly powerful figurative language for the expression of what was specific to the spiritual struggles of pregnant and laboring women. It was particularly common for men and women to construct elaborate analogies comparing the physical processes of birth with the spiritual processes of repentance. Oliver's statement that women must "repent of the miscarriages of [their] lives, if [they] would be provided against the danger of a miscarrying womb" can be taken as typical of the rhetoric as it is used by preachers.[33] Women themselves, however, made use of it in ways that, though they are based upon the same figurative logic, had a different emphasis. Women tended to see their physical processes as manifestations of their own spiritual states: outer signs of inner fitness or failure. They felt and understood their own bodies' reproductive processes as manifest expressions of their own capacities for praise and good works (granted by grace, perhaps smothered by sin, but always on the verge of being reborn).

The fascinating poem that Mary Carey wrote as a devotional exercise on the occasion of a miscarriage in 1657 provides a striking example of how a woman might imagine her reproductive condition. At line 38, she imagines God speaking to her:

[31] John Donne, *The Sermons of John Donne*, eds. George R. Potter and Evelyn M. Simpson, 10 vols. (Berkeley, CA: University of California Press, 1962), vol. V, pp. 171–2.

[32] See Cressy's comments in *Birth, Marriage, and Death*, p. 19.

[33] Oliver, *A Present for Teeming Women*, p. 27. The passage is noted in this connection by Thickstun, "Mothers in Israel," in *Praise Disjoined*, pp. 81–2.

Methinkes I heare Gods voyce, this is thy [the] sinne;
And Conscience justifies ye same within:
Thou often dost present me wth dead frute;
Why should not my returns, thy presents sute:
Dead dutys; prayers; praises thou dost bring,
affections dead; dead hart in every thinge:
In hearing; reading; Conference; Meditation;
in acting graces & in Conversation:
Whose taught or better'd by ye no Relation;
thou'rt Cause of Mourning, not of Immitation:
Thou doest not answere that great meanes I give;
My word, and ordinances do teache to live:
...
Mend now my Child, & Lively frute bring me;
so thou advantag'd much by this wilt be; (lines 37–48, 51–2)[34]

This divine speech comes to her after she speculates that in allowing her unborn child to die, God was perhaps seeking to teach her to value her two living children more fully (she later reveals that she had given birth to seven children, only two of whom were still living at the time she wrote the poem). She then asks God to tell her why He took his rod in hand to punish her. She wants to know what fault He saw in her so she can learn to "kisse" the rod of punishment; that is to say, to embrace it as (and for) her own good. God answers her in a way that echoes the language of preachers like Oliver. Carey, however, goes on for some forty lines in response to God, articulating the terms of her acceptance and concluding with an elaborate (perhaps it is best to say "fertile") development of God's preacherly and chastising reproductive metaphor:

But lord since I'm a Child by mercy free;
Lett me by filiall frutes much honnor thee;
I'm a branch of the vine; purge me therfore;

[34] Mary Carey, "Upon ye Sight of my abortive Birth ye 31th: of December 1657," quoted from *Kissing the Rod: An Anthology of Seventeenth Century Women's Verse*, ed. Germaine Greer *et al.* (New York, NY: Farrar Straus Giroux, 1988), pp. 158–62. All quotations are from this edition. Donna J. Long emphasizes the union of physical and spiritual experience in women's reworkings of elegiac and meditative conventions in "'It is a lovely bonne I make to thee': Mary Carey's 'Abortive Birth' as a Recuperative Religious Lyric," in *Discovering and (Re)Covering the Seventeenth Century Religious Lyric*, eds. Eugene R. Cunnar and Jeffery Johnson (Pittsburgh, PA: Duquesne University Press, 2001), pp. 248–72, especially 260–71. See also her "Maternal Elegies by Mary Carey, Lucy Hastings, Gertrude Thimelby, and Alice Thornton," in *Speaking Grief in English Literary Culture: Shakespeare to Milton*, eds. Margo Swiss and David A. Kent (Pittsburgh, PA: Duquesne University Press, 2002), pp. 153–76 and Raymond A. Anselment, "'A Heart Terrifying Sorrow': an Occasional Piece of Poetry on Miscarriage," *Papers on Language and Literature* 33 (1997), 13–46 and *Realms of Apollo*, pp. 84–5.

father, more frute to bring, then heertofore;
A plant in God's house; O that I may be;
more flourishing in age; a grouing tree:
Lett not my hart, (as doth my wombe) miscarrie;
but precious meanes received, lett it tarie;
Till it be form'd; of Gosple shape, & sute;
my meanes, my mercyes, & be pleasant frute:
In my whole Life; lively doe thou make me:
for thy praise. And name's sake, O quicken mee;
Lord I begg quikning grace; that grace aford;
quicken mee lord according to thy word:
It is a lovely bonne I make to thee.
after thy loving Kindnesse quicken mee:
Thy quickning Spirit unto me convey;
and therby Quicken me; in thine owne way:
And let the Presence of thy spirit deare,
be wittnessd by his fruts; lett them appeare;
To, & for the; Love; Joy; peace; Gentlenesse;
longsuffering; goodnesse; faith; & much meeknesse,
And lett my walking in the Spirit say,
I live in't; & desire it to Obey:
And since my hart thou'st lifted up to the;
amend it Lord; & keepe it still with thee: (lines 67–92)

The rod of punishment has become, in effect, a fertilizing instrument of grace. It may be difficult for modern readers to embrace what might seem to us an excessively masochistic spirituality, but I would argue that this poem provides us with a remarkable example of the imaginative power a woman could wield with instruments that in other contexts were designed to simply admonish her. In this poem, the figurative logic that governs a dour recommendation like Oliver's is turned into an opportunity for the wholesale reimagination of the process of spiritual regeneration in terms of a woman's own bodily experience. Behind the figure of the mended heart as womb (lines 71–4), in addition to the passages from Philippians and Colossians that she herself cites in the margins of her manuscript (Phil. 1:27 and Col. 1:6–10), lies Paul's sense of himself as a mother travailing "in birth again until Christ be formed" in the members of the community he addresses in Galatians 4.19.[35] Her goal, the power she claims, is to evangelize and reform, to give shape to the lives around her. Her figure expresses a desire to nurture, as if in her womb, and then give birth to renewed

[35] See Long, "It is a lovely bonne," in *Discovering and (Re)Covering*, pp. 266–70 for other instances of Carey's reworking of biblical touchstones and meditative tropes.

Christian believers. If God has chosen to close her womb as a figure of her having closed her heart to him, she says, let her recognition of this fact and acceptance of His judgment inspire Him to open that heart again, like a womb opening to a loving husband, so she can be "quickened" and give birth in a Platonic sense to manifest spiritual beauties that can have a social effect. She has exchanged physical for spiritual reproduction, hoping to become again what God tells her she once was, a cause of imitation rather than of mourning (lines 45–6).

The fact that all of this is imagined in distinctly feminine terms suggests a fully articulated female Protestant spirituality that reappropriates Paul's figurative rhetoric in the service of the spiritual self-understanding and self-fashioning of those who inhabit the bodies from which it originally derived. The fact that Paul made use of the figure ratifies it in a sense, but this is nothing compared with the power unleashed by its being used in this far more direct referential context. It is one thing, as a man, to say "my experience is like that of a pregnant or travailing woman." It is quite another to say, as a woman, that you experience the feelings of your heart as both metaphorically and metonymically tied to the action of your womb. The one is merely a way of describing an emotional and spiritual state vividly; the other actually describes a complex and inseparable internal dynamic between the state of the believer's body and that of her soul. If the one turns hard and dead, so does the other; when the one is quickened, the other leaps into life and creates life. Such a way of thinking attempts to account for Carey's "whole life," as she puts it (line 76), as a woman: not just the reproductive aspects, but also not *just* the spiritual, for they are one and the same.

FURTHER REIMAGININGS

The more orthodox Protestant formulae I discussed earlier in this chapter, although they are the ones that appear most commonly in the surviving written records, do not, as we can see from Carey's example, exhaust the religious imagination of the period. The range of biblical references, for example, was much wider than my earlier list of the three most prominent passages suggests. Women could look to a wide range of passages and the interpretive traditions that surrounded them not just for lessons in proper behavior, but also for comfort and even for what we might call today "empowerment." Women remembered God's mercy for Sarah's and Hannah's barrenness, Rebekah's and Tamar's difficulties in the births of their twin sons, Rachel's struggle with barrenness and her suffering and death in the birth of Benjamin. They also recalled the good Hebrew

Midwives, Shiphrah and Puah in Exodus (1:15–25), the painful death of Phinehas' wife in childbirth (1 Samuel 4:19–22), the happy mother of Psalm 113, the travailing women who provided figures of consolation for Micah (4:8–10 and 5:2–3),[36] as well as Isaiah's striking description of God letting Himself cry out with the license of a laboring woman (42:14) and his later characterization of the redemption of Israel as a rebirth that will come without labor pangs (65:23 and 66:7–13). All of these together, and many others that themselves had no direct relationship to childbirth, created a rich body of words, images, and identifications for women.[37] These not only chastened and disciplined, but created within the physical space of the birthing chamber an imaginative space that allowed women to transcend both their physical conditions and the general strictures and responsibilities of their ordinary lives. Allusions and interpretations of this kind – whether made in private prayer, poetry, and meditation or in public sermon or published handbook – transported temporal experiences that profoundly constricted women's freedom of will both physically and socially into realms that embraced all of human history, sometimes transcending the limitations of even that.

The following, for example, comes from one of two sermons preached by John Donne in the 1620s at a churching ceremony for Francis Egerton, Countess of Bridgewater, the mother of the three children for whom Milton would later write his Ludlow masque, a sermon that Milton might have heard, although we cannot be certain. Donne is commenting on a passage from Micah that has no direct application to the childbed: "Arise ye, and depart; for this is not your rest: because it is polluted, it shall destroy you, even with a sore destruction" (2:10). In the first of the two sermons preached that day, Donne had argued that the passage should be understood in a spiritual rather than a simply historical sense. The Israelites were forced to leave their land and go into exile not simply as a punishment, but also to teach them not to rest in material, worldly comforts. So, at the beginning of the second sermon, Donne reasons that Christians are admonished to give up their reliance on the world and realize that they depart from it only to rise to the blessed state of salvation. He then comments that:

[36] See above on the connection between these two passages, John 16:20–1, and the prediction of the Nativity at Matthew 2:6.

[37] Carey, for example, cites twenty-eight different biblical passages in the margins alongside her poem. Most have no immediately obvious application to childbirth, and are not among those I list in this chapter, but she adapts each of them to her occasion artfully (Carey, *Kissing the Rod*, pp. 159–61). See, for example, her adaptation of the request for "quickening" in Psalm 119:37 (p. 159). In the Psalm, the request simply suggests "save me from death" or "keep me living," but Carey uses the word "quickening" as part of an elaborate analogy between physical and spiritual "pregnancy."

the words admit a just accommodation to this present occasion, God having rais'd his honorable servant, and hand-maid here present, to a sense of the *Curse*, that lies upon *women*, for the transgression of the first woman, which is painfull, and dangerous *Child-birth*; and given her also, a sense of the last glorious resurrection, in having rais'd her, from that Bed of weaknesse, to the ability of coming into his presence, here in his house.[38]

In suffering and surviving the birth of her child, the Countess has not only experienced both Eve's curse and Christ's redemptive grace, she has imitated Christ's redemptive act, encompassing figures that bind together the whole of human spiritual history.

Many texts also, despite the protestations of many Protestant divines, included exhortations to the Virgin Mary as an ideal, perfected mother and a comforter of all women in childbed distress. Mary was popularly thought to have given birth without pain and while keeping her virginity intact.[39] Women also remembered that she gave thanks and underwent a purification ritual after the birth of Jesus, and that this rite was understood, for better or worse, as the roots of the churching ritual, adding strong biblical resonance to the culminating event of the rites of childbirth.[40] Bentley's text preserves a prayer in which a woman asks that she be safely delivered as not only Mary had been, but Elizabeth also in the birth of John the Baptist (Luke 1:157–59), and with perhaps another Christological implication, as Jonah had been delivered from the "whales bellie."[41]

The prayer that precedes this one in Bentley explicitly associates the suffering mother with traditions of Christian martyrdom, and this suggests

[38] Donne, *The Sermons*, vol. V, p. 198. This sermon was probably preached after the birth of either John or Thomas Egerton, the boys who played the Brothers in the first production of *A Mask*. Although at present we have no way of knowing if Milton actually heard this particular sermon, Shawcross has recently observed that we can "assume with good reason" that Milton did hear sermons given by Donne "in his formative years and later": John T. Shawcross, *Rethinking Milton Studies: Time Present and Time Past* (Newark, NJ: University of Delaware Press, 2005), pp. 16–17, 19–20.

[39] See, for example, Carolyn Whitney-Brown's account of the *Ludus Coventriae* and *Chester Cycle* nativity plays. She also observes that there were other traditions that insisted Mary travailed like any ordinary woman because she believed in the law, and yet had faith in the saving power of the child she was bringing forth (Whitney-Brown, *Tudor and Stuart Birth Stories*, pp. 2–5, 10–20). See also Sarah Jane Boss, *Empress and Handmaid: on Nature and Gender in the Cult of the Virgin Mary* (London: Cassell, 2000), pp. 187–211. The following *anti*-Marian admonition by Puritan divine Robert Hill is also suggestive of beliefs and practices involving Mary: "If wee were Heathens, we would call upon Iuno: if Idolaters, wee would call upon the Virgin Marie: but seeing thou [God] hast vouchsafed us as to become true Christians, we call upon thee alone to help": see Robert Hill, *The Pathway to Prayer and Pietie* (London, 1609), p. 411.

[40] Luke 2:22–4. See also Cressy, *Birth, Marriage, and Death*, pp. 197–229.

[41] *Monument*, pp. 128–9. The Christological implication comes from the invocation of the "sign of Jonah" as a figure for the death and resurrection of Christ in Matthew 12:38–41.

yet another avenue of elaboration available to travailing women.[42] Many prayers offered, as my earlier discussion of the passages from Timothy and John has already suggested, images of childbirth as a redeeming self-sacrifice. Many of the surviving texts might even be said to exhibit modes of spiritual meditation that framed childbed suffering in ways that affirmed a particularly female spirituality that had roots in medieval women's spiritual traditions, as well as both general Catholic and Protestant traditions of psalmic meditation and *imitatio Christi*. It is particularly telling that one section of Bentley's *Monument* advises that women recite Psalm 22 as part of their childbed devotions when they find themselves "[i]n long and sore labor." He suggests recitation of the traditional penitential psalms as well, but he actually prints an adapted text of Psalm 22, explicitly referring to it by its conventional designation: "The complaint of Christ on the Cross."[43] As a woman recited its opening lines ("My God, my God, why hast thou forsaken me"), she reenacted Christ's despairing moment of humanity. She is, in addition, able – as He could not before He died – to complete the psalm to its consoling conclusion. Of particular interest are the changes Bentley (or his source) makes to the psalm in adapting it to the occasion. For example, the Bentley version adds "and mothers" to verse 4's proclamation in the *KJV* that "our fathers trusted" in God's deliverance. Verse 6, which in the *KJV* reads "But I am a worm, and no man; a reproach of men, and despised of the people," is rendered in Bentley "But as for me, I seeme rather to be a worme than a woman, the dounghill of Adam and Eve, the outcast of the vulgar people." "Brethren" at verse 22 becomes "breethren and sisters." The male "afflicted" of verse 24 is rendered "poore hand-maid." The verses that speak of how the psalmist was dedicated to God from his "mothers wombe" (verses 9–10) take on a different resonance in this context, as do the verses that describe the physical state of the speaker (verses 14–15), which now have an almost uncanny relevance to the severe pains of labor. The concluding promise that the speaker will praise the Lord for his deliverance comes inescapably to echo a woman's hope that she will be able to attend her churching, and the final proclamation that future generations will serve God has special resonance for a woman who was actually trying to bring a member of the next generation into life. Perhaps

[42] Bentley, *Monument*, p. 128. Sharon Howard suggests that Alice Thornton's language, and that of many other women writers who discussed their childbirth experiences, was influenced by the discourses of Protestant martyrology: see Sharon Howard, "Imagining the Pain and Peril of Seventeenth Century Childbirth: Travail and Deliverance in the Making of an Early Modern World," *Social History of Medicine* 16 (2003), 375–6.

[43] Bentley, *Monument*, pp. 109–12.

even more important is how closely recitation of this psalm at this particular point in a woman's experience brings that experience together with the redemptive suffering of Christ.[44]

CONCLUSION

Seen through the lens of such creative uses of important biblical passages and motifs, the enclosed and curtained space of the birthing chamber, with its circle of female witnesses, can be seen as a private theater for the acting out of a spiritual drama, which, it was hoped, would lead to a woman's justification, whether she lived or died. It also offered women an array of positive ways of imagining even the most painful aspects of their spiritual, physical, and even social conditions. The sense of balanced and typological justice articulated in 1 Timothy and John, as well as the heroic, creative, female-centered religious experiences trumpeted in prayers and sermons did not, however, always suffice to rationalize childbirth suffering. In birth, women's greatest spiritual powers and dignities confronted stark physical vulnerabilities that could not fully be explained away as part of a universal condition. This was because, in terms of direct experience, the universality of suffering under original sin diverged sharply along gender lines. As Lucinda M. Becker puts it starkly, the "arena of risk" represented by childbirth is "perhaps the most striking factor in differentiating the male and female experience of death in early modern England."[45] The form that such risks took often seemed too great a price for any – especially any innocent – individual to have to pay for a general condition. The idea of an innocent suffering for others' sins could in some ways be resolved by meditation on the crucifiction, but the sharp divergence of such sacrificial experiences along gender lines was a much more difficult matter. According to Genesis, men and women were vulnerable to two different sorts of dangerous "labor." Men had to work to maintain the material life of humankind; women had to labor to produce humankind itself. Both faced mortality in these

[44] Whitney-Brown's discussion of this text is the only one of significant length of which I am aware. She recognizes that "identification with Christ" here "radically transforms the theology of childbirth pain from punishment to divine participation," but her discussion underestimates the widespread identification women had with Christ's suffering (Whitney-Brown, *Tudor and Stuart Birth Stories*, pp. 74–8). For a history of such identification in women's spirituality, see Caroline Walker Bynum, *Fragmentation and Redemption: Essays on Gender and the Human Body in Medieval Religion* (New York, NY: Zone Books, 1992), especially Chapters 3 and 5. See also Boss, *Empress and Handmaid*, pp. 199–201 and Charlotte F. Otten, "Women's Prayers in Childbirth in Sixteenth-Century England," *Women and Language* 16 (1993), 20.

[45] Becker, *Death and the Early Modern Englishwoman*, p. 34.

tasks, but it was widely recognized that women seemed to pay a higher price (with the significant exception of warfare, in which it was recognized that men suffered harshly – although women were, of course, not immune to what we would today call "collateral damage").[46] Some attempted to resolve the injustice of the matter by focusing on the idea that Eve had been primarily responsible for the Fall, and the fact that her punishment, as I said before, was tied up with her subordination to men. Woman's pain, in other words, could be made to go hand in hand with the justification of patriarchy. This explanation was not, however, universally satisfying, as the examples I have already enumerated and as my discussion of Milton's work will show.

As should be clear from my account, the various discourses that surrounded childbirth in the period (social, medical, and religious) framed the event for people in highly complex and flexible ways. For most women, it constituted a trial of their faith, but also a heroic act of possible self-sacrifice, a chance for a woman, in imitation of Christ, to redeem some small part of the world by exposing herself to pain and death in the name of her child, of human posterity as a whole, and especially in fulfillment of God's command to mankind to be fruitful and multiply. In childbed, a woman became the suffering nexus of a cosmic process by which souls were brought into the world for their own trials, leading either to their own damnation or salvation. This cosmic process was colored by social values, especially those concerning, at the higher levels of society, the maintenance of dynastic lines. At the lower end, it was colored more simply by the desire of men and women to see themselves in their children and to see their families continue to exist in time. Each birth, in other words, drew temporal concerns together with eternal ones. Each was nothing less than a key event in the ongoing maintenance of the cosmic and social fabric of creation, commonwealth, and family.

That fabric could not be kept whole without women's willingness to take on great pain and make, possibly, very great sacrifices, and this fact was of concern to many commentators. Marriage and childbirth (the latter figured heroically, sacrificially, and as a proving ordeal) were thought of as a woman's primary responsibilities, and the demographic information that historians have been able to gather reflects this. Rates of marriage and fertility were relatively high, and as many historians have observed, there were intense ideological pressures at work in the period designed to

[46] The dangers of warfare and childbirth were often compared. See, for example, Nicolas Guy, *Pieties Pillar: or a Sermon Preached at the Funeral of Mistresse Elizabeth Govge* (London, 1626), pp. 51–2.

emphasize familial and reproductive life as parts of woman's role in the social fabric. The sense of danger created by high rates of maternal and infant mortality and the sense of burden that came with the diseases and the often disabling effects of obstetric complications, all of which came along with high fertility rates under contemporary circumstances, gave the increasingly central responsibilities of domesticity and reproduction a tremendous urgency.

As we have seen, documents from the period show that people were well aware that the frequency of maternal mortality was high, perhaps abnormally high, especially in the cities. People were also well aware that reproductive life subjected women to a host of burdensome physical conditions. As we have also seen, interest in the fate of women in childbirth increased significantly in the period, a period that saw the first appearance of prayer collections and devotional handbooks for pregnant and birthing women, and a vogue for tomb sculpture memorializing women who died giving birth. As the seventeenth century wore on, there was also a veritable explosion in the publication of medical texts and practical handbooks. Some authors were concerned that women might feel a desire to control more carefully and perhaps reduce or even avoid their own fertility. It seems in general, however, that while a high rate of fertility may have perceptibly increased women's risks, such risks were accepted by both men and women as both divinely ordained and even desirable (in fact, these were for most people two ways of saying the same thing). While some texts expressed worry that women might attempt to escape maternity by either refusing to marry or by refusing or drastically reducing their sexual activity within marriage, there is no evidence that such refusals were actually widespread. Women perceived themselves as occupying a highly pressured and charged position, one from which there was no honorable escape, or at least no escape that did not deny them things they very much wanted: a life of relative autonomy, even if it was only within their appointed sphere, and salvation at the end of it. They tended, therefore, to work on increasing the honor of the activities they were engaged in, tying their wills to what they had no way of resisting, and intensifying their commitment to a course of events they had a stake in thinking of as inevitable once the more basic choice to obey had been made. It was easier, we might say, to concentrate on how best to face what was "inevitable" than to think about how one's freedom had been curtailed in the first place, especially given that there were no categories for thinking about such freedom in positive terms.

The rites of childbirth and the religious discourses that informed them were constructed in large part to create a space in which the obedient woman could imagine herself as exercising heroic choices, and they arranged that she did so in the presence of others who had already, or would later, make the same ones. The rites tended to make the birthing chamber, the space set aside and externally constrained by the contemporary forms of patriarchy as women's sphere, into what could be felt as a wholly free and creative space, one that gave women powerfully satisfying ways of living out a set of ideal roles perfectly. As we have seen, a great deal of energy was expended in keeping men *out* of this sphere, and while we may see this today as a part of a strategy of control or containment, it was more often seen and experienced by contemporary observers and participants as a constraint on *men*, rather than on women. Its primary purpose was to protect something of inestimable value to the women within the chamber: the social basis of their resources of religious hope and consolation. Any constraining male authority, or even presence, could not only cause the fear that Wilson so pointedly describes in his account of tensions between the midwife and the surgeon, it could also taint the sense of female self-creation produced by the gendered exclusivity of conventional practice.[47]

The texts we will look at in the following chapters show that Milton strove in his art to give a poetic form to his own and his culture's complex process of accommodation with the anxieties provoked by the conditions we have been discussing. As we shall see, there are reasons having to do with the theological and social issues at play in childbirth that made poetic contemplation of the matter very difficult and therefore either very rare or very simple. As we shall also see, however, it was this difficulty that drew Milton to the subject in the first place. Later, as he constructed his essentially Arminian theodicy, he would be drawn to the idea of childbirth as an event that both compromises and empowers the human will. He also found himself profoundly drawn to the narrative and figurative logic of the typology implied by the central intertext of 1 Timothy and Genesis. He made use of the death of Rachel and of Christ's comparison of himself and his anxious believers to the participants in a childbirth in John 16:21 in ways that were colored by their currency in the discourse of birth. When he came to figure his cosmos, when he thought about marriage both early and late in his career, when he came to figure his own ambitions, the nature of sin, the perplexity of the will in the face of severe suffering, his imagination would also always be colored by what he read and experienced of childbirth under painful and fatal circumstances.

[47] Wilson, "The Perils," 14 and *The Making of Man-Midwifery*, pp. 33–8 and 49–53. See discussion in Chapters 1 and 2 (see pp. 27 and 33).

My argument does not utterly depend upon Milton's having extensive book-knowledge of obstetric medicine (he could have derived much of what he knew from lore and common knowledge). Nevertheless, there is evidence that Milton, in fact, had a fair amount of medical learning, and his treatment of birth may have been influenced by his reading as much as by ideas he would have absorbed from the culture at large. As several social historians have shown, most educated people (and, to a less systematic extent, most people in general) had a pretty good idea of how the basic concepts of humoral medicine worked. The bulk of day-to-day diagnosis and treatment was done in the home. Simplified medical handbooks and herbals were also widely distributed and popular, and a good deal of information about symptoms and remedies was passed along orally. Most people only consulted a physician (sometimes only in correspondence) after various self-treatments failed to relieve a chronic condition.[48] Milton certainly would have had access to most of the texts to which I refer. Most were often reprinted and widely distributed. It is also reasonable to assume that he would have had some interest in what these texts had to say, particularly the ones that dealt with general medical matters as well as obstetrics. Most dealt to some extent with both, and Paré's *Workes*, for example, which was among the more authoritative and expensively published of these – and therefore among the most likely to interest a learned man and a lover of books – is a comprehensive medical text and anatomy.[49]

The deaths of Mary Powell and Katherine Woodcock, of course, would have given Milton personal reasons for learning for himself what the leading thinkers of his time thought happened in childbirth, but, as many passages in Parker's biography show, Milton, for other reasons, had a life-long interest in general "physic" and considerable knowledge of basic humoral medicine. Parker notes, for example, that in the early years of his blindness, Milton searched for a cure for his condition, trying several very painful and invasive treatments before giving up on them as more harmful than helpful (Parker, pp. 393, 992). Milton also made the study of physic a part of the curriculum he outlined in *Of Education*, recommending that students should be read to "out of some not tedious writer the institution of Physick; that they may know the tempers, the humors, the seasons, and

[48] Lucinda McCray Beier, *Sufferers and Healers: the Experience of Illness in Seventeenth-Century England* (London: Routledge and Kegan Paul, 1987), pp. 101–28, and Roy Porter, "The Patient in England c1660 to c1800," in *Medicine in Society: Historical Essays*, ed. Andrew Wear (Cambridge University Press, 1992), pp. 91–118, especially pp. 96–114.

[49] Ambroise Paré, *The Workes of that Famous Chirurgion Ambrose Pare*, trans. Thomas Johnson (London, 1634).

how to manage a crudity" (*CP*, 2.392–3). For very young men, such knowledge need not have extended beyond the nature and the care of the male body (Milton, in fact, recommends this as good knowledge for a soldier to have) but one can imagine that Milton himself had the works of medical writers around, and that since most included extensive discussions of generation and birth, he was free to read (or be read to) from them about these matters. If Milton read ancient rather than modern writers on the subject, he would have found many of the same ideas, the moderns mostly having derived their materials from Galen and Aristotle. Finally, Milton was acquainted with some of London's leading physicians, including Theodore Diodati, who had an active practice in London until 1649 and was the father of Milton's good friend, Charles, who was himself studying to be a physician before he died in 1638.

Whatever poems on childbirth Milton might have encountered as he contemplated his own work, whatever sermons he might have heard or medical books he might have read, it will be clear that he used much of the same imagery, made the same biblical allusions, and (for the most part) had the same religious purposes in mind as the prayers, sermons, and private devotions we have surveyed. His work also reflects the practices he would have witnessed and the lore and customs he would have absorbed more informally. In the next section of this study, we will look at some of the ways in which these discourses, practices and customs had already been brought into poetry by the time Milton sat down to write "An Epitaph" in 1631. The poetry of the period offered Milton only a few imperfect and inconclusive models for the adaptation of the art to the requirements of both the birthing chamber and the maternal grave-side. His own early attempt to do so strove, as we will see, to perfect those imperfections and offer a conclusive consolation by overlaying the formal funeral elegy that Ben Jonson had perfected in the decades just preceding and following Milton's birth with a new and elaborate schema of typology and allusion. The poem Milton produced, however, proved too conclusive, too perfect. The later chapters of this book will tell the story of Milton's breaking of that form and of his search for a consolation rooted not in perfections of thought and verse, but in the recognition of their ultimate and inevitable failure. It is in the failure, confronted in a pair of profound personal losses that, as I will argue, Milton will find a different, and I believe much more adequate, strength.

PART II

"Scarce-well-lighted flame": the representation of maternal mortality in Milton's early poetry

CHAPTER 4

"Too much conceaving": Milton's "On Shakespear"

It has been noted, but little discussed, that when Milton sat down in 1630 to write what would become his first publication (a sixteen-line epitaph for Shakespeare in heroic couplets that appeared in the 1632 Shakespeare Folio), he chose to end his poem with a figure that not only described poetic inspiration as a reproductive process, but as a dangerous one.[1] The figure, as we shall see, suggests that the inspiring power of Shakespeare's verse is so great that it not only impregnates the imaginations of his readers, but also causes the deaths of their imaginations, making them give birth – in the Platonic sense – to so many progeny, to so many fancies, that "fancy" itself ultimately dies in the process. The epitaph was only the sixth poem Milton had attempted in English since he had begun writing vernacular poetry about five years earlier, and was only the fifth that he had completed. The others were "On the Death of a Fair Infant Dying of a Cough," written some time in 1628, Sonnet I, "Song: On *May* Morning," "On the Morning of Christ's Nativity," and "The Passion".[2] As many critics have noted over the years, all of these poems, as well as a fair number of the Latin poems Milton had also written by this time, are full of self-conscious expressions of worry over just what sort of poetic identity it would be best for the young poet to establish. The poem for Shakespeare, with its striking final figure, represents Milton's most explicit expression of this worry up to this time, and I would

[1] The poem was originally printed, with no attribution in the 1632 Folio, as "An Epitaph on the admirable Dramaticke Poet W. Shakespeare." Milton gave it its shorter title, "On Shakespear," and dated it 1630 when he published it in the 1645 *Poems*. It was also published in Shakespeare's *Poems* (1640) with the initials "I. M.," in the Third Folio (1664), and in Milton's 1673 *Poems*. There are several variations, some of them significant. See *The Complete Poetry of John Milton*, ed. John T. Shawcross, rev. edn. (New York, NY: Anchor Books, 1971), p. 630.

[2] These last four were probably written in 1629–1630. "The Passion," which was attempted and left unfinished either during or just after the spring of 1630, is the only poem Milton published (in the 1645 and 1673 volumes of *Poems*) as a fragment. Milton had also written one hundred lines of English verse for a university vacation exercise in either 1628 or 1631. On the dating of these, see John T. Shawcross, *Rethinking Milton Studies: Time Present and Time Past* (Newark, NJ: University of Delaware Press, 2005), pp. 181–2, n. 1.

like to suggest the sense it made for Milton to express his anxiety using the figure of the mortal mother.

By emphasizing the image of the reader as a mother dying in the process of giving birth, Milton produced in this very early poem a striking twist on a set of commonplaces (some poetic, some Platonic, and some deriving from early modern theories of physiology and sexual reproduction). Milton was drawn to the figure, I believe, because it allowed him to express anxiety while also asserting his originality in a particularly forceful way. Using the figure allowed him to reflect on matters of vocation that were of immediate concern to him, express worries over uncertainties he felt, while at the same time overcome these worries by producing something new, and not a little uncanny, with what he had inherited. It also pointed the way to a less self-involved or merely self-assertive achievement. We are not sure exactly when Milton wrote the poem. He himself dated it 1630 when he published it in his *Poems* of 1645, and there is no reason to disbelieve him, but we do not know exactly when during that year he actually wrote it. Nor do we know what other poems he wrote at or close to the same time (there are several possible candidates, including "The Passion," but there is little certainty).[3] We do know, however, that some time not long after April 15, 1631, he composed "An Epitaph on the Marchioness of Winchester," which not coincidentally is a poem about a woman who died the way Milton imagines the fancies of Shakespeare's readers dying in "On Shakespear" (in her case while giving birth to her second son). In other words, in a matter of a few months, perhaps a year or so at the most, Milton went from a figurative appropriation of a rather terrible and common female experience to a more serious – or at least differently serious – examination of the implications of such an experience for a woman who actually suffered it.[4]

The nature of Milton's achievement in "On Shakespear" itself and its place in his early development has seemed, however, less than clear to many critics. It has been taken by some at more or less face value, as a youthful poet's conventional encomium for a poet just beginning to emerge as an important figure of the previous generation. Some have thought it modestly good at best, derivative and not all that promising. The poem has also been the site of some extended debate over Milton's larger evaluation of Shakespeare, and has provided opportunities for working out theories of

[3] It may be significant, given the anxieties that I argue it expresses, that Milton might have written the poem to Shakespeare in the wake of his failure to complete "The Passion."

[4] Gerald Hammond is one of the few critics to note a close connection between the poems in terms of stillbirth and maternal mortality (Gerald Hammond, *Fleeting Things: English Poets and Poems, 1616–1660* [Cambridge, MA: Harvard University Press, 1990], pp. 152–3).

literary representation, influence, and history. For some, its praise of Shakespeare has seemed less than straightforward.[5] I myself think it was intended as unambiguous praise, but it is also clear that it indicates a good deal of self-conscious worry. There is no attack on Shakespeare, no ironic undermining of the praise, but the speaker does seem, as I have already indicated, more than a little worried about his own originality and concerned to define his own poetics in contrast to Shakespeare's. Even that last sort of assertion, however, was already a cliché in the still small but growing subgenre of encomia for the dramatist. In using it, as at least one critic has noted, Milton was in danger of too closely following Jonson, whose elegy for Shakespeare – published in both the First and Second Folios – contains one of the earliest descriptions we have of Shakespeare as a poet of natural and easy-flowing verse (a stylistic paradigm that both Jonson and Milton praise, and yet one from which they both distance themselves).[6] The extravagant and unconventional treatment of the poem's final figure could have been Milton's response to this double problem of influence, his attempt to make something strikingly original in a situation fraught with anxiety and from some pretty unpromising and conventional materials.

Whether we see all this in Bloomian terms or we try to understand the poem's multivalence in terms of some other theory (or as simply an unresolved matter of literary biography), it should be clear that the poem's figures, especially its final one, are psychologically and allusively complex. They suggest far more than simple praise or blame, expressing no small measure of wonder (as Paul Stevens has argued), but terror as well, and a deeply self-conscious – and not yet fully assured – ambitiousness. In this particular case, I believe Milton faced down his terror by attempting to express mastery in the act of representing the reader's unmastering. He set

[5] Following remarks first made by E. M. W. Tillyard and later by Leslie Brisman and others, the poem has seemed to some a back-handed compliment. For some, it expresses a Bloomian anxiety over Shakespeare's influence and/or Milton's association of Shakespeare's work with the lower and less rational aspects of the imagination. For others, its admiration has seemed more genuine, or at least unambiguous. See E. M. W. Tillyard, *Milton* (New York, NY: Dial Press, 1930), pp. 50–1; Leslie Brisman, *Milton's Poetry of Choice and its Romantic Heirs* (Ithaca, NY: Cornell University Press, 1973), pp. 50–2; John Guillory, *Poetic Authority: Spenser, Milton, and Literary History* (New York, NY: Columbia University Press, 1983), pp. 18–19, 71; and Paul Stevens, "Subversion and Wonder in Milton's Epitaph 'On Shakespeare,'" *English Literary Renaissance* 19(3) (1989), 375–88. For Paul De Man and Jonathan Goldberg, it provided a key text for the development of a Derridian method of poetic analysis: see Paul De Man, "Autobiography as De-facement," *MLN* 94 (1979), 919–30 and Jonathan Goldberg, *Voice Terminal Echo: Postmodernism and English Renaissance Texts* (New York, NY: Methuen, 1986), pp. 126–58.

[6] Daniel Lanier, "Encryptions: Reading Milton Reading Jonson Reading Shakespeare," in *Reading and Writing in Shakespeare*, ed. David M. Bergeron (Newark, NJ: University of Delaware Press, 1996), pp. 220–50.

about making something strikingly new out of the materials of his own terror, and he found what he needed in the figure of the mortal mother: a terrible and psychologically dense figure for what we might call Platonic self-annihilation.

Milton treats all of the poem's images in a remarkably intense and allusive way, although he does not do so all at once. The conceit that governs the poem is the familiar one that claims that poetry outlasts monuments of stone because there is something more durable somehow in the social processes that preserve valued texts for future generations of readers – something more powerful than those that preserve monuments against the ravages of time. As has been noted by critics and commentators as far back as the eighteenth century, Shakespeare himself had used this conceit in many of his sonnets, and although evidence is slim concerning Milton's knowledge of the sonnets, it is possible that in constructing his version of the conceit, he had them in mind, as well as some lines from William Browne's elegy for the Countess of Pembroke and any number of other possible analogues and sources. The first half of the poem develops this conceit, at least to begin with, in a more or less conventional way over four tightly structured, end-stopped couplets:

> What needs my *Shakespear* for his honour'd Bones,
> The labour of an age in piled Stones,
> Or that his hallow'd reliques should be hid
> Under a Star-ypointing *Pyramid?*
> Dear son of memory, great heir of Fame,
> What need'st thou such weak witnes of thy name?
> Thou in our wonder and astonishment
> Hast built thy self a live-long Monument.

The poet asks his rhetorical question twice (first over two couplets, and then again in one). He then explains in one more very tidy pair of lines why the answer is obvious. "Wonder and astonishment" is a far greater monument than a tomb could ever be, no matter how great or how symbolic ("Star-ypointing") its design. The monument contains the poet's bones, enshrining them as relics, hiding them and pointing beyond them to eternity, but it is a weak witness to the poet's name, to what "Shakespear" really means. Whatever feelings the pile of stones might itself inspire, whatever attachment we might have for the poet's remains (for Milton, such an attachment would have no doubt seemed idolatrous), or for the idea that he had been translated from the time-bound human realm to that of eternal fame, these are nothing compared with the ongoing effect of the poet's *work*. Although it is not said explicitly until the second half of the poem, this effect is, of course, the result of reading, of direct encounters with the texts the dead poet has left behind. The shift from the singular "my *Shakespear*" to the plural "our wonder and astonishment" seems designed to reinforce the distinction, as if the speaker were giving up an individual relationship with the remembered poet for a sense of belonging to a generation of his readers.

Things begin to move beyond these forcefully expressed but relatively conventional sentiments in the poem's subsequent examination of the nature of that collective process of reading. In the first half of the poem, all we are asked to assume is that the present generation, having experienced "wonder and astonishment," will make sure that Shakespeare's texts will survive so that subsequent generations will have access to the same experience. The second half of the poem, drawing on some commonplaces about the nature of Shakespeare's art – those Jonsonian ones I mentioned earlier – then goes on to provide a detailed description of what that experience is like. The lines imply not only that reading Shakespeare will always be as they describe it, but concentrating on a set of dark implications buried in what Milton probably thought of as the actual etymology of the second of his two terms of praise, they elaborate on the opening figure in an unexpected and unconventional way:

> For whilst to th'shame of slow-endeavouring art,
> Thy easie numbers flow, and that each heart
> Hath from the leaves of thy unvalu'd Book
> Those Delphick lines with deep impression took,
> Then thou our fancy of it self bereaving,
> Dost make us Marble with too much conceaving;
> And so Sepulcher'd in such pomp doth lie,
> That Kings for such a Tomb would wish to die.

Here the prosody is looser and more expansive, imitative of Shakespeare's "easie numbers" as one sentence stretches over the four couplets, the first of which is strongly enjambed and "flows" into the second. The clever formal figure is designed to demonstrate what it describes. Shakespeare's lines have made a "deep impression" on "each" reader's heart. The experience is collective in the sense that it is the same for everyone, but individual in each actual encounter with the "unvalu'd Book" (the Folio that the original readers of the poem would have actually had in their hands). It has also, however, clearly made an impression on the heart of the speaker himself, the writer of these particular lines. Having earlier called Shakespeare a "son of memory," Milton now shows what that epithet implies. Shakespeare is a brother to the muses, perhaps even a male, tenth muse himself. He can and does inspire poetry of a particular kind, and the speaker tacitly identifies himself as someone enabled by the power of Shakespeare's example to write his own flowing verses. Some "slow-endeavouring" artists might be shamed in the presence of Shakespeare's easy, flowing example (and it is possible that the speaker does see himself as a slow-endeavourer), but he also demonstrates that he can imitate, in the course of his more carefully and slowly constructed verses, the easy flow itself. Wonder and astonishment has bred in him, in other words, an ability. It has changed him, to some extent empowered him, and in this sense he stands out from the collective generation of admirers. He has the authority to address them, to explain to them the nature of their own experience.

The last two couplets, however, are a surprise, and let us know that there is a dark side, or at least a downside, to this empowerment. Rather than going on to simply further celebrate the power he has acquired, concentrating on how it has resulted in the grateful tribute offered by the poem itself, the speaker extends his description of the psychological effect of wonder and astonishment, producing a figure that elaborates unexpectedly on some up-to-now hidden implications of the poem's account of reading. His elaboration describes the consequences of the process he presented figuratively at the start. People read Shakespeare, they feel wonder and astonishment, and these feelings, expressed in an ongoing way in the course of subsequent history, are what constitute the true monument that Shakespeare has built for himself in the ongoing effects of his work. That much is unproblematic and merely repeats in some new terms what others have already said. However, the new terms also tell us that, in the process, wonder *breeds* something in the minds of these readers, and the process of "conception," described in terms both abstract and physical, leads to an unexpected result. The reader, we are now told, is also turned to stone. "Astonishment," now comes to mean petrification, a sense (really based on a pun) that is suggested by one possible, though probably erroneous, derivation of the word (that it derives from roots meaning "turn to stone").[7] The reader becomes not an inspired individual but a tomb in which Shakespeare is "Sepulcher'd." The poet is therefore figuratively memorialized by the sort

[7] The *OED* cites Milton's line for definition 4 of the word: "Mental disturbance or excitement due to the sudden presentation of anything unlooked for or unaccountable; wonder temporarily overpowering the mind; amazement." The word, according to the *OED*, had been used in similar senses since the later sixteenth century. Its etymology is, however, uncertain. At some point it seems that a figurative sense that one who is "astonished" is turned to "stone" grew out of a pun that connected two sets of words with different derivations. The word itself is probably derived from the root from which we get the word "stun," rather than the one from which we get "stone." See the entries in the *OED* for "astonish" and "astone," as well as both the adjectival and verbial usages of "'stonish" ("like stone" and "to astonish").

of thing that the conceit tells us does not endure adequately, and the reader has become this tomb because of an excess of what we might call Platonic fertility in the process of giving birth to the new poems and ideas that Shakespeare's verse has inspired.

The penultimate couplet is more than a little syntactically obscure. The core of the image can, however, be paraphrased simply: "then our fancy (our imaginative capacity, perhaps only our lower, less rational capacity) turns us to stone." "Of it self bereaving" suggests, in addition, that in the process, "fancy" kills itself.[8] None of the close analogues that have been cited for this figure suggest this idea. The lines from Browne's elegy for the Countess of Pembroke, for example, make grief the cause of the petrification: "Marble Pyles let no man rayse/ To her name; for after dayes;/ Some kinde woman borne as she/ Reading this; (Like Niobe,)/ Shall turne Marble, and become/ Both her mourner and her Tombe."[9] The two other analogues that are usually cited from later poems by Milton also differ significantly. Line 42 of "*Il Penseroso*," for example ("Forget thy self to Marble"), merely suggests loss of self-consciousness in the process of contemplation. Comus' lines about the songs sung by his mother with the Sirens (which he says "lull'd the sense,/ And in sweet madnes robb'd it of it self") are somewhat closer, describing a narcotic effect that can be thought of as causing a loss of both "meaning" and "sensation," but this too is different. In Comus' figure, a "sweet madnes" inspired by the beauty of the song takes away the capacity to think and feel, and he contrasts this with the bracing power that the Lady's song has to inspire what he calls "waking bliss" (*A Mask*, lines 260–4). In "On Shakespear," the lines of Shakespeare's verse seem, however, to spur fancy on to a higher level of intense activity, and it is that activity – a reproductive activity – that kills.

Sixteenth- and early seventeenth-century poetry is full of images of poetic creativity figured as childbirth, a figure that took advantage of the fact that

[8] The 1632 text reads "her self," which was changed to "our self" in 1640. Milton used "it self" in 1645 and 1673, and all editors have followed him. "Our self" was probably a misprint for "her self," but may have been an attempt by the compositor at a clarifying emendation. As the *Variorum* editors note, drawing on Todd and others, "our self" makes easier sense: "the strong impression made on our imagination causes us to lose consciousness of our self." This meaning is closer in sense to line 42 of "*Il Penseroso*" (which has often been cited as an analogue) and to what Comus says about the effect of his mother's song at lines 260–1 of *A Mask*. See *A Variorum Commentary on the Poems of John Milton*, eds. A. S. P. Woodhouse and Douglas Bush (New York, NY: Columbia University Press, 1972), vol. II, Part 1 pp. 211–12. As my reading shows, however, neither of these is an exact analogue of the version in 1645 and 1673.

[9] *The Penguin Book of Renaissance Verse 1509–1659*, ed. H. R. Woudhuysen (New York, NY: Penguin Books, 1993), p. 644. This is the usual way the figure is used in funereal verse. Another example can be found at the opening of Ben Jonson's elegy for Lady Jane Paulet.

the word "conceiving" denoted both a mental process of reproduction and a physical one, as well as the fact that the two processes were seen as analogues for one another in the dominant medical and psychological discourses of the day.[10] One might be of a higher kind than the other, but the relationship was not always, or at least not simply, metaphorical. Mental creativity and physical pregnancy and birth were understood as the same process at work in two different parts of the body and at two different levels of physical and spiritual purity. In other words, when Milton says that reading Shakespeare causes "conceiving" to occur in the mind, he means more or less that the brain, in what were often called its greater and lesser "mothers" or wombs, is impregnated by the spirit contained in Shakespeare's work, and gives birth to ideas.

Seen Platonically, and in a positive light, this process should simply be a matter of what in the *Symposium* Diotima calls "giving birth in beauty";[11] that is, in this case, giving birth to beautiful ideas inspired by love of the true beauty to be found in Shakespeare's texts. The result should then be texts that themselves contain that beauty and continue the process for subsequent readers. Milton's treatment of the figure, however, suggests that the imaginative capacity of the impregnated mind is somehow harmed by the process of impregnation and birth. In fact, his figure suggests that ultimately the birthing process does not happen successfully for long, and that the pregnant imagination ("fancy") dies in the process, presumably – as often happened to women in the period – of a fatal last birth after a long and exhausting series of successful ones. It has not been noted in the critical literature just how unique this suggestion actually is. Milton crucially shifts the referent of his metaphor's vehicle toward a concrete historical condition, and this gives the figure a strangely anti-Platonic bias that allows it to express

10 According to the *OED*, use of the word in contexts relating to reproduction and birth goes back to at least the fourteenth century. The use of the word to denote mental processes is later, beginning perhaps in the sixteenth century. Both usages were current and common in the 1630s. On the figure of poetry as reproduction in Shakespeare and others, see Elizabeth Sacks, *Shakespeare's Images of Pregnancy* (New York, NY: St. Martin's Press, 1980); Jay Halio, "The Metaphor of Conception and Elizabethan Theories of the Imagination," *Neophilologus* 50 (1966), 454–61; Elizabeth D. Harvey, *Ventriloquized Voices: Feminist Theory and English Renaissance Texts* (New York, NY: Routledge, 1992); Katherine Eisaman Maus, "A Womb of His Own: Male Renaissance Poets in the Female Body," in *Sexuality and Gender in Early Modern Europe*, ed. James G. Turner (Cambridge University Press, 1993), pp. 266–88. On the roots of the metaphor in hermetic and quasi-medical discourses, see Anthony P. Russell, "'Thou seest mee strive for life': Magic, Virtue, and the Poetic Imagination in Donne's *Anniversaries*," *Studies in Philology* 95 (1998), 374–410, and "Dante's 'forte imaginazione' and Beatrice's 'occulta virtù': Lovesickness and the Supernatural in the *Vita Nuova*," *Mediaevalia* 22 (1998), 1–33.

11 See *Symposium*, 206b–207a: Plato, *Symposium*, ed. (with an introduction, translation, and commentary by) C. J. Rowe (Warminster: Aris and Phillips Ltd., 1998), pp. 88–91.

an anxiety alien to conventional versions of the figure. This bias, in turn, allows it to overcome that anxiety by making an implicit claim for the appropriate and powerful suggestiveness of what might otherwise seem a serious breach of decorum. The poem implicitly claims that no experience other than the self-annihilation faced by a woman who seeks to do God's will – as well as her own and her husband's – in childbirth can quite capture the danger a young poet faces in setting out to imitate his elders. It also suggests that no other figure could quite capture the equivocal reward: an immortality that comes at the cost of ending an ongoing, ordinary life (either uninspired or childless). This is why the extremity of the figure matters to Milton. It is as if he knew he had to embrace a fate analogous to that of a mortal mother, to accept the possible self-annihilation, if he were going to be able to give figurative birth to a new poem that might bear some mark of originality. Although birthing it might kill him, that poem might, on the other hand, validate his bid for at least some authority. The construction of an anti-Platonic figure based on a reference to concrete mortality makes possible one final Platonic bid for immortality.

Other examples of the figure of poetry as Platonic reproduction from the period are, in contrast, pretty insistently positive, borrowing at most, as in the case of Sidney's first sonnet in *Astrophil and Stella*, a certain dramatic urgency, even a sense of peril or helplessness from women's actual experience of birth, but not the death of the birthing mental faculty itself. As a result, these earlier poems all merely reproduce the positive Platonic logic of the figure's conventional sense. However, I know, of one partial exception. There is no way, as I said before, to establish for sure that Milton knew Shakespeare's sonnets, but his version of the figure does bear a striking resemblance to the figures of Sonnet 86, turning its conceit in a new direction, and the distinction here is again instructive. Sonnet 86 is one of the poems that deals with the speaker's competitive relationship to the "other poet" who has written about his beloved young man:

> WAs it the proud full saile of his great verse,
> Bound for the prize of (all to precious) you,
> That did my ripe thoughts in my braine inhearce,
> Making their tombe the wombe wherein they grew?
> Was it his spirit, by spirits taught to write,
> Aboue a mortall pitch, that struck me dead?
> No, neither he, nor his compiers by night
> Giuing him ayde, my verse astonished.
> He nor that affable familiar ghost
> Which nightly gulls him with intelligence,

As victors of my silence cannot boast,
I was not sick of any feare from thence.
  But when your countinance fild vp his line,
  Then lackt I matter, that infeebled mine.[12]

The connection and the distinction are both clear. Shakespeare's speaker invokes the inhibiting "astonishment" created by the other poet's greatness, figuring it in terms of stillbirth and then simply as a death-blow, only to displace the effect onto his subject matter (or perhaps onto the fact that the young man has been promiscuous when it comes to appearing in others' verses). Milton perhaps took his figure of poetic anxiety and astonishment from this text, suggesting, however, that his experience is one of maternal death (not stillbirth), and that the two things that Shakespeare's conceit distinguishes (the experience of the other poet's great verse and his experience of seeing the young man's countenance in that verse) have become for him one and the same. In Milton's case, after all, it is the other poet himself who is the subject of the encomium, not simply a beautiful person that the other poet has also chosen to praise. Moreover, as a result of his having read the "great verse" of his subject, he has created poems in which he can see only the countenance of Shakespeare; that is, the countenance of the other poet, who is also, in a sense, his beloved.[13] The poems all look like their father. He, their mother, has given birth to too many of them, and in the end has died as a poet in the process.

Although this dynamic might be understandable in Freudian terms, Milton is, I believe, primarily thinking in terms of early-modern natural philosophy. And here, again, we can see the swerving away from Platonic abstractions toward a concern with the concrete and physical, one that in this case is actually Aristotelian. Milton imagines himself as the mother of his poems, and this suggests, according to the dominant Aristotelian account of procreation, that he sees himself here as only a provider of their matter, not the informing power that gives them their unique living shape, which was provided only according to the theory by the father. As a dead mother, in the end, he will have provided material for the forming power of the inspiring poet to work on, but no formative, fatherly power of his own.[14] Only the last one, the one that kills his fancy, bears any mark of

[12] Quoted from the facsimile of the 1609 quarto, printed in *Shakespeare's Sonnets*, ed. Stephen Booth (New York, NY: Yale University Press, 1977), pp. 74, 77.

[13] The implication may also echo Shakespeare's Sonnet 76, which Booth connects with Sonnet 86 (*Shakespeare's Sonnets*, p. 288).

[14] The Aristotelian understanding of the roles of male and female in reproduction, articulated in *De Generatione Animalium*, was widely distributed and accepted, with some minor variations, from

the mother, and in this case the mark is that move to a concrete reference to physical reproduction. The maternal distinction is death.

That the figure has also suggested Niobe to many readers reinforces and extends in another direction this "maternal" interpretation. Milton may have picked up the suggestion from Browne's elegy, but it has more complex resonances in this context. Niobe was turned to stone with grief over the deaths of her children, punished by Latona for claiming that they were finer than Latona's own progeny, Apollo and Diana. The myth explicitly, for example in its Ovidian version, is one among those that meditate on divine envy of human creative power. It was placed by Ovid – along with the story of Latona's treatment of the Lycian peasants – between the stories of Arachne and Marsyas in Book VI of *Metamorphoses*, and Ovid goes so far as to criticize Niobe for failing to learn the lessons that Arachne's tale clearly taught: that human creative power can call down the envy of the Gods, and that human beings therefore need to learn humility, even if they are, in fact, better creators.[15] The fit here is imperfect. Niobe, for example, does not die *in childbirth*, but only of grief over the slaughter by Diana and Apollo of her children. It is as a figure for grief that she is usually invoked in funereal verse. Here, however, in so far as she is recalled, Niobe matters as a figure of the artist as mother (or conversely of the mother as artist). She is conflated for Milton with the Medusan figure that both he and Shakespeare recall from the Petrarchan tradition, and together they are used to represent the rather astonishing figure of maternal self-annihilation we have been discussing. Niobe is annihilated, furthermore, by Gods who, among other things, represent poetic power and inviolate virginity, things that in several other works in the 1630s and 1640s Milton would closely associate with one another (think, for example, of *A Mask* and of the autobiographical digression in *An Apology Against a Pamphlet*).

What redeems the figure of self-annihilation in this context, however, is the fact that it can suggest so much. It turns out to be rather successful in asserting its own originality as an expression of worry over that very thing. What matters most about this strange figure for the present study is the fact that, in hindsight, it is possible to see in it that Milton was already, at this very early stage of his development, meditating on an important theme that

ancient times through the early modern period. See Ambroise Paré, *The Workes of that Famous Chirurgion Ambrose Parey*, trans. Thomas Johnson (London, 1634), pp. 885–6 for one example of its common expression. On Milton's approach to both the traditional and some newer theories of generation, see John Rumrich, *Milton Unbound: Controversy and Interpretation* (Cambridge University Press, 1996), pp. 103–9.

15 See *Metamorphoses*, Book VI lines 146–51: *Ovid's Metamorphoses, Books 6–10*, ed. William S. Anderson (Norman, OK: University of Oklahoma Press, 1972), pp. 42–3.

would preoccupy him later in his more explicit poetry on maternal mortality. As I said earlier, in treating the figure directly and literally about a year later, Milton would not lose sight of the relationship between maternal suffering and his own poetic creativity. He would, however, stop using the subject merely as a vehicle for expressing his own wonder and his own anxieties. Instead, he would use it as an occasion for overcoming those anxieties in a more productive way, by displaying his ability to, in fact, accomplish something far more original and far more ambitious.

Milton would continue for some years to express worry over whether or not his poetic style was, as he put it, playing with figures of poetry and childbirth in Book 2 of *The Reason of Church Government*, "by certain vital signs it had, … likely to live" (*CP*, 1.809). In the course of the 1630s, however, he would prove to himself in no uncertain terms that he was at least capable of accomplishing something of value according to the terms set by his own sense of vocation. He would, in the process, profoundly rethink the relationship – implied by his early metaphor – between women who risked their lives giving birth and poets who hazarded to create and publish works that they hoped would be of value to others (and to "aftertimes"). In the epitaph he would write within a year, he would decide that the value of poetry should be, in part, tested by whether or not it could be made to serve those that suffered in reproduction. Milton still used the occasion to express his own vocational anxieties and hopes, but he also asserted his ambitions in a new way, subordinating his penchant for self-dramatization to the task of creating a poem that might do more than simply announce its own originality or mark the emergence of a new voice from among a set of older ones. The epitaph for Jane Paulet attempts to provide an effective and appropriate consolation to those who faced a death in childbirth. It also, in ways that anticipate Milton's later achievements, gestures toward larger issues of social, political, and religious import. A few years later, Milton would weave some of these same concerns into the story he would choose for the Ludlow masque, a story that would present the trial of a virtuous young woman just arrived at marriageable age, anticipating the future trials of a reproductive life. Only much later, of course, would he be moved to treat his own suffering in the face of maternal mortality, this time in a striking sonnet whose speaker is a bereaved husband, then in the larger scheme of his epic.

CHAPTER 5

"Tears of perfect moan": Milton and the Marchioness of Winchester

On April 15, 1631, Lady Jane Paulet, wife of Lord John Paulet, fifth Marquis of Winchester and daughter of Thomas, first Viscount Savage of Rock Savage, Cheshire, died giving birth to her second son. She was twenty-three years old (about the same age as Milton), just one month short of her twenty-fourth birthday. According to sources close to the family, her son was born dead, and the difficult stillbirth was complicated by a fever and the lancing of an "impostume" on her cheek.[1] She was delivered of her dead son before she died. As Parker notes, the story seems to have touched a number of people, for Lady Jane was mourned in verse by at least six poets whose poems survive; these include elegies by Ben Jonson, William Davenant, an obscure Catholic poet named Walter Colman, and two even more obscure young men: a Mr. John Eliot, about whom almost nothing is known, and, of course, John Milton. There is also a short, anonymous Latin epitaph in William Camden's *Remaines Concerning Britaine*.[2]

[1] The sources are a letter from Katherine, Duchess of Buckingham, to her father on April 16th and a newsletter from John Pory to Sir Thomas Puckering, dated April 21st. What Pory calls an "impostume" we would probably call today an abscess. It may have been the source of the fever: see Parker, pp. 94–6, 766–8 and "Milton and the Marchioness of Winchester," *MLR* 44 (1949), 547–50. Pory may have been the biographical connection that occasioned Milton's composition of the poem and provided him with the accurate biographical information he seems, on the evidence of both versions of the poem (1645 and another found in BL MS Sloane 1446), to have had. John Pory may have been related to Robert Pory, Milton's longtime schoolmate (at both St. Paul's and Christ's) (Parker, p. 722). The family connection between Lady Jane and Henry Rich, Earl Holland, who had become Chancellor of Cambridge University in 1629, may also have been enough to commend the occasion to Milton. See Kate Gartner Frost, "No Marchioness but a Queen: Milton's Epitaph for Jane Paulet," *Milton Studies* 39 (2000), 1–25, especially 6–8 and 12–13.

[2] William Camden, *Remaines Concerning Britaine* (London, 1636), p. 415. Davenant's poem, "On the Death of the Lady Marquesse of Winchester," can be found in Sir William Davenant, *The Shorter Poems and Songs from the Plays and Masques*, ed. A. M. Gibbs (Oxford: Clarendon Press, 1972), pp. 54–5. Walter Colman's poem, "An Elegie. Vpon the Ladie Marchioness of *Winchester*, daughter *to the right honorable* Thomas *Lord* Sauage, etc." can be found in *La Dance Machabre or Deaths Duell* (London, 1632), p. 70. For Jonson's "An Elegie On the Lady Jane Pawlet, Marchion: of Winton," see *Ben Jonson*, eds. C. H. Herford and Percy and Evelyn Simpson, 11 vols. (Oxford: Clarendon Press, 1925–1952), vol. VIII, pp. 268–71. I discuss Eliot's poem briefly below. In his *John Milton: Complete Shorter Poems*, 2nd edn. (London: Longman, 1997), p. 131, John Carey reports an elegy by William Strode and several others to be found in

The poem that Milton contributed to this set, "An Epitaph on the Marchioness of Winchester" (hereafter "An Epitaph"), is not a poem that has attracted the full attention of Miltonists over the years – it has rarely occasioned more than a paragraph or a passing aside. There are a few important exceptions, but most of the essays and notes that have been written concern only a small set of issues (a few biographical riddles, the influence of Jonson on Milton's early style, the poem's concluding reference to Dante, and Milton's flirtation with the possibilities of patronage), and most critics have found themselves apologizing for what they have taken to be the poem's immaturity, its overreaching, and/or its failure to give a weighty enough impression of Milton's engagement with the occasion.[3]

BL MS Sloane 1446 (where a manuscript version of Milton's poem appears). There are a number of elegies in the manuscript, including others on maternal deaths, but it is unclear if any of the others refer to the Marchioness. This fascinating manuscript, however, warrants further study. There is an anonymous epitaph on p. 128 of the manuscript, entitled "On an Infant unborne and the mother dyinge in travell," that may pertain to Lady Jane. However, it contains no clear biographical references beyond the nature of the occasion itself. The infant in the poem seems never to have been born at all, dying instead inside its mother's body, and perhaps being buried along with her that way. The Duchess' letter clearly indicates a stillbirth before the mother's death. Pory's language is less clear, however, and suggests a death before delivery. Milton's poem allows for – perhaps even strongly suggests – that scenario, suggesting that Milton may have drawn on Pory, but we have no way of knowing what Milton – or perhaps the other poet – knew or did not know. Versions of "On an Infant unbourne and the mother dyinge in travell" appear in fifteen other seventeenth-century manuscripts, indicating that it was popular in circles that kept and circulated such collections. It is attributed to "W Davenat" in BL MS Egerton 2421, and A. M. Gibbs prints a version of it from that manuscript in *The Shorter Poems*, though he thinks the attribution erroneous. Gibbs also notes that the poem was attributed to William Browne in two other manuscripts (BL MS Harleian 6931 and Bodleian CCC.328) – it was thought to be his by nineteenth-century editors – and to Richard Corbett in Bodleian Rawlinson Poetical 117. None of these attributions has been established with any certainty by modern editors. See Gibbs, *The Shorter Poems*, pp. lxxxvi–lxxxvii and 278.

3 The earlier criticism is surveyed in *A Variorum Commentary on the Poems of John Milton*, ed. Merritt Y. Hughes, 6 vols. (New York, NY: Columbia University Press, 1972), vol. II, Part 1, pp. 192–202. See also Parker, pp. 94–6, 766–80 and "Milton and the Marchioness"; Michael F. Moloney, "The Prosody of Milton's *Epitaph, L'Allegro*, and '*Il Penseroso*,' *MLN* 72 (1957), 174–8; William J. Roscelli, "The Metaphysical Milton (1625–1631)," *Texas Studies in Literature and Language* 8 (1967), 463–84, especially, 475–6; J. B. Leishman, *Milton's Minor Poems* (London: Hutchinson, 1969), p. 87; and Gerald Hammond, *Fleeting Things: English Poets and Poems 1616–1660* (Cambridge, MA: Harvard University Press, 1990), pp. 145–53. Michael West, "The *Consolatio* in Milton's Funeral Elegies," *The Huntington Library Quarterly* 34 (1971), 233–49 offers a rare bit of praise. G. W. Pigman compares the poem with Jonson's and Eliot's in *Grief and the English Renaissance Elegy* (Cambridge University Press, 1985), pp. 92–3, 106–7. John Rumrich includes some remarks about the poem and childbirth danger in *Milton Unbound: Controversy and Interpretation* (Cambridge University Press, 1996), pp. 78, 97. The following are the few full-length treatments: Gale Edward Wilson, "Decorum and Milton's 'An Epitaph on the Marchioness of Winchester,'" *Milton Quarterly* 8 (1974), 11–14; Louis Schwartz, "Scarce-Well-Lighted Flame": Milton's 'Epitaph on the Marchioness of Winchester' and the Representation of Maternal Mortality in the Seventeenth-Century Epitaph," in *All in All: Unity, Diversity, and the Miltonic Perspective*, eds. Charles W. Durham and Kristin A. Pruitt (Selinsgrove, PA: Susquehanna University Press, 1999), pp. 200–23; and Frost, "No Marchioness." Frost's is by far the most important and comprehensive account, especially in its treatment of what she calls the poem's "pre-modern Augustinian Poetics" (2–3), its social and political contexts, and its startling ambitiousness. See below for my debts and disagreements.

However, the poem is worthy of extended comment. Not only is it the only poem about Lady Jane that actually treats her death explicitly and at length as a death in childbirth, but it is also one of the few full-length elegies in the period as a whole that attempted to structure itself entirely around figures of a catastrophic birth and to provide a consolation specifically adapted to such an occasion. The poem is far more ambitious and original than most critics have thought (much more so than we might expect from a poet as young as Milton was in 1631).[4] In its approach to maternal mortality, it shows a keen awareness of medical and ritual practices. It draws on the rich and complex discourses of childbed consolation that were available at the time, as well as on figures used in the few poems about maternal death Milton might have read, including a remarkable elegy by Michael Drayton that might have provided its most immediate model. The structure and occasion are fully integrated with one another, and Milton has consciously set out to sum up *and better* what other poets had so far achieved (or failed to achieve) in confronting this vexing subject. He deliberately constructed his consolation in a way that conflates signs of his own literary ambitions with a strikingly complex idealization of Jane Paulet's powers (both realized and unrealized) not only as a pious, suffering, and literally self-sacrificial mother, but also as a potential evangelist for the Protestant cause. The poem's act of literary representation is ambitiously designed to recuperate the loss of Lady Jane's potential maternal and evangelizing powers, suggesting not only that these powers were interdependent, but that their recuperation required a wholesale revision of the Jonsonian elegy.

MATERNAL MORTALITY AND THE EARLY MODERN ENGLISH FUNERAL ELEGY

In order to explain more fully how Milton accomplished such a revision, and why he was moved to do so, I would like to address the question of why the epideictic funeral poem, the most significant body of poetry on death in

[4] At this point (at the age of twenty-four), Milton was the author of approximately forty poems, mostly exercises and epistolary poems in Latin (including the seven "elegies"). He had also written a Greek epigram, five sonnets and one canzone in Italian, two psalm paraphrases, and a handful of poems in English ("On the Death of a Fair Infant Dying of a Cough," Sonnet I, "Song: On *May* Morning," "On the Morning of Christs Nativity," "The Passion," "On Shakespear," and the two Hobson poems). He had also written the English verse section of "At a Vacation Exercise" and, perhaps, "*L'Allegro*" and "*Il Penseroso.*" Of these (if we exclude the companion poems), only the Nativity ode and "On Shakespear" have received adequate attention, but these early works show a very high degree of technical mastery and self-conscious ambition. For useful surveys that pay particular attention to Milton's mastery of form, see John T. Shawcross, "Form and Content in Milton's Latin Elegies," *The Huntington Library Quarterly* 33 (1970), 315–50 and *Intentionality and the New Traditionalism: Some Liminal Means to Literary Revisionism* (University Park, PA: The Pennsylvania State University Press, 1991), pp. 141–56.

the period, seems to have largely ignored maternal mortality, or at least failed by and large to treat it with anything but a very narrow set of conventional figures. There are remarkable exceptions to the general silence, but they are relatively rare, and their rarity itself is worth some extended consideration.[5] One brief example of the sort of poem Milton might have seen will illustrate what I mean by the narrowness of conventional treatments. The following is an epitaph written for a woman named Anne Scott who died in childbirth on November 10, 1617. In the early eighteenth century, John Le Neve found it inscribed on her tomb in Great St. Mary's Church, Cambridge, the official church of Cambridge University, and Milton could very well have read it there:

> Under this Marble Stone a Matron lyes,
> Who to gyve lyfe her own did sacrifice:
> The happy womb that gave so many breath
> Became her Infants Tomb, her Infants death.[6]

[5] Michael Drayton's "Upon the death of Mistris Elianor Fallowfield" is a remarkable exception (see below). Only a few other poems that explicitly make reference to maternal mortality predate Milton's, and most fail to construct any extended figures. See, for example, Nicholas Grimald's "Upon the Tomb of A. W." and the anonymous "Of the ladie Wentworth's Death" in *Tottel's Miscellany (1557–1587)*, ed. Hyder Edward Rollins (Cambridge, MA: Harvard University Press, 1928), pp. 109, 166–7. Several elegies on childbed death that mention the subject only glancingly can be found in William Crashawe, *The Honor of Virtue* (London, 1620). Among the other poems on Lady Jane, Eliot's is the only one, other than Milton's, that mentions the cause of death directly. The anonymous epitaphs "On a Lady dying in childe bed" and "On an infant unborne, the Mother dying in travell," collected as numbers 90 and 136 in Sir John Mennes, *Wits Recreations* (London, 1641) are probably earlier than their publication date (the collection contains many poems dating back to the early decades of the seventeenth century and beyond – including seven epitaphs for Thomas Hobson, the university carrier for whom Milton also wrote two poems just a few months before Lady Jane's death). This is also possibly true of the epitaph in BL MS Sloane 1446. That poem and the second of the two epitaphs from *Wits Recreations* are among the more elaborate examples we have. Poems that possibly or certainly postdate Milton's include Robert Herrick's "Upon a young mother of many children," "Upon Batt," "Upon a Lady that died in child-bed, and left a daughter," and "Upon Lady Crew": see *The Poems of Robert Herrick*, ed. L. C. Martin (London: Oxford University Press, 1965), pp. 58, 72, 126, 304; Lady Jane Cavendish's, "On the death of my Deare Sister the Countesse of Bridgewater," in *Kissing the Rod: an Anthology of Seventeenth-Century Women's Verse*, ed. Germaine Greer (New York, NY: Farrar, Straus, and Giroux, 1989), p. 118; George Wither's "An Epitaph upon a Woman, and her Child, buried together in the same Grave," in *The English Spenserians*, ed. William B. Hunter (Salt Lake City, UT: University of Utah Press, 1977), p. 192. Three out of the five elegies appended to the publication of Edmund Staunton's sermon on the death of Elizabeth Wilkinson suggest that she died in childbed: see Edmund Staunton, *A Sermon Preacht at Great Milton in the County of Oxford: Decemb: 9. 1654* (Oxford, 1659), pp. 37–44.

[6] Quoted from John Le Neve, *Monumenta Anglicana: Being Inscriptions on the Monuments of several Eminent Persons Deceased in or since the year 1600. to the end of year 1649* (London, 1719), p. 63. See Parker, pp. 25, 42 and J. Milton French, *The Life Records of John Milton*, 5 vols. (New Brunswick, NJ: Rutgers University Press, 1949), vol. I, pp. 180–9 for Milton's connections with the church. Raymond A. Anselment offers some brief comments on the epitaph and one of the two from *Wits Recreations* in *Realms of Apollo: Literature and Healing in Seventeenth-Century England* (New York, NJ: University of Delaware Press, 1995), pp. 74–5.

Although he used all three of this poem's basic figures (the marble tomb, the maternal sacrifice, and the womb as tomb), we have no way of knowing if Milton saw and was directly inspired by it. He could have come across these figures elsewhere. What matters for our purposes is that wherever he found them, such figures would seldom have been treated more elaborately than this. These and the few others Milton might have come across (for example, the comparison of a dead mother and infant to a tree and its fruit, which he also used in "An Epitaph") might have provided the basis for a rich and flexible discourse of psychological and theological accommodation, should a poet with sufficient ambition and imagination have chosen to take them up and elaborate upon them. Most of the poems Milton could have seen, however, tended to repeat such figures in a starkly lifeless way. In fact, most poets who wrote of women who died in childbed deliberately chose not even to make this much reference to the occasion, choosing instead to ignore the matter entirely.

Some of the causes for this sparing treatment or utter silence are more or less obvious, others less so. For example, it certainly had something to do with the general tendency toward abstraction of the cause of death in conventional elegiac verse. As we know, writers of funeral verses turned more readily to poetic and mythic motifs than to physical or even broadly biographical particulars, and they also tended to treat these abstractly, if they treated them at all. In addition, how the dead faced their deaths – and what they believed happened to their souls as a result – was generally thought, in religious terms, to be far more important than what killed them. In other words, the abstraction of specific physical causes of death was, in part, the result of the pervasive application of Christian Platonic commonplaces and prevailing ideas about pious suffering and spiritual trial in the traditions of the *ars moriendi*.[7] The nature of medical practice may also have had some effect, given that the causes of particular deaths were often unknown or vaguely or misleadingly named.[8] For example, this lack of specificity may have made it unlikely for an elegist to draw on particulars that were simply not available or very well understood. In other words, death in childbirth, in so far as it was understood as a medical matter, may

[7] See Nancy Lee Beaty's *The Craft of Dying: a Study of the Tradition of the Ars Moriendi in England* (New Haven, CT: Yale University Press, 1970); David Cressy, *Birth, Marriage, and Death: Ritual, Religion, and the Life-Cycle in Tudor and Stuart England* (Oxford University Press, 1997), pp. 389–93; and Lucinda M. Becker, *Death and the Early Modern Englishwoman* (Reading: Ashgate, 2003), especially pp. 69–128.

[8] See Nancy Siriasi, *Medieval and Early Renaissance Medicine: an Introduction to Knowledge and Practice* (Chicago, IL: University of Chicago Press, 1990), pp. 123–33.

have gone the way of most medical particulars in the genre. When sickness was evoked at all in an elegy, it tended to become an occasion for the elaboration of one of several generic topoi (declarations of *contemptus mundi*, of faith in God's power to heal the soul whatever might happen to the body, or for satiric remarks about the ineffectuality or inadvertent cruelty of physicians). Fatal childbirth, as a medical particular, may have been treated as simply the "fever" or "consumption" it often occasioned, or it may have been abstracted out of the picture entirely. This may be the case, for example, with Ben Jonson's poem on Jane Paulet, which portrays her death as from an unspecified sickness with no reference to childbirth at all.[9]

We must also keep in mind that, as we saw in Part I, men usually had very little to do with childbirth, and men, of course, wrote most of the elegies we have. Most men, unless they made it their business to read medical or midwifery books, were largely ignorant of what went on in a birthing chamber, and those whose knowledge came only from reading were likely to attain only an abstract and intellectually distanced sense of what actually happened there. This lack of specific, first-hand experience must also be considered in relation to a problem of conflicting decorums. It seems right, as we shall see, that an elegist might wish to portray the death of a birthing mother in relation to any one of a number of conventional themes and topoi (as an instance of pity, an occasion for *contemptus mundi*, as a reminder of original sin, as a heroic deed on the part of the woman in the interest of future generations, as a sacrifice to her husband's desires and the needs of a noble line, etc.). It is easy to imagine how a poet might therefore find reference to childbed suffering poetically decorous, and would have wanted to find decorous ways of treating it. However, the childbed was surrounded not just by an actual curtain and by a female circle of attendants; it was also surrounded by vaguely articulated but palpable taboos about its representation. As we saw in Part I, midwifery books in the period themselves had to fight off the stigma of this taboo, often carrying prefaces from editors and authors warning against their use for prurient purposes.[10] It seems reasonable to assume, therefore, that poets may have been loath to invite their readers into the chamber. They may also have thought many of

9 An abstraction of this sort in a different generic context can be found in the narrative appended to Staunton's sermon on the death of Elizabeth Wilkinson. The narrative account treats the death as if it were from sickness alone, although the epistle that precedes it notes that "*sore paines frequented her in the breeding and bearing of children*," and although several of the poems appended to the text directly suggest a death in childbed. See Staunton, *A Sermon*, pp. d6, 21–44.

10 See Audrey Eccles, "The Early Use of English for Midwiferies 1500–1700," *Neuphilologische Mitteilungen* 78 (1977), 377–85.

the specific details of a painful obstetric catastrophe too awful to be decorously handled, despite their adaptability to the sorts of conventions I have mentioned. In addition, we should remember that women themselves had a significant investment in keeping the rites of childbirth to themselves. This may, in part, explain why so few of even the women poets of the period addressed the issue directly in verses aimed (unlike their private writings) at a largely male audience.

However, for several reasons, ignorance, taboo, the lack of clear medical categories, conventional abstraction, and decorum are not completely satisfying explanations for the silence of epideictic poets. First of all, whatever the actual ignorance of men about the details of birth as it was experienced in the chamber, death in childbirth still should have, and could have, lent itself very nicely to the amplification of various generic topoi. The medical and devotional literature, as well as the maternal deathbed books discussed in Chapters 2 and 3, could easily have provided just the sort of already abstracted and moralized figures a poet needed, yet these materials were rarely utilized.[11] Given the social, psychological, and theological investments the culture had in procreation, it seems unlikely that catastrophic birth would have been simply discarded as an accidental detail poorly fitted to conventional abstraction.

It is true that a sense of the sheer physical ugliness of even a heroic and pious death in childbirth might have kept poets from dealing with it too closely. Still, when other causes of death, often in point of fact just as grotesque, could be specified in an elegy, and they afforded an occasion for praise or the amplification of some commonplace, they very often were clearly specified and described. Sickness, for example, although seldom described with any medical precision, often provided an occasion for a set of appropriate conceits of satire and *contemptus mundi*. For example, many of the hundreds of poems written in honor of Prince Henry refer to his death by plague.[12] In addition, it was not uncommon for a man who died in

[11] Much of the material I discuss in Part I of this study was available by the early 1620s: John Calvin's sermons on Timothy had been available in English since 1579; Thomas Bentley's *The Monument of Matrones: Conteining Seven Severall Lamps of Virginity* had appeared in 1582, Christopher Hooke's sermon in 1590; Phillip Stubbes' commemorative pamphlet about his wife was first published in 1591 and had been reprinted at least ten times by 1603. Robert Hill's prayer for the childbed was published in 1609, and William Crashawe's *The Honor of Virtue or the Monument created by the sorrowfull this band* in 1620. John Donne had preached his churching sermons in 1618 and in the early 1620s. Crucially, the first edition of Elizabeth Joceline's *The Mother's Legacie to her Unborne Childe* had appeared in 1624.

[12] Dennis Kay surveys the elegies on Henry in *Melodious Tears: the English Funeral Elegy from Spenser to Milton* (Oxford University Press, 1990), pp. 124–203, 231–50, 259–64. Milton also addressed death by plague explicitly in "*Elegia Tertia*," his 1626 elegy for Lancelot Andrews.

battle to have that fact made much of in his epitaphs.[13] Things like drownings at sea, which were very common in a maritime economy, were also commonly made mention of or became the crux of important figures. Milton's own "Lycidas," a poem that, as we will later see, has a number of things in common with "An Epitaph," is just one familiar example. However, despite the fact that women frequently died in childbirth, their deaths, unlike these other more general and/or masculine forms of death, never became the source of any really widely used conceit. This suggests that a more complex explanation is required. There was, after all, something very common and highly distressing to elide, something distressing to both men and women, since hardly anyone escaped the experience of birth-related loss, be it of a mother, a wife, a sister, a daughter, an aunt, a cousin, friend, or patron.

In addition, whatever ignorance male poets may have had, a state of ignorance about the realities of a situation should not have been disabling to their imaginative capacity for misconception, symbolic grotesquery, or idealization. In fact, the poems that do treat the subject, even if they are rarely, if ever, as thoughtful and ambitious as Milton's, do show that the poetic tradition (and certainly the discourse found in sermons and set prayers) was perfectly capable of constructing decorous abstractions of the event, and of conveying at least some of its pitiful ironies in ways that fit the epideictic and consolatory purposes of their genre. It is also true that the drama and the satiric traditions of anti-epideixis are rife with figures opposite to those purposes. Grotesque evocations of birth were also, as we have seen, common in the sermons, prayers, and meditations. In other words, rhetorical strategies for dealing with the physical details of birth, whether inspired by anti-feminist rage, denigration of the body, *contemptus mundi*, pious meditation, or a sense of personal and collective sin (even, as for example in Rabelais, a carnivalesque celebration of the physical), were available as a dark twin to the sort of idealizing praise desirable in a funeral poem, and some of this sort of thing did find its way into lyric and narrative

[13] This is particularly true from the 1590s onwards, when, in the wake of the death of Sir Philip Sidney, specificity of all kinds became more common in elegaic verse (Kay, *Melodious Tears*, pp. 10–17). See also Sheldon Zitner's discussion of Surrey's epitaph on the death of Thomas Clere in "Truth and Mourning on a Sonnet by Surrey," *ELH* 50 (1983), 509–29 and Andrew Marvell's "An Elegy on the Death of My Lord Francis Villiers"; as well as the set of elegies published in 1633 on the death of Gustavus Adolphus, which includes poems by Davenant, Carew, et al., Davenant also wrote several other specific elegies. See "Elegie on B. Haselrick, slaine in's youth in a Duell" (Gibbs, *The Shorter Poems*, p. 59), "Written, When Collonell Goring was beleev'd to be slaine, at the siege of Breda" (p. 69), and "An Elegy on the Duke of Buckingham's Death" (p. 272).

poetry.[14] The figure of birth, as we saw earlier, was also commonly used as a figure for the imagination in the poetry of the age. So why should it have been so hard to figure it elaborately for the purposes of praise?

Part of the answer lies, I believe, in the personal specificity of epideictic rhetoric. As I observed briefly in Part I, it was rare for a preacher to claim that either a death in childbed or the sickness of a particular person were punishment for individual sins (in satire, on the other hand, and in "fire and brimstone" sermons, the gloves could come off). The poetic culture may have displayed the same scruples and been loathe to approach the figure as a biographically particular referent because of its close association with the general condition of original sin. Women who wrote about their own experiences (women like Alice Thornton, Elizabeth Egerton, and Mary Carey) could refer all they wanted to their own immersion in original sin because they were confessing their own sinful natures and trying to give themselves over to God's justice and mercy, but a poet may not have wanted to presume to judge, or even seem to judge. I would like to suggest, however, that while this dynamic surely played a role, the primary causes of poetic unease about elaborating too fully on the specifics of maternal mortality were a combination of theological paradox, the ironies that attended the imperative that aristocratic families felt toward dynastic continuity, and male guilt over exemption from this sort of suffering. In addition, certain aspects of the genre itself, its reliance on motifs drawn from both funeral rites and marriage rites, may have in some cases complicated the conventional rhetorical construction of poems that made explicit mention of the childbed. Together, these complicated a powerful and specific kind of grief, and made it hard for the conventional modes of mourning verse to represent it and adequately provide consolation.

For example, the seemingly decorous topics that, as I mentioned before, could be used to accommodate childbed death to the conventions of the genre required a complex discourse on the need for sacrifice, on the fragility of noble lineages, on a web of biblical touchstones, and on the nature of original sin itself, particularly its guilt-laden gender specificity. A seeming symmetry (for instance that men might die on trading missions or in war, etc.) might have seemed not only asymmetrical but also weighted with a peculiar psychological burden when consideration of the relationship of

14 See, for example, Heather Dubrow's discussion of John Collop's grotesque poems in "Foreign Currencies: John Collop and the 'Ugly Beauty' Tradition," *Women's Studies* 24 (1994), 165–87. An even more striking example of this grotesque mode can be seen in the opening episode of Michael Drayton's *The Moone-Calfe*, a long satire published in the same volume as the Fallowfield elegy. The opening of Drayton's poem is indebted to, among many other things, the birth of Gargantua.

childbed death to sexual intimacy with men was added to the picture. This asymmetry took on a further social and ideological complexity when the role played in reproduction by male desires and dynastic hopes, as well as by rape and seduction outside of wedlock and across class lines, was considered with any seriousness. All of these considerations suggest very vexed questions of theology and sociability, and they required more complex forms of theodicy and social reflection than could normally be offered in an occasional poem.

An evocation of death in childbed also brought certain conventional elegiac motifs into conflict with one another, complicating the formulae by which such poems were often written. These motifs, broadly speaking, are those derived from epithalamia on the one hand, and from funeral imagery and ritual on the other (the former as part of the consolation, the latter as part of the complaint). This rhetorical problem may have made it difficult for poets to reach toward the more complex discourses that might have enabled the genre to adequately confront death in childbed. Elegies often made use of motifs derived precisely from the very human rituals (wedding and funeral) that collided in the childbed, where the "ends" of marriage (physical love and procreation) became its end in death, presenting yet another paradox insoluble by conventional rhetorical means.

Milton, as I will show, used a solution to the latter of these problems as a means of solving the former, resolving the generic tension in an ambitious literary and typological allusion. In addition, he accommodated the problem of male guilt to his epitaph's ideologically motivated critique of John Paulet, and resolved the problem of competing decorums by maintaining a high level of mythopoeic abstraction. We can see these processes at work most clearly, however, if we compare Milton's epitaph to Michael Drayton's elegy "Upon the Death of Mistris Elianor Fallowfield." Milton may have known Drayton's poem and used it as a model, but even if he did not, a comparison will allow us to see him ambitiously solving a problem that Drayton courted but could not solve.

DRAYTON'S "UPON THE DEATH OF MISTRIS ELIANOR FALLOWFIELD"

Drayton's elegy provides an indication of some of the anxieties that underlay the subject of childbed death, and put strange demands on a funeral elegy that attempted to deal with the subject. The poem confronts these anxieties more directly than any other early-modern English elegy of which I am aware (Milton's aside), making remarkably explicit use of generic motifs associated with marriage and death, ones that only Milton would put to more successful and rhetorically integrated use. The poem appeared in 1627 as part of "Elegies vpon sundry occasions," a collection of funeral verses and familiar epistles that Drayton appended to the volume containing his long poem, *The Battaile of Agincourt*. The Fallowfield elegy is the last poem of the "elegies" section and concludes the volume. I know of no reason why Milton should not have owned a copy of the book, although I am the first to argue any explicit connection between the elegy and his work.[15] The Lady of Drayton's poem has not been identified, and its occasion is therefore unknown.[16] Given the suggestiveness of her name, it is possible that she is an invention of the poet, but it is also true that the other elegies in the final section of Drayton's volume are all about or addressed to identifiable historical persons, so we can assume that the same is true of this one. In any case, for our purposes, what matters most is Drayton's decision to treat the death of Elianor Fallowfield explicitly as a death in childbirth.

Drayton begins the poem with an attack on death for taking the young and healthy rather than the old, the already sick and dying, the hopelessly indebted, or the enslaved. All of these ask for death, he tells us with an indignant sense of irony, and death never comes to them, visiting instead those who need him least (or at least do not need him yet). Mistress Fallowfield had much to live for. Not only was she young and virtuous, but she was "teeming." Appalled that death has taken both her and her child ("even at once...both flower and seed," line 22), the speaker launches his third verse paragraph with what at first sounds like a threat aimed at death himself. This quickly gives way, however, to a warning to death about the consequences of his actions, not for himself but for humankind as a whole:

[15] In addition to the long title poem, the volume includes several other longish works (a complaint, a pastoral sequence, and three narrative poems). Milton may have adapted line 29 of the fairy narrative "Nymphidia" ("My pretty light fantastick mayde") for line 34 of "*L'Allegro*" ("On the light fantastick toe"). Carey cites the line as an analogue, but does not note that, in addition, the publication of Drayton's volume precedes our earliest estimates for the composition of the companion poems by about two years. The publication date also suggests that the *OED* is incorrect to cite Milton's line as the first example of the combination "light fantastic." The final narrative poem in the volume, *The Moone-Calfe*, comes just before the section of elegies, and commences, as I said earlier, with a detailed description of a monstrous birth. Milton may have derived some of the details he used in the allegory of Sin and Death from this poem, but the connection is not as close as it is in the case of the other more commonly cited sources: Michael Drayton, *The Works of Michael Drayton*, ed. William Hebel, 5 vols. (Oxford: Basil Blackwell, 1961), vol. III, pp. 125, 166–202, and 242–3.

[16] William Hebel indicates that "there was a family of that name in the parish of St Pancras, Soper Lane," and that "Eleanor might be the wife of George Fallowfield, 1571–1617, 'citizen and haberdasher' and son of Edmund (d. 1578)." He is, however, uncertain about this possibility, and offers no evidence of a connection with Drayton. See Drayton, *The Works*, vol. V, p. 218.

But cruell Death if thou so barbarous be,
To those so goodly, and so young as shee;
That in their teeming thou wilt shew thy spight;
Either from marriage thou wilt Maides affright,
Or in their wedlock, Widowes lives to chuse,
Their Husbands bed, and utterly refuse,
Fearing conception; so shalt thou thereby
Extirpate mankinde by thy cruelty. (lines 23–30)[17]

Up to line 25, the passage sounds as if it were leading to a statement like the one Shakespeare's poet hurls at Time in Sonnet 19. Perhaps the poet will immortalize his subject, or perhaps he will give way to *contemptus mundi* occasioned by the death of a young mother-to-be. This might lead to further praise of her virtues and a consoling apotheosis. However, something quite different ensues and, in fact, keeps the poet from ever constructing such an apotheosis. The poet has no intention of threatening death with the eternal power of poetry (at least not yet), or even of drawing some consoling conclusion from the meaning of this particular death. As we can see, beginning at line 26, instead of warning us of the instability of earthly things, he warns death of the consequences of his own actions for one of the primary possible victims of that very instability: the continuity of human social existence.

While Drayton does not make it clear that Mistress Fallowfield died in birth itself rather than of some illness or accident during pregnancy, the difficulty of the child-bed clearly offers the most logical cause of death. There is no reason to assume that this death would have inspired the sort of fear he describes had it not been caused by what turns out to be her last duty in the marriage bed. Causes of death during an earlier stage of pregnancy would have been too vaguely associated with reproduction to have occasioned the direct association the poet makes here, and the poem clearly follows out the logic of this association in its management of the next several topoi. In doing so, the poet makes very clear his concern with childbirth not only as a cause of Elianor's death, but also as the cause of a more general anxiety about human continuity.

It is, in fact, remarkable how long it takes Drayton to take up one of the generically expected strategies for consolation. He does finally choose to immortalize Mistress Fallowfield, but not until the last two lines of the sixty-three-line poem. It is one thing for Shakespeare to hold off until the couplet of a fourteen-line sonnet, but sixty-three lines is quite another

[17] All quotations are from Hebel's edition. Drayton, *The Works*, vol. III, pp. 242–43.

matter. And when Drayton finally employs the eternizing conceit, its effect is strangely anticlimactic. Rather than a conclusive offer of consolation, it seems to be presented as an after-thought, or as something the poet says just to bring the poem to a close, fulfilling a generic obligation without the proper rhetorical preparation or pay-off. In addition, his path to this compromised conclusion is itself far from straightforward. In the next verse paragraph, he swerves away from the usual generic concerns, making the worry of the poet itself the occasion for a remarkable turn on a set of epithalamic figures:

> If after direfull Tragedy thou thirst,
> Extinguish *Himens* Torches at the first;
> Build Funerall pyles, and the sad pavement strewe,
> With mournfull Cypresse, & the pale-leav'd Yewe.
> Away with Roses, Myrtle, and with Bayes;
> Ensignes of mirth, and jollity, as these,
> Never at Nuptials used be againe,
> But from the Church the new Bride entertaine
> With weeping *Nenias*, ever and among,
> As at departings be sad *Requiems* song.

This "anti-epithalamium," drawing on motifs in Ovid and Apuleius (the weddings, respectively, of Orpheus and of Psyche) and unfolding in the midst of a funeral elegy, makes explicit the generic similarity between elegies and epithalamia noted by Celeste Schenck (an imaginative intimacy that here serves a painful purpose, and one that Drayton makes full use of).[18] It also makes explicit what Heather Dubrow has said about the marriage poems of the period themselves: that an association of death and sex preoccupies their authors for very basic reasons. As Dubrow puts it, death "deeply threatens the occasion and the values they are celebrating. The bride might produce stillborn children and die herself in the process. The very hopes that epithalamia express might themselves be stillborn."[19] Drayton's evocation of virgin fears and his extraordinary equation of sexual

[18] See Celeste Marguerite Schenck, *Mourning and Panegyric: the Poetics of Pastoral Ceremony* (University Park, PA: Pennsylvania State University Press, 1988), pp. 7, 10–16. The term "anti-epithalamium" was coined by Virginia Tufte in *The Poetry of Marriage: the Epithalamium in Europe and its Development in England* (Los Angeles, CA: Tinnon-Brown, 1970). As Schenck observes, use of the term should not be confined to examples of full-blown parody, like Donne's "Epithalamion Made at Lincoln's Inne," but should be used to refer to the serious use of antithetical motifs in conventional marriage verses, funeral elegies, and all sorts of what she calls "poems of pastoral ceremony." For more on the use of anti-epithalamic motifs, see Dubrow, *A Happier Eden: the Politics of Marriage in the Stuart Epithalamium* (Ithaca, NY: Cornell University Press, 1990), pp. 121–2.

[19] Dubrow, *A Happier Eden*, p. 120.

refusal with widowhood followed by the imagining of the "funereal wedding" is a forceful, and for this occasion very appropriate, attempt to express fully the anxieties that feed the anti-epithalamic traditions that he is himself drawing upon, anxieties that were regularly combated rhetorically by the authors of commissioned epithalamia.[20] In those poems, the poet often incants a charm to protect the bride and bridegroom from baleful influences, enclosing them in a space in which God and various mythic patronesses of fertility could be invoked.[21] In Drayton's poem, death pervades – has in fact invaded – the poet's imagination because the catastrophe that marriage poems attempt to charm away has overwhelmed one marriage and now, because all flesh is heir to this same natural shock, threatens to overwhelm all future marriages.

Such a catastrophe demands that the poet give full voice to the threat to marriage that female fear of death posed, both before and within nuptial union. Because actual marriages are here ending in death, all marriage becomes proleptically funereal, and the ceremony Drayton describes mourns the destruction of both the marriages that will not occur because of virgin refusal and those that will be destroyed by wives who, "fearing conception," will now refuse their husbands' beds and live like widows, figuratively killing their spouses by refusing to live with them as spouses. Drayton's use of anti-epithalamic motifs in an elegy that specifies death in childbirth throws the threat posed to the institution of marriage by its very own ends (sexual union and procreation) into bold relief, requiring that the twin and yet antithetical modes be used in tandem, but not in the ways they normally work together. Normally, the one is a foil for the celebration of the other, in other words acting like an anti-masque to a masque. In this case, however, the one in effect cancels out the other's ability to repair its damage or charm away its worries. As Schenck observes, epithalamic conventions, when they are used in a funeral elegy, usually come into play in the *consolatio* providing the consoling, figurative counter-ceremony to the funeral procession of the poem's lamentation. In conventional epithalamia, on the other hand, death and lament serve as foils for the nuptial celebration. They are invoked only to be displaced from the ritual of union and exiled to its margins. They may also, as Dubrow notes, find oblique expression in laments about the passing of youth or maidenhood, but

[20] "Funereal wedding" is a translation of Apuleius' phrase "*funerei thalami.*" See *Metamorphoses*, 4:33: Apuleius, *Metamorphoses*, ed. and trans. J. Arthur Hanson (Cambridge, MA: Harvard University Press, 1989), vol. I, p. 247. The motif has a long history in anti-epithalamia. See Schenck, *Mourning and Panegyric*, pp. 73–4.

[21] See, for example, stanzas 19 and 20 of Spenser's self-commissioned "Epithalamion."

they are never allowed to maim the rite of marriage itself, or stain it with real tears.[22]

The purpose of the evocation of such things at all in a marriage poem, as Dubrow puts it, is to "control" and "subdue" the elegiac, making room for celebration *and* assuring all concerned that the couple will enjoy both long life and numerous progeny, despite the fact that these desires often proved incompatible.[23] This is not so far from the funeral elegy's purpose of using epithalamic motifs to control grief and make possible an argument for consolation. However, the actual evocation of childbed death in a funeral elegy for a woman who died that way weights the generic frame with a complex and unbearable crossing. In fact, it hobbles Drayton's poem, which never manages to generate much of a consolation at all.

In the next three verse paragraphs, Drayton moves from the funereal wedding to, first, a complaint against Lucina, Roman goddess of childbirth, for not coming to Mistress Fallowfield's aid (for this he blames a general failure of belief in what had been said of Lucina "by th'olde Poets" and a consequent failure to worship at her altars). He then moves on to an inconclusive philosophical debate over whether "Fortune" or "Nature" is to blame for her death (he finds himself taking one side and then the other, unable to resolve his ambivalence or uncertainty). After this, a reiterative meditation on the fact that all are fated to death returns us to one of the roads not taken earlier (*contemptus mundi*), and this leads to the concluding four-line eternizing conceit. The poem comes to a conclusion never having confronted the terrifying question of what we are supposed to feel in the face of the tragic irony it has presented:

> *Lucina* by th'olde Poets that wert sayd,
> Women in Childe-birth evermore to ayde,
> Because thine Altars, long have layne neglected:
> Nor as they should, thy holy fiers reflected
> Upon thy Temples, therefore thou doest flye,
> And wilt not helpe them in necessitie.
> Thinking upon thee, I doe often muse,
> Whether for thy deare sake I should accuse
> Nature or Fortune, Fortune then I blame,
> And doe impute it as her greatest shame,
> To hast thy timelesse end, and soone agen
> I vexe at Nature, nay I curse her then,
> That at the time of need she was no stronger,
> That we by her might have enjoy'd thee longer.

[22] Dubrow, *A Happier Eden*, pp. 121–2. [23] Dubrow, *A Happier Eden*, p. 122.

But whilst of these I with my selfe debate,
I call to minde how flinty-hearted Fate
Seaseth the olde, the young, the faire, the foule,
No thing of earth can Destinie controule:
But yet that Fate which hath of life bereft thee,
Still to eternall memory hath left thee,
Which thou enjoy'st by the deserved breath,
That many a great one hath not after death. (lines 41–62)

There is no confrontation with the questions raised by the earlier warnings about fear of conception, the funereal weddings, and the failure of poets to keep alive a hopeful belief in Lucina's power to aid teeming women. The conclusion is particularly weak given that the speaker had already figured the possible refusal of women to marry in terms of poetic failure. Not only do they neglect Lucina, but according to the implications of his earlier statement, poets cannot attack death with warnings about poetic power. They are instead merely fated – if death keeps doing to others what he did to Mistress Fallowfield – to reflect, via the painful generic crossing of the funereal wedding motif, a generic aporia that cancels out the power of poetry to celebrate and console. By the neglect of praise, Drayton must have meant poets' failure to praise childbirth and counter fear of it with comforting tales of divine care. In other words, Drayton seems to be complaining about the fact that there are so few poems around like the one he is trying to write. His frustration over this lack is underlined by the fact that, after all of this hand-wringing, he concludes the poem by suggesting we accept poetic eternization as an adequate consolation anyway. But why should we? Poetry has not only failed to do its job, but, as we have also been told, the very grounds of its ability to eternize (the ongoing existence of a posterity to do the reading and remembering) has itself been threatened by that failure. Such an inconclusive offer of poetic immortality – especially in the absence of some more explicit theological statement (the poem makes no reference to the dynamics of sin and redemption, nor reference to Eve's curse or Elianor's heavenly reward) – is therefore no comfort at all. Drayton sees that the occasion demands the release of the elegiac sub-currents of traditional epithalamia, but he also senses that poetry offers no solution to the problems suggested by such a rhetorical move. His poem implicitly recognizes its own helplessness, ironically undermining its final offer of self-praising consolation.

When Milton sat down to write his epitaph, he was faced with similar problems, and perhaps he had read Drayton's poem. He also makes use of the topos of the funereal wedding; he too invokes Lucina and a philosophical debate (actually two debates, one between "Nature and fate," parallel to Drayton's "Nature" and "Fortune" and a second between "blame" and "mischance," who turn out upon reflection to be indistinguishable in a number of senses from the other abstractions). Like Drayton, he also uses the image of death's destroying of both a flower and its seed as a figure for a woman who dies along with her infant. However, Milton extends these conceits as he found them (perhaps in Drayton, perhaps elsewhere) with further fabling. He takes care to weave his treatment of childbirth motifs together with his more conventional figures of genealogy, communal and institutional mourning, personal compliment, and biblical comparison to produce what has emerged in my research as one of the most ambitious and successful poems on the occasion of maternal mortality produced in the period.

MILTON'S "AN EPITAPH"

As I noted at the beginning of this chapter, of the poems written on the death of Lady Jane, only the epitaphs by Milton and John Eliot even mention that she died in childbed, despite the fact that the general circumstances of her demise were, it seems, commonly known.[24] Only Milton's is structured *entirely* around figures of tragic childbirth. Eliot develops a striking conceit based on the manner of the Lady's death (as part of his complaint, he calls for all procreation to cease each year on the anniversary), and he uses the fruit and tree metaphor for the death of both mother and child, ending his complaint with an image of both of them together, like the "*Phenix*," burning to ashes "in their own fire."[25] These images, however, are not integrated with any larger pattern of reference in the poem. Milton, however, figures and refigures the death in a set of complexly interrelated reproductive conceits, then concludes with an apotheosis that places Jane

[24] We do not know how Milton got his information. However, if someone as distant from the Paulets as Milton knew of the circumstances of the Lady's death, along with the other accurate biographical details I discuss below, then we may assume common knowledge within a reasonably wide circle of poets, aristocrats, clergymen, and academics. It seems unlikely that information picked up through the Porys, at least, would have been privileged. John Pory was an indefatigable collector of information about courtly circles. See William Stevens Powell, *John Pory, 1572–1636: the Life and Letters of a Man of Many Parts* (Chapel Hill, NC: University of North Carolina Press, 1977).

[25] The poem ends, like Drayton's, with a weak version of the inadequacy trope followed by the promise that the Lady will be remembered: See "*An Elogie. On the Lady* Jane Paulet *Marchioness of* Winchester, *daughter to the right honourable the Lord* Savage *of* Rock-savage" in *POEMS or Epigrams, Satyrs, Elegies, Songs and Sonnets* (London, 1658), pp. 34–9. This is the first, anonymous edition. Another, attributed to Eliot, and with poems by other "Wits of both Universities" added, appeared in 1661.

where Dante placed Beatrice, next to Rachel in the heavenly rose.[26] He does so not only because he wishes to associate her death and apotheosis with the very highest realms of literary endeavor and theological speculation, but also because Jane, like Rachel, died giving birth to her second son.

The youthful ambitiousness of such a conclusion is not in itself surprising coming from Milton, even at such an early stage in his career. However, its application to this subject matter is. As we have seen, few poets responded to such occasions with such specificity and/or at such length, and we do not know what moved Milton to do so. Parker long ago suggested that all of the poems about Lady Jane (including Milton's) probably had more to do with religion and politics than with the poignant manner of her death. The Paulets were a prominent Catholic family, but Jane seems to have had Protestant leanings.[27] She was also a kinswoman of Henry Rich, Earl Holland, who had become Chancellor of Cambridge just a few years before Jane's death and who was instrumental in resisting attempts by Archbishop Laud to control the University.[28] Frost is probably right that Milton intended the poem as a criticism of the Paulet family, Jane's husband in particular.[29]

If, however, these were Milton's only motives, his poem could have been as devoid of reference to the childbed as the rest of the poems about Lady Jane. One can easily imagine that these were the sorts of concerns that drove the other poets to write on this occasion (in the cases of Colman, Jonson, Davenant, and Eliot, probably from the opposite political perspective). A close reading of those poems reveals a great deal of interest in *how* Jane Paulet faced her death, but hardly any interest in what killed her. The

[26] This allusion was first noticed by James Holly Hanford in *The Poems of John Milton*, 2nd edn (New York, NY: The Ronald Press Company, 1953), p. 79.

[27] Pory's letter states that her death "is lamented as well in respect to her other virtues, as that she was inclining to become a Protestant" (Parker, p. 95).

[28] Frost, "No Marchioness," 4–8. Some have thought that the poem was originally meant for a volume of dedicatory verses for the Marchioness from the University itself, but no such volume has ever been found. See Alberta T. Turner, "Milton and the Convention of the Academic Miscellanies," *Yearbook of English Studies* 5 (1975), 86–93.

[29] The critique would have been relevant in both 1631, when the poem was composed and perhaps circulated in manuscript form, and in 1645, when it was finally published. In a historical coincidence that was not likely to have been lost on Milton, just two days after *Poems of Mr. John Milton* was registered for publication in 1645, John Paulet, who had become one of the most prominent Royalist fighters during the war, was captured by Parliamentary forces after a protracted siege of his family seat at Basing House. He was committed to the Tower to await possible trial and execution. The siege had been going on since August of 1643, and Paulet's stubborn resistance had become famous (or infamous). He would be spared execution, although his estate was confiscated for a number of years. By the time of his capture, he had remarried and had two children by his second wife, Lady Honora De Burgh (*DNB*).

question of why Milton turned his attention so fully to the matter of maternal mortality in addition to matters of politics and religion is therefore central to any just account of the poem, and it is clear to me that he wanted to say something specific about the role reproduction played in a woman's social, physical, and spiritual life. Milton was well aware of the fact that, because of her early death, the political and religious possibilities that Lady Jane represented all proved as tragically stillborn as her poor infant son, and he wants us to understand this as more than just an implied simile. His poem is designed to assert in no uncertain terms that Jane's actions as a laboring woman were bound up with her larger possibilities for spiritual action within her family and the polity. They are also central to the terms of the apotheosis he imagines for her. The considerable originality of the poem rests, in fact, on Milton's having chosen to unite Jane's transcendent and earthly religious virtues with her reproductive activity, making her a heroic, free agent in both matters at once.

Milton accomplishes this unification by organizing the poem around the theme of heroic childbirth. The poem's numerology and typology, its rhetorical structure, its crowning allusions to the story of Rachel and to Dante's *Paradiso*, its treatment of genealogy, its thinly veiled criticism of John Paulet, as well as the way Milton identifies himself with Lady Jane, are all carefully and consistently connected to the central theme. Frost is correct to see that Milton's guiding purpose is to praise Jane Paulet's "moral and spiritual efficacy" and to portray her as "a rich co-creator of the poem."[30] There is no doubt that she rises above certain aspects of her aristocratic identities as wife and daughter. However, far from moving us, as Frost puts it, "beyond" a depiction of an aristocratic woman's "traditional biological role," Milton's poem manages to elevate a key element of her biological function to what he saw as its proper heavenly dignity. In the epitaph, childbirth is presented to us not as a limiting, earthly matter to be transcended but, in line with aspects of the childbirth discourses we examined earlier, as a key way in which women could – and this woman did – *achieve* transcendence.

High birth and graces sweet

Milton begins his epitaph by directly addressing the nature of Lady Jane's moral and spiritual dignity, carefully distinguishing between her true and her superficial virtues before going on to describe how her final actions on

[30] Frost, "No Marchioness," 21–2.

earth made the true virtues fully manifest. The poem begins, conventionally, with an evocation of the Lady's lineage along with a decorous reminder that her essential moral and spiritual virtues were greater than those she derived from that lineage. This is a strategy the poem has in common with the other poems on Lady Jane, not to mention with many other early modern funeral poems for the aristocratic dead:

> This rich Marble doth enterr
> The honour'd Wife of *Winchester*,
> A Vicounts daughter, an Earls heir,
> Besides what her vertues fair
> Added to her noble birth,
> More then she could own from Earth. (lines 1–6)

The "Earth" here is both the earthly mould of the fallen world and the more specific earth to which she owed her *familial* "vertues": the power, prestige, and property she was to inherit and bring over to her husband's family. Until line 6, such virtues are presented as the main order of business. Her personal virtues are merely described in line 5 as what seem at first to be mere additions. She was heir, by default of male issue through her father, to her maternal grandfather's titles (Lord Thomas Darcy was Viscount Colchester and Earl Rivers), and these factors were no doubt prominent matters in the negotiation of her marriage to John Paulet (Parker, p. 766). Such properties and titles clearly had "vertues," and the poet suggests, at least up to line 5, that these can and should coexist with a moral legacy. Line 6, however, pulls the rug out from under this suggestion, pointedly reminding us that, being matters of earth, such virtues are of a relatively low order. The higher virtues, the moral and spiritual ones, can only be expressed in individual actions (things, as we are later shown explicitly, in which Lady Jane was also rich).

The fact that she is buried in "*rich* Marble" (my italics) probably also suggests, in a more pointed way, a direct critique of her husband's family. She was, as I said before, connected on her mother's side to Henry Rich, Earl Holland, the Protestant and anti-Laudian chancellor of Cambridge.[31] The line suggests, therefore, that she has been taken in death into the bosom of the Protestant wing of her family – or at least this is where the poem wishes, figuratively, to lay her to rest. The tomb of "rich Marble" in which Milton imagines her aligns her with what the poet thinks were her proper

[31] Up until the publication of the poem in 1645, Rich was of the Parliamentary party, though he later changed his mind and was executed in 1649 for his support of the King in the second Civil War. See Frost, "No Marchioness," 6–8.

allegiances on earth, ones that point in the direction of her higher allegiances in heaven. The allusion also suggests that even the right-thinking earthly ties she had will be transcended at the end in an apotheosis that, not coincidentally, will suggest the Resurrection as she rises from that tomb of rich marble to take her proper seat in heaven. This will occur, however, only after the poem reveals childbirth to be her defining moral and spiritual act, an expression of her individual virtues and, in effect, her Golgotha.

This first period of the poem's fourteen-line *exordium* is designed, as we can see, to establish the proper hierarchy of virtues while putting in play certain images and motifs that set the stage for both the presentation of Lady Jane's defining action and for the final, triumphant ascension that the action earns her.[32] In the next section of the *exordium*, Milton continues this process by turning to the youthfulness of his subject and the untimeliness of her death:

> Summers three times eight save one
> She had told, alas too soon,
> After so short time of breath,
> To house with darknes, and with death.
> Yet had the number of her days
> Bin as compleat as was her praise,
> Nature and fate had had no strife
> In giving limit to her life. (lines 7–14)[33]

This eight-line passage is made up of two balanced and parallel four-line clauses, the second continuing the thought of the first and starkly contrasting with it. Together, they bring the *exordium* to a conclusion with a figure that elegantly handles youth and untimely death along with further praise of the virtues Milton identified in the first period as her truest legacy. The first numbers her days: she was only twenty-three at her death (this was, as Frost

[32] In my description of the poem's rhetorical structure, I follow Frost's useful schema ("No Marchioness," 13–17).

[33] I quote from Shawcross but, like Frost, follow most other modern editors in accepting 1645's full stop at the end of line 10, where Shawcross uses a comma. Frost cites Shawcross' justification: "I use the comma because the strong stop – particularly a period – separates the thoughts [those of lines 7–10 and lines 11–14] and I think they should not be. The word 'Yet' in l. 11 is a contrastive continuance of the thought." I agree with Frost that the 1645 reading is rhetorically acceptable. I am, however, less sure that it is aesthetically superior. It certainly helps to bolster her numerological reading of the poem, which requires that we see the *exordium* as dividing into three periods, and about which I will have more to say below. Shawcross has, however, added in correspondence with me that part of his concern in using the comma was to allow the sentence beginning "Yet" to function as either "a 'new' sentence OR a continuant." I believe his position has considerable merit, and have tried to register the ambiguity in my account of these lines.

observes, a "traditional number of short time").[34] Yet the second tells us, alluding to the numbering of her virtues, that had her allotment of days been as full as her allotment of virtues (for which she was and is here being rightly praised), she would have lived much longer.

The fact that her time on earth was "incomplete" presents a classic Boethian problem.[35] Why was she not rewarded with long life? Why do the good die young? In order to reinforce the suggestion, Milton here introduces the idea of strife between "nature" and "fate." "Nature," in this context, means not just the natural span of human life (which was for her incomplete), but more precisely what *we* think of as "natural" in a moral sense. We feel not only that the particularly virtuous deserve to be rewarded (at least in a universe governed by a good divinity), but that their continued life is a continuing blessing to a world in need of blessing. Fate, however, in its inscrutable and seemingly meaningless way, has dictated that this particular virtuous person should die short not only of her natural allotment of years, but short even of a space of time like the twenty-four years that would at least have echoed the "compleat" number of each of her days. The incongruity is underlined by Milton's choice to rhyme "days" and "praise." Phonology suggests that these, like virtue and long life, should align with each other, but in this case they did not align, expressing the Boethian problem structurally. Milton's task will be to find some way of realigning these terms by providing a providential vision, and he will choose to do this by showing that the end of her short life had its own perfection, its own completeness. Having done so, the poem will be able to add its "tears of perfect moan" (line 55) to the chorus of praises suggested by line 12, drawing out the thread of perfection in Lady Jane's curtailed but only seemingly imperfect life.

Just how close this task was to Milton's heart, with its implicit praise of the power that poetry has to reveal the hidden perfection of a seemingly imperfect world, is suggested by the other implications of Milton's emphasis on "numbering." There is more to the number twenty-three, for example, than just biographical accuracy and a clever numerological symbol. As has been noted by several scholars, Milton emphasizes the number in order

34 Frost, "No Marchioness," 16.

35 Milton is playing on several senses of "compleat" here. Her allotment of days was incomplete and defective in the sense that we often feel it is "unnatural" for someone to die before attaining at least some significant portion of the number of years usually allotted to human beings (a "complete" number of human years [*OED*, def. 2]). Her "praise," on the other hand, *was* "complete" in a different sense. She had the full complement of human virtues, she carried and expressed them without defect, and she was praised for that by everyone who knew her (she was the "compleat" young aristocratic woman [*OED*, defs. 3, 4, and 5]). In other words, if she had had a day for every virtue numbered in her praises she would have lived a long time, and we would not feel that something was wrong with her dying.

to suggest a significant parallel between himself and Jane Paulet. It is true that there is some record that Jane was herself a poet of modest accomplishment, but we have no way of knowing whether Milton knew this. Clearly more important to Milton is the fact that they were both about the same age, both young and full of incompletely realized potentials within their own spheres of action. As Parker observed, Milton calculated slightly loosely in the poem, possibly in order to make the parallel seem even closer than it actually was. In April of 1631, Milton was eight months short of his twenty-fourth birthday; the Marchioness was just one month short of hers. This means that while they were both indeed twenty-three, it was Milton, not Lady Jane, who had passed "three times eight save one" *summers*. She had actually already passed her twenty-*fourth* summer, had in fact nearly completed her entire twenty-fourth year, while Milton still had the bulk of his yet to live (Parker, pp. 95–6). This is a small matter, but it suggests that it was important to Milton to establish a connection and identification with Lady Jane, even if he had to fudge slightly, and even if it was something only he or the few readers who knew him were likely to notice.[36]

If this were an isolated instance, it would hardly be worth *our* taking notice of it, but it is in fact one of the first examples of what would become a keynote theme in Milton's early poetry (indeed, of much of his poetry well into middle age): the anxiety that death might come before the native talents of a given individual could be manifest in a clear achievement.[37] "An Epitaph" therefore bears the pressure of one of Milton's several moments of self-doubt about his slow progress in his own vocation. I would not want to reduce the poem to the impulse of self-doubt and vocational introspection, but it seems clear that this is an important reason for Milton's finding the occasion congenial to his concerns. In any case, like everything else in the poem, he closely adapts it to the task of accounting for the nature of Lady Jane's accomplishment, spending the rest of the poem detailing the organizing power of what she achieved at the end of her short life, while at the same time presenting the poem as a significant achievement of his own. Her accomplishment, and the poem that clarifies its significance, are together what give shape and meaning to a life that might otherwise have seemed too short and possibly meaningless.

[36] See, also, Frost, "No Marchioness," 14–17.

[37] See Sonnet 7, "Lycidas," and the autobiographical digression in *The Reason of Church Government*. The theme also appears in a more muted way in the anxieties of the lover drawn away by love from his more serious commitments in *Elegia Septima*, the "Canzone," and the first five sonnets, which are all probably earlier, and of course in "On Shakespear." The theme is later expressed in different terms in Sonnet 19 and in the invocations of *Paradise Lost*.

"A Cipress bud"

So far, nothing has indicated the central matter that will bring the two concerns mentioned thus far (individual and dynastic virtue) together and organize the poem's up-to-now rather abstract treatment of virtuous action around one concrete, defining event. Milton's next section, however, clearly introduces Lady Jane's death in childbirth in a way that is designed to do so. He is at pains to make it seem the inevitable, if tragic, conclusion of a life governed by the genealogical and moral virtues he has been praising. At the same time, he significantly revises the inconclusive ways in which the genre has tended to treat the matter.

Again, the poem's numerology is central to Milton's strategy. In introducing the numbering of Jane's days and virtues, Milton had suggested that "numbering" itself might be central to the poem's method for reconciling the short time of her life with her, as yet invisible, eternal reward. Frost has demonstrated that the poem makes use of a complex numerological schema, but it is even more central to, and deeply integrated with, Milton's purposes than she has shown. She notes, for example, that the whole of the *exordium* and *divisio* contains twenty-three couplets, numbering the years of Jane's life on earth, the "short time" that is then juxtaposed with the perfect *twenty-eight* lines of the poem's *conclusio*:

> twenty-eight is not only a female number in its associations with the lunar cycle, but also a perfect number in that it forms the sum of its aliquot parts (1+2+4+7+14) and virtuous in that it hits the mean. Viewed as a triangular number, it symbolizes the perfection of eternity toward which the soul yearns and was traditionally employed for funeral verses.[38]

Frost goes on to note that if the two closely related clauses of lines 7–14 are considered separate periods, as the 1645 punctuation suggests they should be, the *exordium* and *divisio* together consist of six periods (three each). This is, she points out, another number suggestive of earthly imperfection. The *conclusio*, on the other hand, can then be seen as a perfect set of four sevens, constituting a Sabbath of rest that follows, perfects, and completes the six periods that recount Jane's earthly life. The *conclusio* is also made up of a single period, and hence suggests an undivided whole in comparison with the first two parts of the poem, which are both unevenly divided into periods of different lengths.[39] I would add that this numerology also

[38] Frost, "No Marchioness," 15–17.

[39] Frost, "No Marchioness," 19–20. In the structure implied by Shawcross (see above), this would be five periods of six, eight, eight, twelve, and twelve lines. For Frost, it is six periods of six, four, four, eight, twelve, and twelve.

suggests that we think of Jane's earthly existence as a procreative, laboring existence, the period of six days being the period in which God labored to create the universe, crowning it with the creation of the animals and humankind, all of whom are commanded to be fruitful and multiply.[40] Milton will later explicitly assert that the "sweet rest" he wishes Jane in the poem's "Sabbath" section should be thought of as a direct reward for Jane's reproductive travail (see lines 47–52). The figure implied by twenty-eight may therefore be thought of as combining a figure for female reproductive life with a figure for eternity, both the traditional twenty-eight days of the female reproductive and lunar cycles and the constitutive seven of Sabbath rest. This suggests a redemption of the imperfections of earthly reproductive life, not simply a rejection or transcendence of them. Jane enacted them imperfectly in their inherently imperfect material form (expressed by the number twenty-three), but with perfection as regards their spiritual essence (expressed by the number twenty-eight). Milton reveals this both in the numerology and, as we will see, in his description of her final apotheosis.

Frost has also observed that the first period of the *divisio*, in which Milton starts his treatment of the events of Jane's married life, begins with line 15, corresponding to her age at the time of her marriage, and that it ends with line 22, corresponding to her age at the birth of her first son. Line 23, in Frost's schema, signifies the actual year of the Lady's death, echoing the number of couplets in the poem's mortal half. It also begins the first of two twelve-line periods that complete the *divisio* with two descriptions of that death in two different poetic registers. However, there is, again, even more at work in these three periods than meets Frost's very observant eye:

Her high birth, and her graces sweet
Quickly found a lover meet;
The Virgin quire for her request
The God that sits at marriage feast;
He at their invoking came
But with a scarce-well-lighted flame;
And in his Garland as he stood,
Ye might discern a Cipress bud. (lines 15–22)

It is important that in this first period of the *divisio*, Milton inserts the topos of the funereal wedding, the first figure suggestive of death in childbirth to

[40] It may also be of some significance that the births of Jane's two children are figured in the fifth and sixth periods of the *divisio*, aligning them in the hexameral framework with the fifth and sixth days of creation, the days in which the animals and humankind are created and the two days on which the commandment to multiply was uttered.

appear in the poem. It is also important that the eighth line of the period (line 22) not only marks the year of her first birth, but introduces the second of the two central figures of the topos itself (the first is the sputtering torch, the second is the cypress bud). The poignant horticultural image of the cypress bud appears exactly half-way through the line that signifies the Lady's eighth year of marriage (the phrase, "a Cipress bud" takes up the last four syllables of the eight-syllable line). This is almost exactly when she gave birth to her first son, an event that Milton seems to have known occurred after what may have been an extended period of infertility, although we have no idea how he knew about it (this possibility, as we will see, is even more clearly suggested in the Sloane Manuscript version of the poem). In addition, the figure, as it is deployed here, foreshadows the death that lies ahead, and, importantly for Milton, it is both a reproductive and a poetic image, a figure of natural fertility that, in the topos, also figures the intrusion of the funereal into epithalamic celebration. The virgin choir sang an epithalamion, but the garlands of the wedding they celebrated contained, in still unopened form, the figure for epicede, a figure for the kind of poem we are actually now reading. The bud, which we must assume was picked by mistake in the making of the wedding wreath (a figure that will be echoed in the mistaken plucking done by the "unheedy swain" of the *divisio*'s third period), is also one that will never actually open, therefore signifying, by decorous suggestion, not only death in general and the poetry of death, but also the later stillbirth.[41]

The purpose of the first eight lines of the *divisio* is to introduce us to reproduction within marriage as a consequential sphere of Lady Jane's moral and spiritual agency, and the *exordium* is carefully constructed to lead us directly to an apprehension of this idea. Lines 7–10 are linked with the first period (lines 1–6) by an amplification of the speaker's original remark about Lady Jane's higher virtues. Lines 11–14 pick up where that first period leaves off, giving us a more detailed discussion of what lay behind the title Milton uses to name the Lady at line 2: "honored wife of Winchester." In other words, line 15 (the beginning of the *divisio*) brings together both of the major thematic threads of the *exordium* ("high birth" and "graces sweet"), establishing that they are integral, and that together these attributes led Jane directly into the next stage of her life. In this context, the

[41] Wedding wreaths were usually made up of flowers. While some evergreen branches were also used (particularly myrtle), cypress was usually associated only with funerals. See Cressy, *Birth, Marriage, and Death*, pp. 363–7 and James Patrick McHenry, "A Milton Herbal," *Milton Quarterly* 30 (1996), 64–5.

"meetness" of the "lover" that her birth and graces found for her (John Paulet) should be understood as a meetness *both* of lineage *and* of personal virtue. This may seem to trouble Frost's insistence that the poem is critical of Paulet, but as we will shortly see, something does go wrong, and Milton's treatment of the catastrophe upholds her position. In the meantime, the ensuing description of the wedding represents a logical narrative demonstration of Jane's dual virtues. Chronologically, it comes next after the discussion of her tender age, and it continues to expand upon the two governing topoi of personal grace and high birth.

It is at this point that the poem turns to its first direct confrontation with the problems of maternal mortality. And it is now worth observing that these problems are, of course, tied up with what the poem had been concerned with from the start: personal virtue and lineage (virtue in so far as Jane faces childbirth, indeed embraces it with piety; lineage in the sense that there can be – to put it bluntly – no lineage without it). The way Milton handles the matter is, again, biographically particular. "Quickly," in line 16, has biographical resonance, indicating that Milton knew that Jane married young. As an extension of the praise he has already offered, the line tells us that it did not take her long to attract a good husband. The connotations of "quickly," however, make it a slightly odd word in this particular context, given that Jane did not give birth to her first child until 1629, after seven years of marriage. Her birth and graces found her a husband quickly, but she was not herself particularly "quick" in the sense of fertility (or, for one reason or another, the marriage was not "fertile" – at least in those years). It is, of course, possible that the fertility problem was her husband's, but this would not have occurred to anyone as a cause. However, the fact that Jane did give birth to two children in about two years after the first seven suggests that the reasons for the "infertility" had more to do with her young age at the time of the marriage than with any particular physical problem. Paulet may have waited several years before consummating the marriage with his very young wife. She might have refused his bed on those grounds, or she might have reached puberty late. It is also quite possible that once they did begin having sexual relations, it may have simply taken a while for her to get pregnant for the first time. There might also have been earlier miscarriages we know nothing about.

All of this is, of course, speculation. We may, however, have access to what Milton made of the seven year delay. The manuscript version of the poem, which may represent an earlier authorial and not a corrupted or altered scribal version, describes the wedding from the point in time of the first and explicitly long-awaited birth. Here is the relevant passage as it is found in 1645:

Her high birth, and her graces sweet
Quickly found a lover meet;
The Virgin quire for her request
The God that sits at marriage feast;
He at their invoking came
But with a scarce-well-lighted flame;
And in his Garland as he stood,
Ye might discern a Cipress bud.
Once had the early Matrons run
To greet her of a lovely son,
And now with second hope she goes,
And calls *Lucina* to her throws; (lines 15–26)

As we can see, there is no indication of a delay before the birth of a first child, which seems to follow closely on the wedding just as the second birth seems to follow closely on the first. Lines 15–19 of the manuscript, however, read as follows:

Seauen times had the yeerlie starre
in euerie signe sett vpp his carr
Since for her they did request
the god that sitts at marriage feast
(when first the earlie Matrons runne[42]

These lines completely replace lines 15–23 of the 1645 version (note also that line 20 of the manuscript reads "her" rather than "a" lovely son, as in line 24 of 1645). The poem then continues on more or less the way it does in 1645, although with some significant smaller variants that I will discuss below. The 1645 version, as we can see, focuses on the wedding in its ordinary narrative place, rather than retrospectively (she finds a mate, marries him, and has a child in seemingly quick succession). Reference to the reproductive delay survives in the later allusion to Rachel (lines 63–8), but Milton elides all mention of it in the earlier section. It is worth noting here that while we do not know the reason for the delay, the later lines on Rachel in both versions of the poem do suggest that Milton or his sources assumed barrenness. More importantly, the comparison is built on four details: (1) the years of barrenness, (2) the birth of a "highly favored" first son, (3) death in the birth of a second son, and (4) a high position in heaven. It seems that, at one point, Milton might have contemplated providing a more explicitly dark and sad rendering of the events of Jane's life in order to set

[42] "On the Marchionesse of Winchester whoe died in Child bedd," in BL MS Sloane 1446, ff. 37b–38. See also Shawcross' transcription of the lines in *The Complete English Poems of John Milton*, p. 552.

the stage for the later revelation of the also sad, but ultimately redemptive, biblical allusion. In any case, only in the manuscript version are we invited explicitly and early on to contemplate the fact that Jane got pregnant twice in relatively quick succession and then died while giving birth to the second child after seven years of marriage with no issue. At some point, Milton may have rethought that strategy and decided to submerge reference to this sequence of events – with its biographical accuracy and fully typological resonance – in the elaborately and more obliquely suggestive figure of the funereal wedding.

The substitution matters a great deal to the logic and structure of the 1645 version, which is far more suggestive and ambitious than the one in the Sloane Manuscript. Milton's description of the wedding not only allows the biographical and numerological readings to work, but the figure forces us to think of the wedding of Jane Savage and John Paulet as proleptically funereal. The figure serves at once to push the narrative forward, complicating matters by pushing them toward an unfortunate end. The figure, as I have already noted, works in ways similar to those imagined by Drayton in the Fallowfield elegy (it suggests the appropriate collapse of epithalamion into epicede), but there is a significant difference. Jane, unlike the women imagined by Drayton, chose to marry despite any anxieties that might have turned her mind to death in the midst of her celebration, anxieties that in this case proved horribly justified. Milton's wounding of the wedding like this, with these allusions and at a point in the poem that would normally be reserved for an uncomplicated account of the Lady's life, is surprising from a generic standpoint. By doing so, Milton is certainly praising Jane for her decision to embrace marriage and motherhood, but in anticipating the fatal collapse of epithalamion into epicede he also gives his *divisio* a distinctly uncomfortable tension. The figure undermines the celebration of the union of two noble houses, reminding us of death and of the fact that such unions (indeed all married unions) have a cost and a danger. The match of Jane and John was "meet," in one sense, but the *meeting*, if you will, was fatal.

Milton courts this difficulty because he intends to move directly to an account of the death. This is the very heart of his revision of the typically incomplete elegiac treatment of maternal mortality found in most, if not all, poems he would have encountered on the subject. While, in the 1645 version, he does gloss over whatever it was that kept the Paulets from having children earlier, he does not elide the birth of her first child, describing it in lines 23–5 with just enough detail to suggest a significant and ironic parallel with the second birth: "Once had the early Matrons run/ To greet her of a lovely son,/ And now…" Here we have funereal wedding immediately leading to one birth (the delay in time removed). This birth, we are also told, was successful (Charles Paulet was a healthy, living child in 1631, and he would live until 1699). The poem, however, almost immediately follows this with an account of the unsuccessful second birth:

> And now with second hope she goes,
> And calls *Lucina* to her throws;
> But whether by mischance or blame
> *Atropos* for *Lucina* came;
> And with remorsles cruelty,
> Spoil'd at once both fruit and tree:
> The haples Babe before his birth
> Had burial, yet not laid in earth,
> And the languisht Mothers Womb
> Was not long a living Tomb. (lines 25–34)

Up to this point, the narrative sequence has been highly compressed. Jane is married "quickly," but with foreboding, at the end of line 22. Seven years and a first birth pass in two rapid and enjambed lines (the period of no "quickness" passes and ends rather quickly in the poem). Then, at the head of line 25, we are thrust into the historical present tense as the Lady calls on Lucina in preparation for her second birth. It is only now that things slow down. The calling of Lucina parallels the choir of virgins that, at her request, once called on Hymen for her wedding. In both cases, the invocations go ironically awry, and it is only the first birth, sandwiched between the other events, that is auspicious (I will discuss the significant parallels and distinctions between the two births below). Hymen came to the wedding unprepared and with a sloppily and inappropriately wreathed garland and a sputtering torch. For the second birth, Atropos comes instead of Lucina and performs a botched bit of obstetric surgery ("fatal" in more than one sense). The parallel seems designed to suggest a connection. There must have been something wrong, we are invited to think, with the wedding, the marriage, and the motives behind the union – figured in the cypress bud and the "scarce-well-lighted flame" of Hymen's torch. In other words, something about the nature of the union must have caused the birth attendance to go so disastrously wrong. This invites us to some uneasy and critical speculation about the "blame" side of the speaker's indecision about whether blame or chance was the cause of death.

In light of this, Frost's suggestion that Milton deeply disapproved of John Paulet makes some sense. He was, as it turns out, only seemingly "meet" for his Lady, and the frail fertility of their union perhaps signifies the spiritual disunion that Milton might have imagined was at play in the marriage.

There is more to it, however, and the implications get darker as the *divisio* unfolds. Milton, it seems, thought John responsible for his wife's death in a way that was rooted in the dynastic ambitions of a theologically and politically "incorrect" aristocratic house, but also in the tragic disjunction between the way men and women were subject to original sin; that is, as a result of the way "blame" was writ large in the human sexual condition after the Fall.

As I said before, at lines 27–34, things slow down and concentrate. Milton, in fact, takes far more time to concentrate directly on the childbed than he does on anything else in the poem. The first long sequence of concentration stretches from line 25 to line 52, when he turns for ten lines to matters of literary production, only to return to the implications of the childbed for a second sequence of lines (line 61 to the end). In other words, from line 25, the childbed is established as the connecting thread of most, if not all, of the poem's figures. Even the lines about literary production are intimately connected with it. The concentration on the childbed as a governing figure serves rather forcefully in the *divisio* to bring one side of the poem's opening concerns to a head: genealogy and marriage, it turns out, have led together to a pitiful death. It becomes clear, however, by line 51 that this is also true of the thread about personal virtue. She has perfected herself at her imperfect end by facing her sorrows with heroic piety, shortening her "own life's lease" in order "to give the world increase." We are then reminded that the poem, now called a "perfect moan," mirrors this action, by providing a perfected representation of the virtue manifested in her actions, and these lines do so while also reminding us of the political and religious arena of the *poet's* actions (the poem is sent from Cambridge – devoted to Jane's "virtuous name" and governed, as we know, by her kinsman, Henry Rich – in resistance to the predations of the Archbishop). The poem, then, in its conclusion, returns to the way she died, showing how the manner of her death determined the nature of her apotheosis, not coincidentally allowing the poet to assert his power to reveal the full truth about her.

Atropos for Lucina

It should be clear by now that the whole *divisio* unfolds with this larger trajectory in mind. Everything is heading toward an apotheosis that will reframe our understanding of the Lady's death, and Milton's placement of a pair of parallel birth accounts at the heart of the *divisio* is therefore a key element in the poem's larger structure. The few details Milton chose to give us for these births are in line with what we know about the norms of seventeenth-century childbirth, indicating that Milton wanted them to resonate realistically with common human experience. In the first birth, the "early Matrons," her gossips, run to Jane as she gives birth with no complications, prepared, we must assume, to initiate the establishment of the female ritual space of the lying-in chamber and its ritual time-table. The positive and ritualized aspects of this first birth are further emphasized (by way of contrast) by the second half of the sentence, where Milton gives us a parallel statement describing how, at her second birth, she called Lucina "to her throws." The invocation of divine aid and the way Milton indicates "throws" in the second case, but not the first, suggests a significant difference between the first and second births. In the first, in a strong enjambment, "the early Matrons run/ To greet her of a lovely son."[43] The birth seems to have happened not only without incident, but just as they arrived or perhaps even just before. It all happened smoothly and quickly, "naturally," we might say, without any sort of aid, and with no mention made of even ordinary labor pains.[44] In the second case, however, Lady Jane calls Lucina "to her *throws*" (my italics), and we are invited not just to imagine the throes themselves, but to imagine that they were the kind likely to inspire a woman to pray for aid. Invocations of Lucina are common in both classical and Christian birth literature, but the figure is usually introduced when the woman is, or believes she is, in some danger.[45] The invocation also expands on the allusion to Psyche implied earlier by the figure of funereal wedding (in Apuleius, Psyche famously calls upon Lucina – who is an aspect of Juno – during her wanderings and is refused aid). In other words, we are

[43] If Shawcross is right in his note to lines 23–4 that the reference to "early Matrons" is meant to suggest the Matralia, a festival held in ancient Rome by the matrons of the city every June 11th in celebration of birth and child care, then Milton's intention might have been to reinforce the celebratory feeling of the lines. We do not know when Jane's first son Charles was born, but it was some time in 1629, perhaps before June or at least in very early June, making the matrons who would have normally held their festival on June 11th "early" in the sense that their celebration of the birth of Charles anticipated the soon-to-be-held festival.

[44] The sense of "greet" here is probably, as Carey notes, one Milton derived from Spenser (see *OED*, def. 3e: "to offer congratulations on [an achievement, etc.])." It may also be a variant of the verb "to great"; that is, to "aggrandize or magnify," with connotations, especially in this context, of its intransitive sense, "to grow ripe or pregnant." The *OED* cites examples up to the very early seventeenth century of the former sense, which must be primary. The intransitive sense may have disappeared from ordinary usage by then, but Milton may have been aware of it and meant it to color the verb in this context. The aggrandizing or magnifying of a woman concerning the birth of a son, however, might also suggest Gabriel's hailing of the Virgin at the Annunciation.

[45] See, for example, the birth of Amoret and Belphoebe to Chrysogone in *The Faerie Qveene*, 3.6.27: Edmund Spenser, *The Faerie Qveene*, ed. A. C. Hamilton (London: Longman, 2001), p. 345. Since Chrysogone gave birth *without* pain, the poet tells us that she did not need to "implore/ *Lucinaes* aid." In the epitaph, Lady Jane does so precisely *because of* the pain. Refusal *by* Lucina was commonly used as a figure for a birth that had gone awry. See Shakespeare's *Cymbeline* (5.4.43–7).

being explicitly asked to think of this second birth in contrast to a first that stands as an almost absurd example of how things can sometimes go spectacularly well. In the second, however, things actually go from bad to worse. Lucina does not come, the Lady's prayers being answered by the arrival of Atropos instead, a reemergence, in other words, of the "fate" Milton had invoked earlier, and that he has as yet failed to explain away. The figure of Atropos and her actions then gives us a gruesome glimpse at just how the debate between nature and fate actually worked itself out in the event. Milton reimagines the midwife's cutting of the umbilical cord as a "slitting of the thin-spun life" of Jane Paulet by the Fate. Lucina, had she come, would have, like a good midwife, cut the cord that would have allowed the *new*-spun life of the child to separate from the body of his mother and live independently. As it turns out, the slitting takes away the lives of both, leaving them bound up with one another in death.

It is important to Milton's symbolism that the death of both be treated together, and the two figures that follow (as well as the long one that takes up the last twelve lines of the *divisio*) assert this painful union. In the first of these figures, we are told not only that both the mother and infant proved mortal, but that the mother's body became a tomb in which her new-born infant both died and was figuratively buried. The image ties the birth to the opening figure of the poem, suggesting that Lady Jane, for a space, became to her infant what the "rich Marble" tomb in which she would later be laid to rest was to her. It also suggests that Milton wished to fold the child's significance into the significance of his mother's suffering (the infant is not given his own elegy; having never had time to *do* anything, he cannot be treated as himself an object of praise).[46] The figure also, not coincidentally, ties the Lady's death to "On Shakespear," suggesting a continuation of the parallel between Milton as poet and the Lady as mother.

Milton clearly employed a fair amount of ingenuity in framing the figure. The rhyme pair "birth/earth" is not only the only pair used twice in the poem (both here at lines 31–3 and in the description of Lady Jane's virtues at lines 5–6), but its semantic force is paralleled by the use of "Womb/Tomb" in the couplet that follows the second iteration (lines 33–4). This has the effect of tying the mother's virtuous actions (which "[a]dded to her birth" and were more than "she could own from Earth") very closely to her giving birth to her child. The irony of the fact that the infant was not laid in *earth* first

[46] He didn't even have a chance to bewail his entrance to the world. Even in this small detail, Milton suggests that Jane's sufferings and how she faced them *were*, on the other hand, examples of laudable action.

upon his death, but first found burial in the womb that nourished him and from which he should have emerged with Lucina's aid into the light, furthermore helps to keep the otherwise predictable rhyme of "birth" and "earth" from having too simple a semantic force. That our attention in lines 33–4 is drawn in such a thematically integrated way to the process of the mother's body going from living – if languishing – womb to a lifeless tomb in any case helps to give the figure the kind of fresh force it does not have in poems like the one Milton might have read on Anne Scott's tomb in Great St. Mary's Church.

It should also be noted here that the sequencing implied by Milton's treatment of the stillbirth is consistent with what we know from both of the letters that provide what little historical record we have of the event – although, again, we do not know how Milton came to know any of it. The Duchess says that Lady Jane "was delivered before shee died of a deed boye." Milton's imagery seems to suggest that he knew the infant died before the birth ("The haples Babe before his birth/ Had burial"). The language of the next lines, however, suggests uncertainty about just what actually happened: "And the languisht Mothers Womb/ Was not long a living Tomb" could suggest, in line with the Duchess' letter, that he knew "shee was delivered…of" the dead child before she herself died; that is, she was alive and suffering in labor over a dead infant, a living tomb to it, then gave birth to it or had it extracted from her some time before her own death. She stopped being a "living Tomb" because she no longer contained the body of the child. It is possible, however, for Milton's lines to refer to a woman who died while still containing the dead body of her infant. In other words, she became a dead tomb to her dead son. There is a detail, however, in the pastoral image that follows in the next period that suggests that it was the second of these scenarios that Milton imagined. The swain, we are told, sought to "crop" only the flower (line 39), but in his unheediness took the whole slip. This suggests an attempt on the part of the birth practitioners to save the mother by extracting what they knew was a dead infant. The procedure went awry, however, and she was also killed. The image of the plucking echoes the harvesting image of the Atropos figure, and both in this context are suggestive of surgery. However, both also, as agricultural or horticultural images, carry on the theme of genealogy.[47] It is unlikely, of course, that Milton would have imagined a killing of the infant to save the mother's life. Atropos and the "unheedy swain" represent figures of death

[47] Frost also notes the connection between the images ("No Marchioness," 18–19).

and ill fate who took away the child; that is to say, they are figures for his dying. On another level of reference, however, they represent a failed attempt to rescue the mother by another kind of cutting and plucking.

In the case of the "fruit and tree" figure, an image of careless harvesting that kills the fruit-bearing tree, we can see Milton experimenting with a technique for rethinking a commonplace figure in a concrete, referentially specific way. Here he conflates the harvest image with the implied image of Atropos' shears, which the Fate used to cut the thread of a newly born life to its appointed length. The mythic trope of replacing Lucina with Atropos, which is, as far as I can tell, original to Milton, fits perfectly with the typical gathering of gossips and midwife in the lying-in chamber of the mother in labor. The switch suggests, in those terms, the arrival of the wrong midwife, or the arrival of some woman unknown to the mother and untrained in the problems of a difficult birth. Note that Milton makes no direct mention whatsoever of the lanced impostume and the surgeon who must have done the lancing. His lying-in chamber retains the traditional character of a completely female world (a man does not enter until the figurative "unheedy swain" is introduced in the next section, and I will discuss the possible significance of that below). Here, the connection of Atropos with midwife and gossips via the substitution with Lucina is a close and resonant one. The Fates (*parcae*, from "*parere*," "to bring forth") were always thought of as birth attendants, spiritual gossips presiding over and determining each life at its beginning. One held the thread, another the distaff, and the third (Atropos) drew out the thread of life, cutting it to its fated length. The cutting of the umbilical cord, usually performed by the midwife, was closely associated with the determination of fate. In Milton's figure, the clipping of the thread and the instrument used to do so is buried in the fruit and tree figure, which is given a striking freshness by the requirement that we imagine Atropos using her shears to carelessly damage a tree that would have been better off left alone to bear its fruit naturally.

What little information we can gather from the two brief accounts we have of her death suggests the probability that Jane was not allowed to bear naturally at all, that some sort of obstetric surgery did take place in the last hours of her life. This seems especially likely in light of the fact that the female world of the chamber may already have been compromised by the entrance of the surgeon who performed the lancing. Stillbirth was a very messy business and a key cause of several fatal obstetric complications. It is likely, therefore, that birth complications, not the lancing, were the direct cause of her death. Pory's remark about the humor oozing from the impostume having run down her throat and dispatched her is in line with what some physicians believed about the humors that collected in such abscesses. It is, however, hard to believe that such fluids could have actually killed her.[48]

In addition to the lancing, however, Jane may very well have had her infant removed by crochet, a terrifying and dangerous procedure commonly performed in cases of obstructed stillbirth. It involved the dismemberment of the dead infant and its removal piecemeal from the uterus (see Part I). It is highly likely that whoever did the lancing would also have been equipped to perform such an extraction, which could often lead to laceration of the uterus and severe infection and/or bleeding, and is at least as likely as the impostume and its lancing to have caused the fever that the Duchess claimed killed Lady Jane. The language of the Duchess of Buckingham's letter, on the other hand, does suggest a way in which the impostume may have in fact been the original cause of death: "my Lady Marques who dyed with an impostome in her checked [cheek], and the extreemity of that putt her in a fever. Shee was delivered before she died of a deed boye." This implies the following sequence of events: the impostume appeared on Jane's cheek some time late in the pregnancy but prior to labor. At some point, still prior to labor, it got bad enough to cause, or was accompanied by, a fever. The phrase "the extreemity of that" may be the Duchess' way of referring to the lancing, or it may be simply her way of saying that the impostume itself got so bad that it gave her a fever. This fever may have created the weakened condition that kept Lady Jane from surviving her pregnancy. We would have to assume this if we did not also have Pory's letter. However, from what Pory says, we may assume that the "extreemity" of the impostume was such that it required the lancing.

How close to the actual birth this was, we cannot say, but both accounts seem to agree that Jane reached some point of extremity before she gave birth to her dead son, and that she died sometime shortly after that. Could the infection represented by the impostume have killed her? It is certainly

[48] Pory wrote: "The Lady Marquess of Winchester ... had an impostume upon her cheek lanced; the humour fell down into her throat, and quickly dispatched her, being big with child." The syntax is a bit ambiguous, but he seems to be saying that a toxic fluid from the abscess killed her, given the weakness of her condition; that is, her "being big with child." Pory here makes a common and reasonable association of childbirth with a vulnerable state of health, although he does not tell us of the stillbirth, suggesting the possibility that he thought Jane died undelivered. His assumption that the humor killed her derives from humoral ideas about the fluids contained in various sorts of pimples, warts, boils, and abscesses. See, for example, Ambroise Paré, *The Workes of that Famous Chirurgion Ambrose Parey*, trans. Thomas Johnson (London, 1634), pp. 249–54. A slightly different sequence of causes and effects is suggested by the Duchess' letter, which identifies the impostume and the fever it caused as the direct causes of death.

possible that it did so either by weakening her enough to make her unable to survive the rigors of a difficult birth, or it might have done so directly if the infection was severe enough. It is also possible, however, that the infection killed her by spreading to the uterus. As Irvine Loudon points out, most cases of puerperal fever are caused by streptococcal infections, but also often from a combination of organisms, including in many fatal cases an organism called *staphylococcus aureas*, which is also the cause of boils and carbuncles.[49] If Jane's impostume was caused by this bacterium, as is possible, it is also at least possible that the lancing of it was itself responsible for transmission of the infection to her uterus, causing a fatal case of puerperal fever. This would have been especially possible (though of course we have no way of knowing for sure) if the surgeon who did the impostume also tended to her obstetrically. All he would have needed to do was perform a manual obstetric examination shortly after tending to the lancing (he would not, of course, have thought to wash his hands or his instruments). For all we know, he might have performed an extraction by crochet. Milton does not mention the impostume at all, but the details he chooses to include concerning Atropos and, as we will see, the unheedy swain of the last period of the *divisio* both suggest he had some surgical procedure in mind, and worked out these figures in order to evoke it decorously. In both cases, the figures serve to connect the physical realities of the event with abstractions that then connect those figures with the poem's thematic preoccupations. In the case of Atropos, the physical is tied to fate; in the case of the swain, as we will see, it is tied to aristocratic genealogy. In both cases, these are significant parts of the fallen world that conspired to destroy both mother and child. They are also things that the mother's heroism allowed her to transcend, redeeming the maternal while leaving a mistaken vision of the universe and of its proper values behind.

The "unheedy swain"

The final discrete period of the *divisio*, which reintroduces these themes in a new poetic register, brings all of the poem's various thematic elements together:

> So have I seen som tender slip
> Sav'd with care from Winters nip,

[49] See Irving Loudon, *Childbed Fever: a Documentary History* (New York, NY: Garland, 1995), pp. xxx–xxxv, lix and *Death in Childbirth: an International Study of Maternal Care and Maternal Mortality, 1800–1950* (Oxford: Clarendon Press, 1992), pp. 77–9, 534–41.

The pride of her carnation train,
Pluck't up by som unheedy swain,
Who onely thought to crop the flowr
New shot up from vernall showr;
But the fair blossom hangs the head
Side-ways as on a dying bed,
And those Pearls of dew she wears
Prove to be presaging tears
Which the sad morn had let fall
On her hast'ning funerall. (lines 35–46)

The death in childbed is now refigured in a tragicomic pastoral figure related to the bumbling mistake of Winter in "On the Death of a Fair Infant." Here, however, the blundering of a divine being becomes the homely blundering of an overenthusiastic shepherd, who expected to take only the flower (that is, the infant son) but instead pulled up the entire slip (the mother as well).[50] That Jane was "Sav'd with care from Winters nip" suggests the actual season at the time of the birth: springtime, after the dangers of a pregnancy whose central months – from the quickening to the seventh month – stretched across the winter of 1630–1631. The child would have been born just as the first flowers were rising with the April rains. The "Pearls of dew" suggest the Lady's youth again and are re-imagined as presaging tears.

Most importantly, however, this pretty pastoral allegory draws us back to the theme of genealogy. The image here is not, as some commentators have had it, of a plant planted in the soil, but of a "slip," a cutting, containing the best offered by one plant, cut off and then grafted into the stock of another. This image reflects on the nature of both childbed and dynastic

[50] The reproductive experience of Milton's sister, Anne, whose second child he mourned in that earlier poem (written some time in the late winter or early spring of 1628), may have affected Milton's imagination, lending some personal urgency to his treatment of Lady Jane's childbed suffering. By the time Milton composed "An Epitaph" in the spring of 1631, his sister had given birth to four children, three of whom had died in early childhood. She gave birth to her first child in January 1625 and her second in January 1626. She then lost that second child (the one Milton mourned in the poem, a daughter named for her mother) in January 1628 (at age two) before giving birth to a third child in April of that year. She then lost the first (at age four) in March 1629, and the third in February 1631, a couple of months short of what would have been the child's third birthday. This last death (the child was buried on February 19th) came just two months before Lady Jane's death on April 15th (the child's birthday would have fallen just a few days or a week earlier, had she lived). Some time in the previous August (1630), Anne had also given birth to a fourth child, a son named Edward. He was still living in April and would in fact live to adulthood, later becoming Milton's pupil and biographer. For more details, see Edward Jones, "Select Chronology: 'Speak of things at hand/ Useful,'" in *A Concise Companion to Milton*, ed. Angelica Duran (Malden, MA: Blackwell, 2007), pp. 220–3 and Parker, p. 738. I am also grateful to Professor Jones for his comments and suggestions in conversation and correspondence.

expectations. That the child is a flower on a "slip," "the pride of *her* [that is, her mother's] carnation train," should remind us both of the opening lines of the poem and of lines 15–16. The botanical image is a way of describing what made *Lady Jane* a "lover meet" for John Paulet within the context of the genealogies of the noble houses that bred both of them. One does not have to remember Shakespeare's Sonnet 15 or Perdita's speech from *The Winter's Tale* to see what Milton is getting at here, although it is perfectly possible that Milton had these passages in mind. The name "carnation" suggested to herbalists at the time both flesh and crown ("*carn*-ation" and "*coron*-ation" were both thought of as possible roots). McHenry suggests that carnations were particularly associated with the *coronae*, or garlands, used at funerals. In addition, carnations were almost always thought of as cultivated flowers.[51] The figures of the unheedy swain and the carnation are therefore extensions of the opening figure of genealogy at the same time that they extend the figure of fatal (deadly and accidental, but also malevolent, even punitive) harvesting we saw in the Atropos passage. The Lady is a slip, taken from the stock of the line of Savage and grafted with clear expectations into the line of Paulet, bringing her carnation train ("carn" connoting flesh) to bloom at Basing House. In the last few lines of this passage, we see the hopes and expectations of the "morn" (personal and dynastic) give way – with the force of a foreshadowed fate – to the hastening funeral at evening. The passage also lays a far darker burden of blame on the earthly intentions behind this sort of dynastic grafting.

The "Winters nip" might also have suggested the seven years of possible barrenness, this second son being only the second flower to be carefully raised from the weak and uncertain transfer of the maternal slip that had been tended with care for some time before it bore its first. Such a reading is perfectly in line with Frost's contention that the poem – and this passage in particular – constitutes an explicit critique of Paulet. Milton is not blaming the husband directly for the death of his wife, but he casts a cold eye on the dynastic significance of the event that killed her, treating it ironically. The earthly means by which earthly gain is preserved and passed on from one generation to another are here shown to be pitifully fragile, and if this were all that were involved in a birth like this one, it would remain, from a higher religious perspective, tragically meaningless. However, this is not for Milton all that animated the sad event, and the next sections of the

51 They also show up in the flower catalogue in "Lycidas" as "pinks" (McHenry, "A Milton Herbal," 58). Perdita calls them "gillyvors" in *The Winter's Tale* (Act 4, Scene 4).

poem will resolve the irony of the first half by making Lady Jane an exemplar of both self-sacrificial courage and the Protestant cause.

Frost makes the intriguing suggestion that winter here represents the Catholicism of the old Catholic aristocracy. I suggest only a slight revision. Lady Jane is not, I think, described as a member of the retinue of winter itself. "Winters nip" can only, therefore, refer to what threatens the process that the passage describes, and these are defined by the poem's agricultural images as natural forces that may be (although only sometimes) escaped or sidestepped by human acts of cultivation. In this sense, as I said before, it clearly refers to the literal winter of the past year with its risks of disease, but it might also be thought of more figuratively as the religious or ideological beliefs (the wintery spiritual condition) that threatened to make the ongoing life of these dynastic houses spiritually barren. Lady Jane is the pride of her train of flesh, her dynastic line, and had been chosen by the swain and cared for during the winter for one primary purpose: the production of hybrid flowers. She has already produced one, but dies producing a second. He is "unheedy" of her well-being, perhaps thinking primarily of the sons she produces. As it turns out, however, this was also *her* primary concern, but what for her husband, the poem imagines, was a selfish desire for offspring – and at her cost – becomes for *her* a heroic self-sacrifice, and this is precisely the virtue most carefully cultivated by the advice books, prayers, and sermons we examined in Part I. The children would, however, have also been of central importance to Lady Jane as her special spiritual charges, and as a mother she would have been the one to tend to their early religious upbringing, perhaps – to Milton's mind – in the redeeming sunlight of her Protestant tendencies. It is her tragic failure to fulfill that responsibility that Milton will seek to redress in the poem's *conclusio*.

"After this thy travail sore"

It is only at this point, after the end of the *divisio* and at the start of the *conclusio*, that Milton's speaker is moved to turn for the first time directly to the Lady, now in her grave, the funeral over. He wishes her the peace and quiet that, as we have been invited to remember and imagine, were not her lot in the last days or hours of her life:

> Gentle Lady may thy grave
> Peace and quiet ever have;
> After this thy travail sore
> Sweet rest sease thee evermore,

That to give the world encrease,
Short'n'd hast thy own lives lease; (lines 47–52)

It is in these six lines that Milton moves for the first time to construct a positive argument for the value and meaning of Lady Jane's death.[52] He does this by treating the death as a heroic self-sacrifice, presenting her as an exemplar able to teach from beyond the grave. The implications of "sweet rest sease thee" are worth some comment. By using so active, even aggressive, a verb for a state of passivity, Milton gives his line an oddly oxymoronic force. In this sort of context, "sease" is usually associated with a sudden or violent death, but here Milton deliberately reverses the disquieting effect of a sudden death by making it equivalent to achieving rest.[53] "Sweet rest" also underlines the numerological suggestion that her rest is a Sabbath granted after her difficult procreative work (she obeyed the commandment of the sixth day, did her part in creation, and now rests as God rested). It is also striking that the poem, in wishing the Lady rest in her grave, should so clearly oppose the unquiet bed of her labor with the quiet bed of her grave. The "this" in line 49 makes it quite clear that Milton has the immediate event of her struggle in childbed in mind, and it is a strikingly specific reference for a poem of this kind.

The passage also returns us to the physical location of the poem's opening: the tomb of "rich Marble." In doing so, the poet reminds us of the noble houses he mentioned earlier, but he now presents Jane's action as part of a project of human "encrease" far larger than the one encompassed by the narrow designs of her class. The sacrifices and rewards demanded and conferred by the imperatives of dynastic marriage are now universalized and sacralized. The poet thus prepares us for what comes next, as he turns to his own motives for writing the poem and the larger world of mourners outside the noble houses, including the specific community of mourners of which he is himself a part.

Given the pointed political and religious associations that the tomb of "rich" marble has with the University, it is important that it is from Cambridge that the poet finally speaks of and for himself:

Here besides the sorrowing
That thy noble House doth bring,
Here be tears of perfect moan

[52] John Shawcross has suggested to me in correspondence that the Sloan Manuscript indentations at lines 47 and 53 may be significant, emphasizing the rhetorical shift, isolating the intervening lines as a unit, and marking the poem's turning point.

[53] West, "The *Consolatio* in Milton's Funeral Elegies," 242.

Wept for thee in *Helicon*,
And som Flowers, and som Bays,
For thy Hears to strew the ways,
Sent thee from the banks of *Came*,
Devoted to thy vertuous name; (lines 53–60)

Milton now, in a sense, names himself, aligning himself with the university community, whose "perfect moan" he brings to chorus with the "sorrowing" of the noble families as the funeral processes in his imagination to the gravesite. He also identifies that "perfect moan" with what is offered by poetry itself (figured by Helicon). These are the lines that have led, probably erroneously, to speculation about Milton's poem having been written for a collection of Cambridge verses on the death of Lady Jane. It is clear, however, that the speaker presents his poem as the spontaneous reaction of the learned community and the traditions of poetry (or as the reaction of one exemplary member of that community who has taken on the responsibilities of those traditions). This is not, in other words, simply a piece of commissioned work, or even one composed in response to a collective invitation.

I think it is likely that the poem was exactly what Milton says it was: a direct reaction to the occasion. However, it was clearly motivated more by aesthetic, didactic, and ideological concerns than by personal feelings of sorrow. "Perfect moan" suggests the young Milton's evaluation of his own achievement. He apparently considered this a very good poem (in any case, he completely eschews any commonplace protestation of inadequacy). The laurels and bays suggest quite plainly that Milton assumed Lady Jane's actions won her a victory over death and fear, but they also suggest his own victory over both the aesthetic challenges the occasion set for him and his own vocational anxieties. He also seems to have considered the poem a "moan" of a higher (more perfect) kind than anything he imagines came from the aristocratic mourners, who are described as "noble," but also as bringing mere "sorrowing." His mourning is of a higher kind not because he feels more pain, but because of the larger mission of his sponsoring powers: poetry and learning.

It is through these sponsoring powers that the victory is offered on behalf of all readers of the poem. Before he turns to his final description of Lady Jane's apotheosis, the poet is careful to conclude this section of his long apostrophe by specifically proclaiming Cambridge's devotion to Jane Paulet's "vertuous name" (the phrase rhymed pointedly with "*Came*," the river from which the university took its name). These lines conclude the topic of Jane's personal virtue with reference to the place that will now be primary in its preservation. Her last act sealed her worthiness, but it is the poem and the community of the learned that will remember that act. Poetry, learning, and the Lady's action dovetail in a design meant, however, to do more than merely facilitate remembrance. The poet now moves on to reveal a truth about this death, a revelation that he believes will rob it of its fearfulness by taking us out of the limited dynamics of time and memory. As he imagines the apotheosis of Lady Jane, he takes her out of her tomb, at once redeeming her from her earthly death-in-birth and enacting his own escape from the death he imagined for his own imagination in "On Shakespear." Both tombs are "marble," but here Milton's "conceaving," newly empowered by his contemplation of Lady Jane's virtues, finds life in the aftermath of bereavement.

"No Marchioness, but now a Queen"

As the final lines of the poem unfold, we are told that the deceased herself now sits above all the mourning and pain her death has occasioned, above the memory of it, and even above the praise her embrace of it has won her. We are now allowed to see, with perfect clarity and outside of time, the nature of her *true* reward. Her body may now have rest in the grave, and the grave may proclaim her proper familial allegiances and her virtuous actions, but it is the special role of the poet to reveal to us a vision of what has happened to her soul in its final and eternal state:

> Whilst thou bright Saint high sit'st in glory,
> Next her much like to thee in story,
> That fair *Syrian* Shepherdess,
> Who after yeers of barrennes,
> The highly favour'd *Joseph* bore
> To him that serv'd for her before,
> And at her next birth much like thee,
> Through pangs fled to felicity,
> Far within the boosom bright
> Of blazing Majesty and Light;
> There with thee, new welcom Saint,
> Like fortunes may her soul acquaint,
> With thee there clad in radiant sheen,
> No Marchioness, but now a Queen. (lines 61–74)

With this conclusion, Milton ties all the threads of the poem together into a consolatory apotheosis that transfigures all the terms of Jane's life, experience, and actions. He provides her, using a complex literary and typological scheme, with a counter-lineage to the earthly one with which he began the poem, and he gives her a new title, one that is above the earthly, Catholic, and marital pinfolds suggested by "honour'd Wife of *Winchester*," "Vicounts daughter," and "Earls heir."

The entire structure of the poem is designed to climax in the biblical and literary allusion to Rachel via Dante's *Paradiso*, Canto XXXII, lines 7–10. The choice to end with an apotheosis is conventional. However, Milton's manner, and the motive behind his choice of figures and allusions, makes the topos operate in a wholly original way. The analogy between Jane's experience and Rachel's, along with the fact that she now sits next to Rachel in the heavenly hierarchy, serves to expand on the gestures that began the *conclusio* by suggesting that: (1) Jane is not only saved, but that the form of her self-sacrifice has achieved for her a place of *particularly* high glory, and (2) her manner of death has typological resonances of rather wide application. Milton makes the analogy between Jane and Rachel, not just the former's ascent itself, at once the tragic and recuperative conclusion of his poem. Lines 67–8 are particularly powerful in this regard. Note that Milton chooses to assert that it is "*through* pangs" (my italics) that both Rachel and Lady Jane "fled to felicity." The term not only identifies the pangs themselves as the process *by which* the apotheoses were achieved, but also suggests that they were an obstacle to overcome, something the women had to move through against some resistance. Both women passed through their pangs, in one sense, as one simply passes through any experience, but also as one passes through a test or trial.

The lines are prosodically rich in ways that reinforce this reading. The comparison begins at lines 61–2, when Milton places the Lady next to Rachel, though he does not name the matriarch right away. Instead, the comparison is stated as a likeness in "story," and Milton develops the comparison by briefly presenting the biblical account, choosing details that parallel the ones he chose earlier in telling Jane's story. This parallel is far stronger in the manuscript version of the poem, which explicitly mentions the seven years between Jane's wedding day and the birth of her first child, but the 1645 version does nothing to keep an attentive reader, especially one who knew something of the Paulet's married life, from making the connection. Rachel is named by a sort of biblical/pastoral title, paralleling Milton's earlier use of titles to refer to Lady Jane, and the years of barrenness are here explicitly invoked as a detail of the comparison. We are then told of the successful first birth of a highly favored son, then (in this case with a brief glance to the husband, Jacob) of the second, tragic birth. At lines 60–1, the comparison had been initiated with the phrase "like to thee." At line 67, we get a variant repetition, "much like thee," and the syntax pushes us through a significant enjambment whose tension passes us *through* "through" in the next line to the resolution of the rhyme and the crux of the comparison itself: "Through pangs fled to felicity." "Felicity" is what gives meaning to the comparison, moving it from worldly circumstance to heavenly reward, retrospectively re-identifying and redeeming the "pangs" as productive trial rather than simply a reproductive catastrophe. Without the pangs, there would have been no felicity, for the felicity is a reward for having faced and passed through those pangs with faith intact.

The poem's forward syntactic movement does not stop there, however, but goes on to invoke Dante's vision of Paradise with a number of explicitly feminizing emphases. Here, not only is it explicitly "through pangs" that both Rachel and Jane achieved heaven, but we are told that they "fled," presumably from the earth, into the welcoming "boosom" of "Majesty and Light." There Jane becomes a "new welcom Saint" in an explicitly female company, and the poem alters the comparative formula of "like thee" (lines 61 and 67) to "with thee" (at line 71 and repeated for emphasis and symmetry at line 73).[54] It is not that Milton imagines a heaven without masculine souls. The very fact that he sees all of this aligns him with the important male figures of Dante's episode: Saint Benedict, who reveals and guides, and, of course, Dante himself, who sees and records. Still, the suggestion of an upward leveling of female experience rooted in an equivalence of spiritual experience is dominant. It also has epithalamic overtones – the installation of Lady Jane as a queen clad in radiance not only resembles the decking of a bride, but the fact that she becomes a "Queen" certainly implies the presence of a King (in this case, of course, the bridegroom Christ). Milton's apotheosis, however, is more concerned with her coming into the bosom of female fellowship than with figures of heavenly marriage, and the elision of any explicitly masculine figure for the divine is deliberate. In this vision, the heavenly society of saintliness echoes the female world of the lying-in chamber. Here, women, we are told implicitly (whether they are simple shepherdesses or privileged members of the aristocracy), become queens, and are granted their special place.

In addition, Milton deliberately appropriates the typological scheme that Dante employed as part of his praise of Beatrice, focusing our attention on a

[54] It may be of some significance that "fled" derives from the old Germanic word "fliohen," which means "to escape," and has no original connection to the verb "to fly." Milton may have been aware of the word's etymological resonances. See, for example, *PL*, 4.1014–15 and 9.53 and 394. I am grateful to Shawcross for the observation. Milton would again make use of a conjunction between fleeing and sainthood in Sonnet 23. See below.

particularly female part of the arrangement of the Heavenly Rose. His purpose is to connect Lady Jane's placement in the Rose to traditions of Christian consolation – and specifically Christian childbed consolation – via a connection with Mary. Milton connects Jane to Mary by placing her in the spot Dante had reserved for Beatrice. It is Mary that Dante is gazing at when he is told by Benedict that the radiant women he sees just below the Virgin are, first, Eve, who "opened" and "pierced" the "wound which Mary closed and anointed." Then, below Eve, is Rachel. Beatrice is on her right, and in gradations below the matriarch come Sarah, Rebekah, Judith, Ruth, and then all the Hebrew women "who follow in succession, dividing all the tresses of the flower." This line divides the seats of the rose between those who "believed in Christ yet to come" and "those who turned their faces to Christ already come."[55] As a pre-Christian Israelite who is later saved (and here appears in heaven), Rachel can suggest the fate of woman after the curse of Eve (she is a woman who gave birth in pain and danger, and died). By her position in the rose, she can also suggest the one birth that makes it possible for her to transcend this curse: that of Mary, who according to tradition (as we saw in Chapter 3), gave birth without sin and therefore without pain or danger, and whose child made it possible for those who suffer in faith to be redeemed from their suffering. Milton may not have himself accepted the full Mariological implications of the traditional figure of the Virgin (later in life, we know he rejected the Immaculate Conception and other aspects of Mariology). However, Milton's allusion to Dante's arrangement of figures in the Heavenly Rose, his specificity about where Jane is sitting in the Rose, does suggest that he considered the arrangement significant from the point of view of childbed death, especially given its typological implications. Placing Jane at Rachel's side, on the Christian side, makes her occupy a position in the rose that is on the cusp between the two dispensations, the line that both divides and makes them one (both piercing and closing the wound).[56] Rachel is there below Eve (and, oddly, before Sarah), not just because she – as the earlier dream of *Purgatorio*, Canto XXVII tells us – represents contemplation, but because in motherhood she

[55] *Paradiso*, Canto XXXII, lines 1–18. Quotations are from Dante Alighieri, *The Divine Comedy*, ed. and trans. Charles S. Singleton, Bollingen Series LXXX, 3 vols. (Princeton, NJ: Princeton University Press, 1975), vol. III, pp. 358–61.

[56] Singleton notes, referring to Niccolo Tommaseo's 1869 study of the *Commedia*, that the dividing line "both separates and unites: between the Old and New Testament these women are a bond, a bond of maternity, of expectation, of love." Singleton also notes the importance of the fact that Mary, whose life spanned both dispensations, is at the head of the line. On the male side of the rose, the matching line begins with John the Baptist, whose life also spanned the gap (Dante, *The Divine Comedy*, vol. III, pp. 536).

represents the wound of painful fallen existence. Rachel's death in Genesis is a wound that never quite gets healed in the course of the Hebrew scriptures,[57] although it is healed for Christians by Mary. In fact, contemplation of Rachel's fallen pain becomes a vehicle for its own transcendence by typological contemplation. Rachel is, for this reason, as we saw in the chapters of Part I, a significant biblical touchstone in discussions about painful and dangerous birth in the period. On the opposite side of the rose in Dante's description is a male line leading from John the Baptist down through Saints Francis, Benedict, and Augustine. This line, symmetrically one space over into the Christian side, just as the line leading from Mary is one space over into the Hebrew side, represents the great figures of Saintly life and theological insight that open the door to an understanding of "Christ already come." Milton's choice to place Jane next to Rachel not only places her on the Christian side, but on the Christian side near the sign of a parallel and wholly female spiritual way into the grace of Christ, one associated explicitly, as I said before, with female suffering in labor pangs. These pangs, faced piously, not only proved the faithfulness of generations of individual women, but allowed those generations themselves to exist over the course of sacred history linking Abraham to Jesus.[58] It is through those pangs that women like Lady Jane achieved their justification before God and attained their reward. It is perhaps this way of thinking that pushed Milton to make use of Dante's divided rose. It provided him with a figure of heavenly female society and lineage that could be used to balance the dangers of earthly, dynastic marriage and allow him to hold birth imagery and epithalamic imagery in productive tension with each other. Rachel's appearance at so important a point in Milton's poem is, for all these reasons, more deeply integrated with Milton's larger purposes than has been suggested in the criticism.[59]

[57] Her death is one of the prominent features of Jacob's account of his difficult "days and years" (Genesis 47:9). She is, significantly, the only one of the biblical Patriarchs and Matriarchs who is not buried in the cave of Machpelah, but in a roadside tomb (Genesis 35:19–20). She appears again later in that place in one of Jeremiah's visions, weeping for her exiled children (Jeremiah 31:15).

[58] Dante's figure and Milton's adaptation of it restores the women left, for the most part, out of the genealogies of Jesus as set forth in Matthew 1 and Luke 3:23–38.

[59] Brooks and Hardy, for example, found the comparison accidental and forced. See *Poems of Mr. John Milton: the 1645 Edition with Essays in Analysis*, Cleanth Brooks and John E. Hardy, eds. (New York, NY: Harcourt, Brace, and Company, 1951), p. 122. Parker thought it perhaps impoverished the Lady, noting that Benjamin lived, and that Jacob had other children by Leah and his various maidservants (Parker, p. 96). Wilson felt that the figure was appropriate, but mainly because of its "elegant straining of the truth" (Wilson, "Decorum and Milton's "An Epitaph," 12). Frost, "No Marchioness," 20–1 treats the figure positively, but discounts the importance of its reproductive resonance.

CONCLUSION

Milton's choices, seen the way I am suggesting, show him to be dealing in a very complex and conscious way with the consequences of birth under contemporary conditions in every aspect of the poem. His choices cannot simply be explained by recourse to inherited rhetorical theory or his motives concerning ideological polemic, although, as we can plainly see, the theories and *topoi* Milton learned so well were the scaffolding upon which he built the poem, and he did mean to marshal his depiction of childbed suffering in the service of an ideological position that would later give birth to the anti-prelatical cause.

Milton's sense of Jane Paulet's "moral and spiritual efficacy" within the religious politics of her family would have been centrally a matter of two spheres of activity: childbirth itself and her influence on the religious education of her children. Upon her death, however (and this is the crisis the poem addresses), her power to influence the children would have become solely a matter of how her exemplary death could and would have been understood. The central task of the poem is to show just what that death exemplified, so that both Jane's manifest and potential virtues could be preserved in the act of mourning. Furthermore, these virtues and the spheres in which they operated would not have seemed to Milton to be strictly personal or domestic in nature. They had political dimensions. By 1645, when he finally published the poem, it would have been abundantly clear to Milton that John Paulet's remarriage after Jane's death and his support of the King's cause in the Civil War had unfortunately confirmed the religious and political allegiances of the family. Jane's death would have seemed by then the marker of a lost opportunity, one with some rather tragic dimensions, particularly given the strength that Paulet was providing for the Royalist cause. Jane's death, like Edward King's after her, had left the world at the mercy of wolves, and while it was true that by 1645 those wolves were being captured or driven away, this was only being accomplished with what Milton would call in Sonnet 12, great "wast of wealth, and loss of blood."

Like Edward King within the Laudian Church, in 1645 Lady Jane would have seemed, even more clearly than she did in 1631, just the sort of young person the pre-Civil War aristocracy had needed (had there been more of them, things might have gone differently). As John Paulet was being committed to the tower after the collapse of his spectacular resistance to the siege of Basing House, Milton must have felt both saddened and prophetic as he oversaw his early poem's first appearance in print, and we therefore have warrant to imagine the poem along the lines suggested by the head note he appended to "Lycidas." In both cases, we encounter lamentation over the loss of a young person who might have played a role, if even a small one, in the happier unfolding of painful historical events, and in both cases the occasion for lamentation is turned into an opportunity for the assertion of poetic power on the part of an equally young poet determined still to play his own small but hopefully effective role. The events of the early 1640s would have confirmed Milton's hope that ideals could win out on the stage of history, and that poetry could help the memory of the dead have the sort of power he would in his later sonnet ask God to give the scattered blood and ashes of the massacred Waldensians. The memory of people like Jane Paulet and Edward King might inspire people to fly the "*Babylonian* wo" of Royalist power.[60] Both early poems, in their different and admittedly limited ways, were symbols of support for those faithful to the cause that by the mid 1640s was finally defeating the corrupt clerical and political order that at the time of both deaths had been in its height. Both poems also make their claims about the power of poetry to act in ways appropriate to present historical exigencies by ambitiously reworking their respective subgenres in ways that allow each to address – and then in new and audacious ways gesture beyond – the particulars of their occasions. And in both poems, the deceased is granted an active role in the world after his or her apotheosis. Lycidas becomes "the Genius of the shoar" (line 183) and Lady Jane a queenly figure in heaven who, via the allusion to Dante, also functions, as Frost suggests, as a "psychopomp," a sponsor of poetic power.

To some extent, what we also have in the Marchioness' epitaph is a concrete examination, in mythical and occasional terms, of the vehicle of the metaphor for poetic anxiety that Milton used in his poem on Shakespeare. Here we have a young, accomplished woman who died in the very way Milton imagined the "death" of the fancies of Shakespeare's readers and the threat posed to his own creative powers by the "Delphick" reproductive force of Shakespeare's achievement. The triumphant poem on the Marchioness is poised, in fact, between two very worried poems: "On Shakespear," written the year before, and Sonnet 7, which Milton would write some eight months later about his own failure by the age of twenty-four to produce something of great worth. Despite whatever limitations it might seem to have in comparison with what Milton would later produce (or might have seemed to have under his own impatient and self-evaluative gaze several months later), the epitaph was a serious and ambitious

60 Sonnet 18, written in 1655.

accomplishment. Milton may have feared creative annihilation in the arena of life he had chosen as his own sphere of meaningful moral and spiritual action. But for Lady Jane, whose sphere of significant action was the childbed, the possibilities for annihilation were far more concrete. In his poem, Milton overcame his poet's anxiety about what he felt he had yet to accomplish by setting aside what Lady Jane had *yet* to do and concentrating instead upon what she actually *did* accomplish in her act of dying. In the process, he ambitiously reworked a limited set of conventions in order to provide a fitting consolation for a premature death in childbirth. What remained undone by Lady Jane's death is, indeed, given new life by the way the poem empowers the memory of her to go on working. What would have been as stillborn as her child is transformed into a living legacy with powerful poetic, religious, and political implications. Even at this early stage, in what is only ostensibly a simple piece of occasional verse, Milton is clearly aiming at some point just above the peak of the Aeonian Mount.

CHAPTER 6

"Farr above in spangled sheen": A Mask *and its Epilogue*

As the rest of this study argues, Milton never discarded his early interest in mortality, and later in life he found himself, for personal reasons, returning to his earlier thinking on the subject. There is therefore something chillingly prescient in the choices he made in constructing his early exercise in Jonsonian verse (though he need not have been a seer to understand his chances of seeing a wife die in childbirth). There is also something surprisingly sensitive and searching in these choices, and they, in part, laid the ground work for the even more remarkable poetry Milton would produce later as he meditated on his personal losses in the context of the Fall, and remembered, with perhaps no small temptation to bitterness, God's words to Eve in Genesis 3:16.

Milton's later approach to maternal mortality would be darker and less resolved than the one articulated in "An Epitaph on the Marchioness of Winchester" (hereafter "An Epitaph"), and it would be even more ambitious, attempting to dramatize irresolution itself while still giving voice to the promises of Christian consolation. Before we turn to that later poetry, however, one other important work requires some comment. *A Mask*, written just a few years after the epitaph for Jane Paulet, contains reproductive images that have not been adequately glossed. They are not all directly concerned with maternal mortality, yet several of them show that Milton had the figures of the mortal mother and of childbirth as a spiritual trial very much on his mind as he conceived his tale of a young woman's trial in the dark woods along the Welsh border.

Indeed, the scattered and seemingly inconsistent reproductive images in *A Mask* represent Milton's most elaborate attempt to grapple, in verse, with problems related to human reproduction between "An Epitaph" in 1631 and Sonnet 23 and *Paradise Lost* more then twenty-five years later. A full study of the meaning of these reproductive images lies outside of the scope of this book. It will be useful, however, for us to look closely at parts of Comus' seduction speech to the Lady, and at the Epilogue that Milton added to the versions of the masque published in 1637 and 1645. The former speech, perhaps inadvertently on Comus' part, includes a striking image of maternal self-annihilation, while the latter evokes maternal death in a way that is intimately connected with Milton's earlier imagination of Lady Jane's apotheosis. I believe the task of meditating on the psychological and spiritual pressures of the situation he imagined for Lady Alice Egerton prompted Milton to begin imagining a more complex account of the difficulties that attended childbearing than he had been able to present in the epitaph for Lady Jane. The experiences of the two Ladies became linked in his imagination, each representing a particular stage in the social, physical, and spiritual experience of a woman's reproductive life.[1]

The masque is a text that has given critics no end of trouble. This is perhaps because it tries to accomplish a number of not particularly compatible things. The result is Milton's most overdetermined work, reflecting a fertile but transitional period in his artistic and intellectual growth. In the years of the masque's composition, Milton moved in a complex social milieu that we are only now beginning to fully understand in detail.[2] He contemplated a number of possible career paths, read voraciously, made sketches for future projects, and seems to have come to a first formulation of the radical political ideas that would later shape his adult life. The complicated context of the masque's commissioning, composition, and eventual publication, as well as the nature of such a period of rapid and complicated intellectual growth – the very difficulty of pinpointing and describing a fixed or definable "Milton" for the decade of the 1630s – all suggest several sometimes incompatible, or at least seemingly unrelated, intentions. The masque has therefore been read in many different ways.[3]

[1] Lady Jane was fifteen when she married, about a year older than Lady Alice was when she played herself in the original performance of *A Mask* in 1634. Although there was every reason to believe, at the time, that Lady Alice would marry relatively soon, she did not marry until July 1652 at the age of thirty-three (this was about two months after Mary Powell's death). Alice had seven sisters who were married at the time *A Mask* was performed. Three had married in the previous year, so matrimony was certainly in the air. Three other older sisters had died before marriage, two of them in infancy (Parker, p. 791).

[2] For some examples of the way new information is complicating our sense of this period in Milton's life, see Edward Jones, "'Church-Outed by the Prelats:' Milton and the 1637 Inspection of the Horton Parish Church," *Journal of English and Germanic Philology* 102 (2003), 42–58; "'Filling in a Blank in the Canvas:' Milton, Horton, and the Kedermister Library," *Review of English Studies* 53 (2002), 31–60.

[3] The following studies have been particularly useful: Cedric Brown, *Milton's Aristocratic Entertainments* (Cambridge University Press, 1985); John Leonard, "Saying 'No' to Freud: Milton's *A Mask* and Sexual Assault," *Milton Quarterly* 25 (1991), 129–40, "'Good things': a Reply to William Kerrigan," *Milton Quarterly* 30 (1996), 117–27, and "'Thus They Relate, Erring': Milton's Inaccurate Allusions," *Milton Studies* 38 (2000), 96–121; Leah Marcus, "Justice for Margery Evans: a 'Local' Reading of *Comus*," in *Milton and the Idea of Woman*, ed. Julia Walker (Urbana, IL: University of Illinois Press, 1988), pp. 66–85; Julia Walker, "The Poetics of Antitext and the Politics of Milton's Allusions," *Studies in English Literature* 37 (1997), 151–71; and John Rumrich, *Milton Unbound* (Cambridge University Press, 1996), pp. 70–93.

My own reading is best situated in the context of those studies that have attended to what we might call the masque's "proto-epithalamic" function: its presentation of Lady Alice as a young woman just arrived at marriageable age. Such readings take a particular interest in the social and psychological situation of Lady Alice as a sexual being who must make choices in a narrative situation that in several ways threatens not only to compromise her ability to do so with any spiritual clarity, but perhaps even threatens to rob her of any choice at all. Concentration on these aspects of the masque's presentation of the Lady allows us to register the role childbed anxiety played in Milton's imagination of her situation. In line with most of the childbed discourses he would have known, Milton certainly thought of the bodily experiences of childbirth as confronting the will with a particularly acute form of trial, and this seems to have affected the way he imagines Lady Alice's situation. She is first confronted with objects that deceive her, then with objects designed to excite her desire, and finally with physical coercion (binding and an implied threat of rape). She overcomes the first stage of her trial: after Comus reveals his initial deception, she rejects his offered pleasures. Then, after being bound, she produces a short speech of striking internal self-possession, asserting that Comus cannot affect her will, no matter what he does to her body: "Thou canst not touch the freedom of my mind/ With all thy charms, although this corporal rind/ Thou hast immanacl'd" (lines 663–5). In the second half of her later response to Comus' seduction speech, she claims, even more strikingly, that utterance of the secret of her inner virginity, the inviolate core of her will, would shatter all of Comus' "magick structures rear'd so high" (line 798). Comus takes this as a real threat, but continues with his seduction, resolving to "try her yet more strongly" (line 806) before the brothers enter and interrupt the scene.

Up to the end, Comus' primary interest remains the Lady's will, rather than simply the use of her body (he wants her to chose to use her body in a particular way). However, as a number of critics have suggested, Comus' allusion to Apollo and Daphne at the beginning of the exchange, along with the anxious conversation that the brothers have in the scene just before, and the possibility that Comus' last offer to "be wise and taste" from his cup might be accompanied by a forceful physical gesture, all suggest that rape hovers over the scene as a final threat. Because the Lady is rescued, however, we never find out how she would have continued to hold out against whatever stronger forms of trial Comus had in store for her (how, for example, might sexual violence have affected the "freedom of her mind"?). The masque instead goes on to portray her unbinding, followed by a celebratory reunion scene and a final allegorical speech from the attendant spirit, all of which only partially resolve the tensions and uncertainties the plot has raised. Not only is the Lady silent in the final scenes, but the images of those scenes leave her future unclear. Some have felt that the conclusion projects a future life governed by an inviolate vow of virginity, a Neoplatonic transcendence of the physical. The proto-epithalamic readings, on the other hand, imagine a married life for the Lady. I believe, however, that the ambiguity of the allegorical tableau, its cycling from time-bound to transcendent resonances and back, allows the conclusion to operate on both levels at once. It suggests not only a final apotheosis, but also the possibility of an ongoing series of trials that must be faced before a final release can be guaranteed. However, it is important, that these trials are not trials of desire, but trials that will come as a result of desires fulfilled, even when they are *properly* fulfilled.

In the "proto-epithalamic" readings, Milton is thought to present the Lady as a paradigm of the chaste, talented, and, above all, *marriageable* young aristocratic daughter, and in this view, the masque can be seen as an explicit celebration of her marriageability itself. It makes sense, therefore, that fertility should figure prominently in the masque's schema, and given what we know about reproductive anxiety in the period, and of Milton's engagement with it in his earlier poems, it makes sense that his attention to fertility should be marked by a set of darker apprehensions. All five passages in the masque that have some significant reproductive resonances are parts of passages that express significant anxiety about sexuality in general, and all have in common a sense that sexuality can disfigure an otherwise perfect and inviolate physical form. The first of these is Comus' puzzling but certainly terrific and grotesque reference to "the dragon womb/ Of Stygian darknes" that "spitts her thickest gloom/ And makes one blot of all the air" in his invocation to Cotytto at lines 128-42.[4] This image, with its suggestion of a primal, underworld reservoir of darkness (perhaps simply an inner cavity,

[4] See B. J. Sokol, "Tilted Lees: Dragons, *Haemony*, Menarche, Spirit, and Matter in *Comus*," *Review of English Studies* 41 (1990), 309–24, who sees this image as primarily reproductive. It is possible, however, that Milton might have meant "dragon" in this case to suggest a giant squid or cuttlefish, the womb being its ink-sac rather than its uterus. I am grateful to Harold Skulsky for making the suggestion in private correspondence and for pointing out that Pliny describes such creatures in ways that may have suggested Milton's figure. See Book 9, Chapter 45 of the *Naturalis Historia*. Pliny, *Natural History with an English Translation in Ten Volumes*, trans. H. Rackham (Cambridge, MA: Harvard University Press, 1940), vol. III, pp. 218–19. "Womb," of course, could have meant any hollow within a body. Still, the sexual context (the darkness is meant to conceal Comus' orgiastic revels) suggests a reproductive resonance.

perhaps a point of origin) spitting some liquid element of darkness over the earth associates the sexual pleasures that the night promises for Comus with some disquieting principle of monstrous, originary disorder. This is perhaps exciting to him, but it stands in counter-distinction to the Lady's sober certainties, the ordering power of her song and the very different eros it inspires in him (lines 244–65). Similarly grotesque images juxtaposed with an image of inviolate chastity attend the brothers' discussion of the danger of rape, climaxing in the Elder Brother's somewhat naive and gently ironized allusion to Minerva's "*Gorgon* shield" at lines 447–52. This climactic allusion has seemed, at least to some critics, not only to suggest the power of chastity in its display of the disfiguring consequences of its rejection, but also to offer an ambivalent figure for the disfigurement that comes with rape and/or reproduction.[5]

Of more direct interest for my own analysis, however, is the extravagant imagery of nature smothered by her "wast fertility" in Comus' speech to the Lady in the debate itself (lines 717–20 and 728–9), and the allusions to Venus and Adonis and Cupid and Psyche in the Spirit's epilogue (lines 992–1011). In both cases, Milton's evocation of mortality is much clearer. In the first passage, Comus suggests – with perfect illogic – that mortality is a danger courted by those who refuse to indulge their desires. The Lady's response, however, represses the fact that death remains a danger in sexual activity, even when Comus' logic is righted and desire is fulfilled properly. It is possible that she would have addressed this matter if she had been given a chance to utter her full "sage and serious doctrine." I agree with Leonard that Milton had good dramatic reasons for portraying her refusal to do so and for then cutting off the scene before letting her have her say.[6] I would like to argue, however, that the final allegorical passage of the masque does give utterance to this aspect of the doctrine, therefore expressing more than just the Neoplatonic idealism that many have read into it. Milton's allegory attempts to bring the masque's reproductive theme to a proper close, and its mythic allusions are designed to evoke and then control the fear of death that Comus himself accidentally brings to the surface. It is possible that the Lady herself has not yet fully confronted this fear. It is also possible that she was simply never given a chance to show her own control of it. Either way,

[5] See Walker, "The Poetics of Antitext"; Rumrich, *Milton Unbound*, pp. 76–80; and Leonard, "Thus They Relate, Erring."

[6] Leonard, "Saying 'No' to Freud," 133–4. My reading expands on Leonard's account of the epithalamic suggestions of the Epilogue in "Good Things," 124–6.

Milton wanted the masque to display and contain these fears in a way that marks an advance beyond the consolations of "An Epitaph."

Let us look more closely at the way the speeches exchanged by the Lady and Comus prepare us for this conclusion. It is no coincidence, I believe, that Milton has Comus' argument for sensual indulgence climax with the image of nature as a mortal mother. It is part of Comus' careful rhetorical scheme that these images lead directly to the frank eroticism of his concluding exhortation of *carpe diem*. Comus' logic is, however, perfectly skewed. Responding to the Lady's figure of a "well-govern'd and wise appetite" (line 705), he accuses her of preaching "abstinence," and offers an argument for indulgence that makes appetite itself a principle of governance. Without indulgence of appetite, he claims, nature would kill herself by her own abundance:

if all the world
Should in a pet of temperance feed on pulse,
Drink the clear stream, and nothing wear but freise,
Th'all-giver would be unthank't, would be unprais'd,
Not half his riches known, and yet dispis'd,
And we should serve him as a grudging maister,
As a penurious niggard of his wealth,
And live like natures bastards, not her sons,
Who would be quite surcharg'd with her own waight
And strangl'd with her wast fertility;
Th' earth cumber'd, and the wing'd air dark't with plumes,
The herds would over-multitude thir Lords,
The sea o'erfraught would swell, and th'unsought diamonds
Would so emblaze the forhead of the deep
And so bestudd with stars that they below
Would grow inur'd to light (lines 720–35)

Once it is abstracted from Comus' persuasive goal, the passage is itself "o'refraught," not only with the incestuous sexual implications that have interested Freudian critics, but with the imagery of fatal birth and even of obstetric surgery.[7] The image of Nature as a mother dying under the weight of her own progeny is striking enough. The final image of "th'unsought diamonds," however, also recalls his earlier image of the earth as a mother who has deliberately "hutched" ore and precious gems in her loins to be

[7] William Kerrigan, *The Sacred Complex: on the Psychogenesis of Paradise Lost* (Cambridge, MA: Harvard University Press, 1983), pp. 22–72 offers the most elaborate Freudian reading of the masque.

drawn out by her children (lines 717–20).[8] Comus' language represses the ugly image of just how those things are to be removed from the maternal body, especially after refusal to extract them has caused them to glow with a light that seems to echo, somehow, the repressed desire for them itself. However, imagining that extraction, alongside the passage's more explicit call to "nature's sons" to devour what their mother brings to birth in order to save her from smothering, gives the inverted moral logic of the speech an uncannily uncomfortable psychological density (that is, if we can shake off the siren-voice of its poetic power).

It is at this point that Comus presents his *carpe diem* argument, which he characterizes as a matter of economic exhange, as a mutual partaking of physical gifts designed to be "currant" (line 740). The implication, of course, is that this sharing will again bring order to natural abundance. However, the concentration is on "workmanship," on the aesthetic pleasure offered by the conspicuous, social display of physical beauty (lines 745–7). The Lady, of course, has no trouble unraveling the logic of Comus' argument, but her response leaves out important elements of its extravagant field of implication. It makes sense that she should counter Comus' two-part speech with a two-part scheme of her own. Her image of Nature as a "good cateress" counters the image of Nature as a helpless and self-smothering mother, whose body must be torn open and whose offspring must consume one another if her life is to be saved. The "good cateress," whom Rumrich suggestively associates with Milton's image of his own mother, represents charity and chastity, forms of love understood as both regulative and regulated.[9] Her job is to harness and evenly distribute Nature's wealth according to principles of love or care, so that everyone will have enough of what is necessary to life. The Lady then makes a move to poise "the sage/ And serious doctrine of Virginity" (lines 786–7) against the *carpe diem* half of Comus' argument, but cannot bring herself to utter a word about it in the presence of someone as unworthy as Comus. Having identified her subject, however, she makes it clear enough where her logic is heading. Virginity represents these regulative and regulating principles as they are embodied in the actions of a young woman. Her withholding of sexual availability, her refusal of sexual activity (at least until she finds the "good" man worthy of it), is for her a presage of how she imagines her own fertility will be later manifested.[10]

8 Rumrich, *Milton Unbound*, pp. 74–5. 9 Rumrich, *Milton Unbound*, pp. 70–5.

10 Leonard, "Saying 'No' to Freud," 133–6 and "Good Things," 123–4.

The image of Nature as "good cateress" implies, without her actually saying so, a regulated personal fertility. She is, in a sense, imagining herself in a maternal future. Like Nature, she will be "no whit encumber'd with her store," an inviolate and generous giver, a mother at ease with what she generates and eased of it unproblematically. The Lady has, of course, carefully removed all sexual responsiveness from her own speech, unwilling, as Leonard has suggested, to offer any implication to Comus that she will engage him on his level (any engagement might offer him titillation even in her refusal). The maternal, however, manages to emerge in the argument she makes, even if how one gets to it is elided, and the speech suggests that a regulated sexuality – and the nature of her response at this point is a sign of her own self-regulation – promises a regulated fertility, one without negative consequences, one that will instead offer continued avenues for chaste and charitable action.

What she ignores or remains unaware of is the fact that in the fallen world, regulated sexuality does not fulfill that promise. Milton is, however, aware of this irony, and he weaves an awareness of the problem into the allegory he created for the masque's conclusion. The passage has been read in many different ways, and I doubt that what I have to say here will end debate about its mysteries. However, the passage is clearly bound up with Milton's ongoing attempts to imagine the spiritual drama of female reproductive life. Let us begin with what I think almost everyone who reads the passage agrees on: in lines 999–1011, Milton is clearly alluding to Spenser's description of the Garden of Adonis in *The Faerie Queene* 3.6; in doing so, he means Venus and Adonis to signify in some sense the realm of human sexual reproduction in its natural, earthly state; in removing Cupid and Psyche from the bower of the garden itself and placing them somewhere "farr above" it, Milton revises Spenser's allegory, suggesting that he means the latter two mythical figures to signify something more transcendent of mortal, mutable human experience than Spenser meant, at least at that particular point in *The Faerie Queene*. Most, if not all critics, also agree that Milton means the tableau that the attendant Spirit describes to translate the major themes of the masque into some clarified discourse that can be understood by those whom he identifies at line 997 as mortals whose ears are "true." Such good listeners are meant to hear in these lines some revelation of the true nature of the reward offered to the virtuous. It has also been clear to most readers that Milton's decision to allude to Venus and Adonis and Cupid and Psyche (and hence his evocation of Book 3 of *The Faerie Queene* itself) is directly related to the situation and experience of the Lady. The reward the passage envisions is, in other words, a reward specific to the virtues of a young woman (or perhaps any young person) tested in matters of sexual chastity, and it gestures toward some more general statement (whether framed in scriptural or Neoplatonic terms) about human virtue and the possibilities we have of transcending our sinful natures.

In light of Milton's attention to childbed suffering up to this point in his career, it is of some interest that the couplet that constitutes the fulcrum or hinge of the allegorical tableau itself, the point at which Milton shifts our attention from Venus and Adonis to the place "farr above," uses the same rhyme pair, reversed, that he used to conclude his epitaph on Lady Jane. Here is the passage from the masque:

> *Iris* there with humid bow
> ...
>   drenches with *Elysian* dew
> (List mortals, if your ears be true)
> Beds of hyacinth and roses
> Where young *Adonis* oft reposes,
> Waxing well of his deep wound
> In slumber soft, and on the ground
> Sadly sits th' *Assyrian* Queen;
> But farr above in spangled sheen
> Celestial *Cupid* her fam'd Son advanc't
> Holds his dear *Psyche* sweet intranc't
> After her wandring labours long,
> Till free consent the gods among
> Make her his eternal bride,
> And from her fair unspotted side
> Two blissful twins are to be born,
> Youth and Joy; so *Jove* hath sworn. (lines 992–1011)

And here, again, are the final lines of the epitaph:

> There with thee, new welcom Saint,
> Like fortunes may her soul acquaint,
> With thee there clad in radiant sheen,
> No Marchioness, but now a Queen.

In addition to the rhyme pair itself, "*spangled* sheen" recalls "*radiant* sheen" (my italics), and the epithet Milton uses for Venus echoes the one he used for Rachel a few lines earlier in the epitaph ("*Assyrian* Queen" echoes "*Syrian* shepherdess"). The occurrence of these three echoes suggests, I think, more than a coincidence, especially given that this particular couplet plays so important a role in the Epilogue. It is hard not to imagine that Milton would have been thinking carefully about what he was reusing. This is, after all, a heavily revised passage that seems to have cost him considerable trouble in composition. Together, the echoes give us warrant at least to suspect that something more is going on, and given the subject matter of the earlier poem, I believe we have warrant to ask whether that something has to do with maternal mortality. It is also of some significance that Milton here chooses to conclude the masque with an allusion to the celestial wedding that concludes the myth of Cupid and Psyche, when he had earlier used their first, false and funereal wedding as an important part of his treatment of Jane Paulet's earthly life.

The couplet clearly marks both a point of allusion and revision. As most commentators on the passage have noted, it is here that Milton makes his key revision of the Spenserian original, taking Cupid and Psyche out of the garden and placing them above it. The passage at the end of the epitaph is similar in this sense. It is also the climax of an elaborate allusion (in that case to Canto XXXII of Dante's *Paradiso*), and it also revises its original text (Milton's placement of Lady Jane in the spot that Dante had reserved for Beatrice). In addition, both passages describe apotheoses. The couplet in the masque's Epilogue, divided as it is by the semicolon at the end of line 1002, is the point where Milton chooses to move our attention from the realm of earthly desire and fertility (as represented by Venus and the wounded Adonis) to a place that stands above it. In the epitaph's couplet, Milton distinguishes climactically between Lady Jane's earthly, married title of "Marchioness" (the product of her doomed earthly marriage) and "Queen," the eternal title she has been given in heaven (one that implies remarriage to her eternal bridegroom in Christ). She also exchanges a false – or at least limited – bond with an earthly husband for a sororal bond with a powerful, redeemed woman (Rachel) who can comfort her because she knows and understands her pain directly.

It is interesting that Milton chose to identify the place that he calls "farr above" in the masque with an incipient marriage and birth, one gained by long trial on the part of a pregnant young woman (that is, on the part of Psyche). At this point in the masque, no marriage having yet happened, Milton's purpose is to suggest that one is coming, and that it will be the Lady's reward for having carefully preserved her chaste inviolability. It should be clear, however, that Milton cannot simply mean by this an earthly marriage. To mean that would consign the Lady to a merely mortal fate. Still, his evocation of the epitaph implies that he acknowledges the fact that one way the Lady might reach her ultimate reward is by entering into an earthly marriage, which will entail, perhaps more than once, her undergoing a trial like that experienced by Lady Jane.

This suggests a narrative like the one Milton articulated earlier in "On the Morning of Christs Nativity," a projection forward to an achievement that is only secured after a considerable trial and in a self-sacrificial act. Milton, as Nancy Lindheim argues, concludes his masque by evoking a Christian teleological vision of time as opposed to pagan visions of historical recurrence or cycles of rebirth (the latter represented by Venus and Adonis, the former by Cupid and Psyche).[11] The referent of his allegory, however, is not only the larger vision of a providential history that should contextualize any believer's life. It also embraces the details of a more particular (or at least gendered) life narrative, one that moves first through a trial in which internal physical desires must be tempered and external sexual violence must be faced with spiritual confidence in anticipation of the earthly reward of motherhood in a chaste marriage. The narrative then continues on to another stage in which yet another trial is confronted, this time, however, in the childbed that constituted the reward of the first one. It is only after *that* trial that a final reward (framed again as a marriage, but this time purely of the soul, a genuine apotheosis) may be attained.

Notice, however, that the emblem seems to give us only two rather than the three stages that I have just outlined. Milton's figure works, I would suggest, by superimposing the last two stages of the narrative, taking advantage of the theme of recurrence suggested by his allusion to Spenser. On one level, Venus and Adonis represent the dangerous realm of natural desire and fertility, and Cupid and Psyche represent chaste earthly marriage. On this level, the emblem can be read as recapitulating the narrative of the masque itself, suggesting also its earthly sequel. On another level, however, Venus and Adonis represent the conditions of human fertility *within* marriage, and Adonis' wound represents the suffering and mortality that in large part defined those conditions. Cupid and Psyche can then represent the redemption offered *after death* to the long suffering and mortal mother should she face her trial well. If the woman does not die, the pair may also signify a *remarriage*. In this sense, echoing the content of rituals surrounding the Churching of Women, they represent a woman's re-entering the bonds of earthly marriage with its cycles of desire and fertility. In other words, as Lindheim has suggested, the realm of Venus and Adonis can, as it does in Spenser, cycle over and over again (these aspects of human experience are "eterne in mutability"). They give way from youthful trial to the chaste marriage represented by Cupid and Psyche, while at the same time suggesting a movement from childbed suffering to the "joy" (expressed in John 16:21–2) "that a man is born into the world," followed by the reunion

[11] Nancy Lindheim, "Milton's Garden of Adonis: the Epilogue to the Ludlow Masque," *Milton Studies* 35 (1997), 21–41.

of husband and wife after lying-in, before then cycling back again to the trial of reproductive suffering. Cupid and Psyche, however, because they are removed by Milton from the bower and placed "farr above," also represent the possibility of escape from that cycle into redemption after death. The Epilogue, in other words, is closely associated in Milton's mind with the human fertility cycle as it might actually have been experienced by a woman in the early years of her marriage.

And there are other matters here as well. For example, it has never been entirely clear to scholars why Milton changes the offspring of Psyche to "Youth and Joy" rather than retaining Spenser's and Apuleius' "Pleasure" or "Voluptas." However, I think the change may have been determined for Milton by the possible double meanings of "Youth and Joy." These terms can signify both transient, time-bound states of existence or mood (the younger years of a woman's life, the early years of a marriage untouched as yet by loss) or transcendent states of existence (the "eternal youth and joy" to which most commentators have thought the lines referred – eternized versions of particularly desirable states of earthly experience). Milton must also have thought that "Pleasure" would have too fully tied his emblem to traditional allegorical readings of the myth. In other words, he is prodding us to read his version differently.

At the end of the masque, in invoking Cupid's and Psyche's transcendence of Venus and Adonis, Milton hopes to suggest that the Lady might too one day pass from "pangs to felicity." But what is striking is his insistence on reminding us of the "pangs" at this moment at all. His imagination was, I believe, drawn back to the pangs that Lady Jane experienced and that he knows Lady Alice Egerton would likely experience or at least face should she marry. The emblem suggests a narrative exposition that is therefore both cyclical *and* teleological. Wounds will be gotten, perhaps more than once, and their healing may not be possible within the world. An exposition of the full difficulties of bearing with those wounds, however, would have to wait until Milton's mind returned to the subject in the later, more difficult, poetry that is the subject of the next part of this study.

PART III

"Conscious terrours": the problem of maternal mortality in Milton's later poetry

CHAPTER 7

The wide wound and the veil: Sonnet 23 and the "birth" of Eve in Paradise Lost

In the twenty or so years between 1637, when he composed "Lycidas" and published the full-length version of *A Mask*, and the late 1650s, when he entered the final, relatively intensive periods of work on *Paradise Lost*, Milton wrote a fair amount of poetry, but it is probably fair to say that it was not his central preoccupation. During these years, he wrote five Latin poems, four Latin epigrams, two sets of psalm paraphrases, a scattering of passages translated for use in several prose tracts, as well as seventeen sonnets, and he seems to have worked intermittently on a longer work about the Fall of Man, at first conceiving of it as a drama and only later reworking it into what became the epic.[1] He was also, however, busy with a number of other things. He traveled on the continent, took on several private pupils for varying lengths of time, and published most of his important prose works (the anti-prelatical and most of the anti-monarchical tracts, as well as *Areopagitica, Of Education*, and the four divorce tracts). In 1649, he also began working as Secretary of Foreign Tongues for the Council of State, producing over the following ten years a substantial number of official documents of various kinds, mostly diplomatic

[1] He may have also written all or parts of *Samson Agonistes* (or an early version of it), as well as parts of what became *Paradise Regained*. *Paradise Lost* seems to have had a long gestation. Milton began planning and composing material for a drama about the Fall in 1640, and he probably worked on it on and off until the mid-to-late 1650s, when he seems to have begun to work at it more assiduously, deciding also at some point (John Shawcross believes between 1655 and 1658) to turn the work into an epic. The final period of composition probably stretched from 1661 to 1665, when the poem, as we have it, was substantially completed. We do not know with any certainty which parts of the poem were composed when, but some rough conclusions are possible, among them the high probability that Milton decided to turn the play into an epic in the years just following the onset of his blindness and the deaths of Mary Powell and John Milton, Jr. It is also probable that important aspects of the poem's final form, including some of its larger structural and numerological devices, were introduced just after the death of Katherine Woodcock and her infant in early 1658. At the very least, their introduction must have coincided with the courtship and the very brief marriage: see below. On the dating of the epic, see Allan H. Gilbert, *On the Composition of Paradise Lost* (Chapel Hill, NC: University of North Carolina Press, 1947) and John Shawcross' useful overview in *With Mortal Voice: the Creation of Paradise Lost* (Lexington, KY: University of Kentucky Press, 1982), pp. 173–7.

correspondence and translations. Above all, during these years, Milton married twice and raised a family, in the process confronting the death of first one wife and then the other, as well as the deaths of two of his five children.

During these years, Milton wrote extensively about marriage as an institution, but we know very little about what went on in his own domestic life or how he felt about it. He comments on his home life only briefly in a few places, and while we can gather some important things from the documentary evidence, the record is frustratingly incomplete, especially when it comes to the births and deaths of the children. Furthermore, during these years, Milton paid very little direct attention in his published works to human reproduction. It makes itself known in the various prose tracts in only a few passing metaphors (for reading and writing, for the creation and publication of laws, for the pain attendant upon the processes of reformation within the church, etc.). He makes one snide remark about the Churching of Women in *An Apology Against a Pamphlet* (hereafter *An Apology*), where he attacks it as smacking of papist superstition. His translation of Psalm 7 takes some time to elaborate on an image near the end of the psalm that describes the wicked as giving birth to trouble and lies. The divorce tracts themselves, which, of course, have an interest in reproduction as an aspect of married life, have little to say about it beyond their emphatic and everywhere-prosecuted contention that reproduction is not the sole or central purpose of marriage as it was ordained by God for humankind. In other words, procreation does matter in Milton's argument about divorce, but it is carefully subordinated to what he argues are the higher purposes of married life: mutual solace and spiritual support, companionship, etc.[2]

When we come to the poetic products of the later years, however, the picture alters considerably. While Milton remains just as reticent as ever about his own biography, marriage itself not only becomes a central concern in *Paradise Lost*, *Samson Agonistes*, and Sonnet 23, but in both *Paradise Lost* and the sonnet, reproduction is closely integrated with the treatment of other aspects of married life. The physical consequences of procreation are shown to create their own specific moral and spiritual burdens for married partners, ones that will require the poet to justify not just God's ways to men but His different ways to men and to women. The connection between Milton's life experiences and the aspects of the poetry that deal with married

[2] It is also interesting that in *Of Education* (1644), Milton recommends that students read Euripides' *Alcestis* because it "treate[s] of houshold matters" (*CP*, 2.397–8). See B. J. Sokol, "Euripides' *Alcestis* and the 'Saint' of Milton's Reparative Twenty-Third Sonnet," *SEL* 33 (1993), 135.

sexuality and childbirth also becomes more intimate or more direct, as Milton – this time with a far more personal and immediate motivation – works his way back into the task of finding a poetic mode capable of responding to maternal mortality.

I am particularly concerned with Milton's poetic response in the late 1650s and early 1660s to the four deaths that took place in his immediate family in the course of the previous decade. The first and second of these happened at about the same time, the third and fourth followed closely upon one another about six years later. Mary Powell, the poet's first wife, died on May 5, 1652 due to complications in childbirth just three days after giving birth to her fourth child. The infant, Deborah, was healthy and lived. About one month later, however, John Jr., John and Mary's third child and their only son, also died (just a few months after his first birthday). Edward Phillips, Milton's nephew, attributed the latter death "to the ill usage, or bad constitution of an ill-chosen nurse."[3] Katherine Woodcock, Milton's second wife, died on February 3, 1658, about three months after giving birth to her first child, a daughter named for her mother. The child had been born less than a year after the wedding, and died just six weeks after her mother.

We have very little direct evidence of how Milton was affected by these deaths. There are no heart-rending confessional letters or journal entries, just one sonnet and its echoes in Adam's account of the creation of Eve (*PL*, 8.462–3, 478, and 482). Many have even thought that the sonnet has only the most tangential biographical significance. There is, however, ample circumstantial evidence that the deaths must have affected Milton very deeply, not simply as a man but as an artist. Indeed, several of the critical conundrums offered by the sonnet and its echo in the epic can be solved by a detailed accounting of their vexed biographical contexts.

In the following section of this chapter, I will examine the referential ambiguity of the poem – the problem of "which wife?" – in some detail, tracing the various ways in which biographical circumstances can help us to understand the sonnet's striking originality as a literary response to maternal mortality. I will also show how the poem's theological and philosophical implications are rooted in the ways in which it gestures symbolically not only toward the quotidian or particular, but also toward the actual biographical and historical circumstances that drove its author to compose it. The poem's relationship to the conventions of the Petrarchan sonnet sequence and its related visionary traditions can be best understood, I believe, if we seek to unravel the way it reworks some of the basic conventions of the

[3] *The Early Lives of Milton*, ed. Helen Darbishire (London: Constable & Co. Ltd., 1932), p. 71.

genre by including biographically particular figures of marriage and reproduction. In addition, the fact that the sonnet either echoes or is echoed by a crucial moment in *Paradise Lost* suggests the key role that it and maternal mortality played in Milton's conception of the epic.[4] The echo is, I believe, a marker of Milton's desire to link his sequence of sonnets with his epic, repeating the gesture toward Dante that concluded the epitaph for Jane Paulet. The sonnet is therefore not only crucial to our understanding of how Milton's approach to childbed suffering developed in the later 1650s, but is also crucial to our understanding of his most important poetic project.

MATERNAL DEATH AND THE BIOGRAPHICAL PROBLEM

Although it has complex implications, the biographical problem presented by Sonnet 23 can be simply put: while most critics agree that it refers to the death of a wife, there is no certainty as to which one, or even if it matters which one. Some critics, Parker in particular, have thought the poem might have been written some time shortly after the death of Mary Powell.[5] Most, however, have accepted the traditional and more likely possibility that it was composed after Katherine's death, some time in 1658, although there has been an increasing tendency to accept that the poem also makes significant reference back to Mary. Some critics have argued against all autobiographical readings.[6]

Part of the reason for all this debate is the fact that the poem suggests a complex autobiographical subtext while making very few references that are *necessarily* autobiographical. The speaker seems careful to specify his status

4 Since we do not know exactly when the lines from Book 8 were written, it is impossible to know if Milton echoed the creation of Eve in the sonnet or the sonnet in the epic. See Gilbert, *Composition*, pp. 19–20, 44–6, and 152 for an intriguing, if inconclusive, argument for the relative earliness of *Paradise Lost*, 8.457–520. However, there is no question that Milton invested Adam's account of Eve's creation with a great deal of significance. Lines 465–71, at almost the exact center of the description of Eve's creation (which begins at 452 and ends at 485), are the golden section of the poem. See John T. Shawcross, "The Centrality of Book 8 in *Paradise Lost*," *ANQ* 14 (2001), 45–55.

5 William R. Parker, "Milton's Last Sonnet," *Review of English Studies* 21 (1945), 235–8.

6 The earlier years of the debate are covered by the *Variorum* notes, although they leave out some important notes and studies. Since the late 1960s, there have been only a few substantial contributions. Anthony Low, "Milton's Last Sonnet," *Milton Quarterly* 9 (1975), 80–1 and Dixon Fiske, "The Theme of Purification in Milton's Sonnet XXIII," *Milton Studies* 8 (1975), 149–63 both argue against Parker's claims for Mary. Sokol's, "Euripides' *Alcestis* and the 'Saint'" combs through Euripides for evidence in Mary's favor. See also my own "'Spot of child-bed taint:' Seventeenth-Century Obstetrics in Milton's Sonnet 23 and *Paradise Lost* VIII: 462–78," *Milton Quarterly* 27 (1993), 98–109. For the most part, however, the consensus that E. A. J. Honigmann described in *Milton's Sonnets* (New York, NY: St. Martin's Press, 1966), pp. 190–4 still holds: the bulk of the evidence, such as it is, is in favor of a later composition and of Katherine as the poem's primary referent, but the poem's ambiguities make it impossible to entirely dispose of Mary's claims.

as a widower, for example, but his language merely suggests the possibility, not the certainty, that he is blind, and nothing in his account explicitly suggests a particular woman, that he may have been married more than once, or anything about how the "late espoused saint" might have died. In describing how she seemed, what she seemed about to do, and then his own painful awakening back to a dark reality, the speaker draws on a complex of allusions to biblical, literary, and philosophical sources, none of which, again, suggest anything explicitly or necessarily autobiographical. The speaker tells us only that in the dream his wife seemed brought back to him just as Alcestis was brought back to Admetus, and that she looked as he imagines the women in Old Testament days must have looked after they had undergone their rituals of childbed purification. He also tells us that she was wearing a white dress and a veil, and that to his "fancied sight" she looked like he imagines she will when he sees her again with "full sight" in the afterlife. There's no necessary reason to assume that the dress suggests more than the purity of his anticipatory vision of her, or that the veil, which hides her face, suggests anything more than the imperfection of "fancied sight" in comparison with the sight he will later have of her ("face to face," as Paul famously put it in 1 Corinthians 13:12). Her attire in fact suggests the attire of the saved as they are described in Revelation, as well as the attire or spiritual status of the women to whom the speaker has already alluded: Alcestis and the women who underwent purification in the Old Law. All of these details suggest a long list of literary and biblical, as well as more abstractly theological or philosophical, analogues: the conventional Petrarchan and epic apparitions, allegorical figures like Spenser's Dame Nature, and behind these a long tradition of Christian Neoplatonic visions. The fact that her face is hidden, and that she disappears before the veil is ever lifted, might suggest the speaker's physical blindness (Milton never saw Katherine's face in life), but because this is not made explicit, it seems more immediately to refer to various states of figurative blindness: his fallen state, his mortality, the fact that he is subject to the illusions of the material world and/or the illusions and limitations of his own fancies and desires, etc.:

> Mee thought I saw my late espoused saint
> Brought to me like *Alcestis* from the grave
> Whom *Joves* great son to her glad Husband gave
> Rescu'd from death by force though pale and faint.
> Mine as whom washt from spot of child-bed taint
> Purification in th' old law did save,
> And such, as yet once more I trust to have
> Full sight of her in heav'n without restraint,

Came vested all in white, pure as her mind:
Her face was vail'd, yet to my fancied sight
Love, sweetness, goodness in her person shin'd
So clear, as in no face with more delight.
But O as to imbrace me she enclin'd,
I wak'd, she fled, and day brought back my night.

The poem is remarkable for the way it balances a complex of intense emotions (awe, regret, guilt, grateful praise, hope, and despair) with an almost pedantic display of learning. Who but Milton, we might ask, would have thought to praise a woman, whether a wife or a symbol, in terms of the Levitical laws concerning purification after childbirth? Or we might ask that question if the effect were not so surprisingly moving. Much of the poem's affective power is, in fact, the result of how these distantly fetched allusions serve to intensify the speaker's account of his dream, suffusing it with images that place his experience in the wider context of human striving toward the divine. However, as the history of commentary on the poem shows, it is also the result of how these same allusions resonate with autobiographical contexts that the author must have known at least some of his readers would perceive. In other words, if we know the poet was blind and bereaved etc., we cannot help but be drawn into a process of autobiographical reading. In fact, the more we know, the more the details of the poem seem to irresistibly line up with details in the poet's life. The allusive structure actually seems designed not only to express the gulf that opens in human grief between subjective uncertainties and higher truths, but also to set particular and personal experiences in a tensely unresolved relationship with such truths. The time-bound and uncertain nature of human self-knowledge is here both fused with and juxtaposed with modes of knowing drawn from the impersonal realms of literary representation, philosophical speculation, and scriptural revelation. It is, I believe, in this complex sense that the poem can be best understood as "autobiographical."

However, in order to get a handle on just how the dynamic works, we need to examine closely what we know and can safely assume about Milton's life in the crucial decade of the 1650s, paying particular attention to the crises and difficulties he experienced as a husband and father. His domestic circumstances both early and late in the decade were, to say the least, rather dark. The deaths I have mentioned were themselves, no doubt, bad enough, but they also brought with them a train of both direct and indirect practical and emotional complications. It seems likely, for example, from what we know of the circumstances surrounding the deaths of Mary Powell and John Jr., that ambivalence and regret must have been painfully mixed with the sadness and shock we would expect from anyone who had suddenly lost both a spouse and a child. Mary's death, in addition, brought with it a number of practical and familial difficulties, and, given that the difficulties themselves might have indirectly caused the baby's death, more than one occasion for self-recrimination. It is, of course, safe to assume that the death of his only son and namesake would have been particularly difficult for Milton, especially coming so close on the heels of the death of the infant's mother. However, if Edward Phillips was right about the cause (or at least if his statement reflects what Milton and most of those in and around the family at the time assumed), Milton probably also blamed himself for not more carefully overseeing, or not being able to oversee, the care of his children. A wet-nurse or nurses had to be hired to care for both John Jr. and Deborah. How this was done or by whom we do not know, but if a nurse that he hired had something to do with his son's death, Milton surely would have regretted not having made a better choice. If Milton had had to rely on his mother-in-law (and there is good reason to believe he would have had to), or on someone else trying to be helpful, he may have regretted his failure to take charge of the situation himself. If it was Mrs. Powell who took charge, he may have, in addition, worried about how his home life and his relationship with his living children would have been affected by the fact that his relationship with her had never been good. Over the past year, he and Mrs. Powell had been locked, in fact, in a bitter legal dispute.[7]

The lack of documentary detail concerning Mary's death suggests, in addition, some form of disruption or dislocation in the family's domestic life at the time. We do not, for example, know where Mary was when she gave birth to Deborah, nor do we know where or how she or John Jr. were buried. The family had moved to new quarters about five months earlier, and we do not know how the move, which entailed a change of parish, might have affected the way the family would have handled birth, lying-in, and funeral arrangements. Although, in a letter, Milton gave his own health as the primary motive, it is possible that the pregnancy also motivated the move. Mary was in about her fourth month, and they perhaps needed

[7] Anne Powell sued Milton over income that he received from property he had taken possession of after Richard Powell's death as payment for a debt long owed to his father. For details concerning this complicated dispute, which got quite ugly at times, see Parker, pp. 397–400. Transactions concerning the debts Richard Powell owed to Milton's father may have brought with them their own emotional complications, given that, as Shawcross suggests, it may have been financial transactions between Richard and John Sr. that led originally to the marriage between Milton and Mary, which may have been arranged. John T. Shawcross, *The Arms of the Family* (Lexington, KY: The University Press of Kentucky, 2004), pp. 40–1.

more space for the coming child.[8] This does not, however, mean that the new house would have been the best place for the birth itself. No church records concerning the birth of Deborah or the funerals of her mother and brother have been found, and this suggests that the birth took place in a parish other than the old one or the new one. It is possible, as Barbara Lewalski speculates, that Milton might have been associated at this time with a congregation other than that of either his old or his new parish church, perhaps one with practices "more to his liking." If so, we have yet to locate that congregation, whose records, in any case, might have been lost or never properly preserved.[9] It seems even more likely that Mary, in line with common practices, went to stay with her mother as her time approached, in order to give birth with her in attendance. We have also been unable, however, to discover where Mrs. Powell was living at the time. As Parker noted, the day we find her address may be the day we find the burial and baptismal records (Parker, p. 1009).

The possibility is, in any case, as intriguing as it is likely. If Mary went to stay with her mother in preparation for the birth, it is also probable that Mrs. Powell did indeed have charge not only of the infant care immediately following the birth, but also over the hiring of the midwife who oversaw the birth itself. The possibilities for blame in that case would have been tempting for Milton on two counts, and it is hard to believe that such a temptation – whether or not he or others gave into it – did not increase the tensions that already plagued his relationship with his mother-in-law, despite the grief they also no doubt shared.

How Milton would have felt about such a temporary move on his wife's part, if it happened at all, we can only guess. He might have been relieved to be free of domestic pressures and the noise and bustle of a busy household, free, for example, to get his government work done more easily. The children, after all, would probably have gone with their mother – the oldest was only about six. For a good year or so leading up to the birth, Milton's public responsibilities had been on the increase, despite the also increasing difficulty he was having with his sight and the health problems that stemmed from his attempts to treat it.[10] It was probably by February or

[8] Parker suggests that there was some pressure from Parliament, which wanted to use the apartments in Whitehall, one of which the Miltons occupied (Parker, pp. 392–3). See Milton's letter to Mylius (*CP*, 4.2.835) and Barbara Lewalski, *The Life of John Milton: a Critical Biography*, rev. edn. (Oxford: Blackwell, 2003), p. 260.

[9] Lewalski, *Life*, p. 280.

[10] In December 1651, the Council almost failed to reappoint Milton, perhaps due to concerns about his health. They did, however, reappoint him, and his work-load continued to be heavy, especially for a

March of 1652 – just a few months before the birth – that his sight finally failed completely. If Mary did move away temporarily, these practical matters might also have been an important motivation. On the other hand, relief would only have been part of the picture. Did he feel guilty? Was he anxious about the birth or about dealing with his now complete blindness? Did he feel abandoned? Lonely? We have no idea, at least no specific idea, but it is hard to believe that he was not assailed by complicated and not altogether consistent emotions. This was not, after all, the first time Mary had gone home to her mother. She had done so shortly after the wedding and, much to Milton's chagrin, had stayed away then for almost three years. Her failure to return to him on this second occasion would therefore no doubt have been fraught with a painful irony, given that this time she was not having second thoughts about the marriage, but had died fulfilling one of its primary ends. In the wake of her death (a stark failure to return to him yet once more), the situation would have been ripe for both blame and self-blame, especially if Mrs. Powell did take charge of the birth as well as the childcare after her daughter's death.

As I said, we do not know for sure that the separation even happened. However, we cannot discount the high probability that Mary and John Jr. both died while Milton was temporarily apart from them and the rest of the children, a time that was tense for the family as a whole and both physically and professionally trying. We should also not forget that because he had gone completely blind during the pregnancy, he was denied a last sight of either Mary or his only son before they both died, and that he, of course, could never have seen the daughter Mary gave birth to in May, even if he had indeed been there at the birth. It is therefore certain, at the very least, that Milton's situation in 1652, even before the deaths that came that spring, was heavy with what we would today call "emotional baggage." In the wake of the deaths, the congregated effects of this "baggage" was in fact enough to plunge him into what is widely recognized by his biographers as a period of depression. In one of the few references he ever made in print to his family life and personal problems, he acknowledged that this was a particularly dark period. In a passage of the *Pro Se Defensio*, explaining why it had taken him so long to respond in writing to the extravagant attacks he had received in the wake of his *Pro Populo Anglicano Defensio*, he said, perhaps a little laconically: "at that time, especially, infirm health, distress over two deaths

man in ill health who had to dictate and be read to in order to compose and translate. His attendance at council meetings and at diplomatic exchanges became less frequent, and he tended, more and more, to work at home. Lewalski, *Life*, p. 260 and Parker, pp. 403–4.

in my family, and the complete failure of my sight beset me with troubles" (*CP*, 4.2.703).[11]

Milton had been on his own for about four years with his three remaining children – the oldest of whom, Anne, was about ten years old – when he married Katherine Woodcock. The years leading up to the wedding had seen his life return to some measure of calm. His health had improved, and he had become reconciled to the permanent loss of his sight. He also engaged again more fully in writing and correspondence, in addition to his work for the council, which he found easier to handle. When he married Katherine in 1656, he had every reason to be optimistic about what the coming years would bring. However, he would never know how things might have turned out. In an event that mirrored the death of Mary terribly closely in certain significant details, Katherine died only fifteen months after the wedding (in February 1658) of a condition she seems to have contracted in the childbed the previous October. Her newborn daughter, as I noted earlier, died six weeks later.

Just as in the case of Mary, there are uncertainties concerning Katherine's death. For example, we have only two sources of information about its cause, and they do not agree. Phillips, as makes sense for a number of reasons, connected the death in retrospect to the childbed, associating it with Mary's death. Discussing the eight years Milton spent in his house in Petty France (the house the Miltons moved to in December 1651 when Mary was pregnant), Phillips wrote: "In this House his first wife dying in Childbed, he Married a Second, who after a Year's time died in Childbed also."[12] Because of another recollection, however, and because of the three months that separated the birth and the death, many have tended to disassociate Katherine's death from the birth of her daughter. Milton's granddaughter, Elizabeth Foster (Deborah's daughter), claimed in an interview – also years after the fact – that Katherine died not in childbed but "of a consumption,"[13] and many scholars have held that while the death might have had some connection with her weakened condition, the fact that Katherine died well after the Levitical period of purification referred to in

[11] See Lewalski, *Life*, pp. 280, 291. Shawcross, *Arms*, p. 244 suggests that the work Edward and John Phillips – Milton's nephews – did for him in 1651 to 1652 should be seen "alongside" his difficult domestic circumstances. Milton may have had to rely a good deal on others during this period, and this no doubt added to his general feeling of despondency and, perhaps, guilt.

[12] Darbishire, *Early Lives*, p. 71.

[13] Parker, "Milton's Last Sonnet," 237. Foster's statements were reported by Birch (1738) and Newton (1749).

the poem suggests that hers was not in any meaningful way a death "in Childbed."[14]

Despite what seems to be an obvious difference, however, these two accounts of the same event and its causes are not incompatible. The birth occurred on October 19th, the death very early the following February. That it was attributed to a "consumption" by one witness (a general term for any lingering disease, rather than a reliably specific diagnosis) and to childbirth by another allows for the possibility that Phillips and Foster were simply emphasizing two different aspects of a situation that included both causes. It is likely, in fact, that Katherine contracted her condition in the birth or late in the pregnancy, and then lingered until early February before succumbing. It is possible, in other words, that she simply never got up from her bed.[15] In other words, Phillips may not have been mistaken in claiming that Katherine died "in Childbed," even if she did not die as the immediate result of a catastrophic birth. Instead, it is possible that he was making a reasonable inference given common experience, and it may very well have been a widespread inference within circles close to the family. It is, of course, possible that Katherine got up normally from her childbed toward the end of November, and then some time later – say in late December – took unexpectedly ill and lingered until her death in early February. This would

[14] Leviticus 12:5 prescribes a purification period of 80 days after the birth of a daughter, and Katherine died about 100 days after giving birth to hers. This puts her death well outside both the Levitical period and the traditional month of lying-in. The timing has been an important crux in debates over biographical context, but it can point to either wife. Katherine's death made her more like the Levitical women at the time of her death, but the intervening months might have disassociated her death from the childbed. There is also less reason to think Milton would have associated her outright with the Levitical rites. Mary did not live long enough to have been like the Levitical women in a strict sense, but her death is more closely and securely associated with both childbirth and its rites. Also, the espoused saint's state of purity, which the poem states is merely *like* that of the Levitical women, is something the speaker is imagining of her in the afterlife. He might very well have done so in Mary's case even if she – or perhaps *because* she – was not like those women at the actual moment of her death (especially given that, as I argue below, she might have been very much like them on three earlier occasions – see the discussion of Mary and churching later in this chapter). For the original debate on these issues, see Parker, "Milton's Last Sonnet"; Fitzroy Pyle, "Milton's Sonnet on His 'Late Espoused Saint,'" *Review of English Studies* 25 (1949), 57–60; and Parker, "Milton's Last Sonnet Again," *Review of English Studies*, New Series 2 (1951), 147–54.

[15] A similar argument was made in defense of Katherine's claim on the sonnet by Pyle in his second rejoinder to Parker. He suggests that Foster was not "dissociating Katherine's death from the effects of childbirth," but correcting the date that Phillips' account implied (that Katherine, like Mary, died *shortly* after her daughter was born). See Parker, "Milton's Last Sonnet Again," 153. Thinking, no doubt, of the common nineteenth-century meaning of "consumption," Pyle thought Katherine had tuberculosis, which is possible, of course, but impossible to substantiate. It is unlikely that she died of puerperal fever, which usually manifests itself soon after the birth, quickly becomes severe, and usually kills within forty days (or of a hemorrhage in the birth, which kills even more quickly). Given the rapidity of her death, it is possible, however, that Mary died of one of these causes. On the causes of maternal mortality, see Chapter 2.

have given people reason both to identify the cause of death as a consumption and to disassociate it from the birth. A consumption was, by definition, a condition that lingered, but it is unlikely that people would have differentiated between a condition that lingered for three months and one that lingered for a month and a half. Elizabeth Foster, in any case, was not an eyewitness to these events. She would have perhaps heard the story from her mother, who *was* a witness but who was also not quite six at the time and may have later had reason, for all we know, to reserve the distinction of a maternal death for her mother alone. Phillips, on the other hand, although he was no longer living with his uncle at the time of Katherine's death, was in his late twenties. He was also a man who remained, as Shawcross puts it, "in close contact with his uncle and with his uncle's world" throughout his adult life.[16] Even if his language was imprecise in a different way than Mrs. Foster's, he is more likely to have reflected Milton's own perception of the matter, and it is with Milton's perception, of course, that we are primarily concerned.

Milton had more reason than most for associating Katherine's death closely with that of Mary, and I believe he did so even if he knew, rationally, that the circumstances differed. It is the closeness of the association, in fact, that accounts for the ambiguities that have plagued scholarly attempts to determine once and for all the referent of Sonnet 23. The sense of *déjà vu* that Milton must have felt at the time he wrote the poem clearly affected his choices of image and allusion. The fact alone that in both cases an infant died close to a month after the mother would have had this effect even if the loss itself were not already its own echo. The timing, however, would have associated the two deaths with each other in another way. Partisans on the side of Katherine have often pointed to the fact that only she lived long enough after the birth to have been purified according to the Levitical timetable suggested by lines 5–6. Her name, indeed, suggests "purity."[17] However, both deaths, as it turns out, occurred in circumstances that could have suggested the Levitical rites and their relation to later Christian ritual practice. Mary has the name of the woman most famous among Christians for having undergone the Levitical rite itself (see Luke 2:22–4),[18] but she

16 Shawcross, *Arms*, p. 94.

17 From the Greek *katharos*, or "pure": Edward Le Comte, "The Veiled Face of Milton's Wife," *Notes and Queries* 199 (1954), 245–6.

18 Luke's reference to the Virgin's purification, which she underwent when she brought Jesus to the Temple to be presented as a first-born, is strikingly exact, detailing the sacrifices she offered (there were two different ways to do it) in accordance with Leviticus 12:8. The verse is not a reference to any sacrifice necessary for the presentation of Jesus, which required none (see Exodus 13:2 and 12).

also, as I will discuss in more detail below, is much more likely than Katherine to have actually undergone the related rite of churching after the births of her first three children, and Milton may have been recalling those churchings in his dream/poem – along with the sad fact that the last time she gave birth she did not live long enough for the rite to have been celebrated. Milton would have thought of purification in spiritual rather than physical terms, and "child-bed taint" would have been a sign of original sin rather than of some physical impurity. Given the swiftness of her death, Mary could only have been "purified" of that sort of "taint" in her ascent to heaven, or in the resurrection that the speaker anticipates at lines 7–8. In the dream, her purified state would have represented, therefore, the redeemed version of the common association that churching had with remarriage. Like Julia in Herrick's poem (see Chapter 1), she has become in the speaker's imagination a pure bride again, but the bridegroom would have to be Christ, rather than the mortal, still-tainted husband. She had returned to Milton, in other words, as a new bride after three earlier births, but the last time she took to her bed she only attained her purity in a way that separated her from her husband more radically than any period of lying-in.[19]

On the other hand, we cannot discount the symbolic significance Milton might have attributed to the fact that Katherine died one day after the Feast of the Purification, which fell on February 2nd and actually celebrated the Levitical purification of the Virgin.[20] Katherine would have been free of "childbed taint" in terms of "th' old law" on Twelfth Night, the winter in which she died (exactly eighty days from the date of the birth), long enough from the date of her death some twenty-seven days later to disassociate it from the rite of churching. That she died, however, on the day after the feast that traditionally celebrated the Virgin Mary's celebration of the Levitical rite (the rite that underpinned the churching ceremony) could not have failed to strike Milton, and would have, in different ways, brought both her and Mary to mind.

After all, we are not dealing here with strict factuality, but with memory and symbol. Even if the sonnet primarily refers to Milton's second wife, it is also clearly overlayed with figures and allusions that powerfully recall his

[19] On "taint" as a matter of original sin, see Anna K. Nardo, *Milton's Sonnets and the Ideal Community* (Lincoln, NE: University of Nebraska Press, 1979), p. 39. See also Marilyn Williamson, "A Reading of Milton's Twenty-Third Sonnet," *Milton Studies* 4 (1972), 141–9. On Milton's mortalism and how it may have affected the poem's sense of the wife's present existence in heaven, see George H. McLoone, "Milton's Twenty-Third Sonnet: Love, Death, and the Mystical Body of the Church," *Milton Quarterly* 24 (1990), 8–20.

[20] The date was first noted by Pyle, who used it to defend the case for Katherine. See Parker, "Milton's Last Sonnet Again," 153.

first.[21] What the poem maintains is its ambiguity, refusing to distinguish itself from either biographical circumstance. It also refuses to completely detach itself from biography, despite its allusive abstraction. Most importantly for our purposes, figures of childbirth link the poem's three levels of reference at almost every point. The questions "which wife?" and "no wife?" therefore need to be rephrased. I agree to some extent with Annabel Patterson's suggestion that "the sonnet's reticence, not to say coyness, on the crucial question of its subject, permits every reader to indulge her personal fantasy as to how Milton resolved his relations with women."[22] I would add, however, that this reticence *also* allows a reader to follow a critic like Leo Spitzer into the aether of a purely literary and philosophical reading of the poem.[23] In fact, I think it should be clear that the sonnet's "reticence" (its feints, equivocations, and ambiguities – whether deliberate or not) actually makes nonsense of any attempt to fix its referential "problem." Better to recognize that it is not a problem at all. The only intention we can safely posit for the reticence – and it is a far more productive one than most of the others that have been posited, however narrowly illuminating they have been – is a desire to allow the poem the widest possible range of reference within the literary, theological, philosophical, historical, *and* biographical realms it *simultaneously* suggests. We can then freely explore the implications of one area of reference or another, and do it for whatever purposes we deem important: personal fantasy, if that is what motivates us, or historical or theoretical arguments (which are different from fantasies, although they might be colored by – or even inspired by – a desire to rationalize a particular one).[24] The poem, in any case, is an

[21] Elizabeth K. Hill, "A Dream in the Long Valley: some Psychological Aspects of Milton's Last Sonnet," *Greyfriar* 26 (1985), 3–13 argues that the ambiguity is the result of what Freud called "condensation," where two or more images or feelings are superimposed upon one another in a dream. See also John Hollander, *The Work of Poetry* (New York, NY: Columbia University Press, 1997), pp. 83–6. Hugh J. Dawson, "The Afterlife of the Widower's Dream: Rereading Milton's Final Sonnet," *Milton Studies* 45 (2006), 21–37 offers some useful distinctions regarding the relationship of the original dream Milton may have had to the poem he composed.

[22] Annabel Patterson, "That Old Man Eloquent," in *Literary Milton: Text, Pretext, Context* eds. Diana Treviño Benet and Michael Lieb (Pittsburgh, PA: Duquesne University Press, 1994), p. 36.

[23] Leo Spitzer, "Understanding Milton," *Hopkins Review* 4 (1951), 16–25.

[24] Patterson's point, of course, is that we are likeliest to avoid mere fantasy only if we attend to what the poem really does and does not allow us to fantasize *about*. In other words, we cannot, in this case, indulge in the fantasy that the poem, for example, expresses Milton's unequivocal love for Mary Powell directly in the wake of her death. It may express love for her, but it must also express it along with any number of other things: for example, his love for Katherine – not to mention disquieting things like regret for having married Mary in the first place, which, human psychology being what it is, could certainly have coexisted with a deeply felt thankfulness for their time together after their reconciliation. The fundamental issue for literary interpretation is the fact that the poem's language will not allow for an *exclusive* referent and meaning.

account of what it itself calls "fancied sight," and it therefore makes the problematic relationship between desire and truth, which the word "fancy" always suggests, explicitly thematic. As a literary account of a tantalizing fancy that ends in a return to darkness (this is itself, of course, a literary motif), it is designed to ask questions about the relationship between truth and desire more than it is designed to answer them. An examination of any one of the areas of implication I have listed can and should be used to illuminate, rather than to contradict or disqualify the others. Theology, art, memory, and fantasy are each there to query the others so that it might be possible for a reader to gauge the role that each plays in the experience of grief. The poem is therefore a nexus for Milton's engagement with any number of issues of deep and abiding concern to him, not the least of which is the relationship between autobiography, theology, and poesis, a concern that could only have forced him in the late 1650s either to repress completely or to find some new way of approaching the subject of childbed suffering. It is clear to me that the poem is the product of his choice to do the latter.

MATERNAL MORTALITY, MASCULINE GUILT, AND THE MYTH OF ALCESTIS

Although there has been no shortage of theories, there has been little agreement about exactly why Milton chose to accomplish his ends by alluding to Old Testament purification rituals and Euripides' *Alcestis*, along with the long list of lyric and narrative poems more immediately suggested by his choice of motif (the dreamed vision of a veiled, beloved woman). Attention to childbirth as a key context, however, can help us to understand how these allusions work together, as well as how they work with the poem's biographical concerns. For example, one of the biggest problems presented by the allusion to Alcestis is the moral ambiguity of the figure of Admetus. Critics have had some difficulty in coming up with an explanation as to why Milton would have chosen, as the logic of his allusion to Alcestis requires, to associate himself and/or his speaker with Admetus, who, especially in Euripides' portrayal, is a decidedly unattractive figure. Despite his graciousness as a host (no small matter in traditional Greek culture), he is also childishly selfish, a coward, and he has a startling lack of self-awareness. One can understand how and why the final scene of the play would come to the mind of a grieving widower in the wake of this sort of dream (or how it might have informed such a dream), but any such extended contemplation of the story would inevitably lead to rather uncomfortable regions of self-recrimination.[25] It has also been unclear exactly why Milton – who was not only a Christian but one with a distrust of church rituals that smacked of papist superstition – would have been attracted to an image that suggested not only Old Testament purification rites, but also the churching, a contemporary ritual dear to high-church Anglicans, and about which he himself actually made some unambiguously negative remarks in *An Apology*.

So why would Milton both put himself in Admetus' position and imbue an image of superstitious temple and church rituals with a sense of personal nostalgia? One way of answering this question is to note that the sonnet expresses guilt as well as grief, and then to accommodate the allusions to Alcestis and Leviticus to the logic of a consistent typological reading. Leo Spitzer's understanding of the poem, for example, consigned both of these figures to the two lower rungs of a ladder that has the Pauline "full sight" of Christian heavenly redemption at its top. The movement is from a classical fantasy of wish fulfillment to an "old law" that can only serve to reveal the human state of sinfulness, but not redeem it, and then to the true redemption offered by Christ's sacrifice.[26] Neither of the first two allusions – which are rooted in the past, but brought to the speaker's mind by his present condition – is sufficient to alleviate that present condition, but their historical placement suggests that the present is, of course, supplemented by Christ's grace. This is what allows the hopeful gesture toward a future redemption, which is the poem's only hedge against the ongoing darkness at its end. What is at stake is the meaning of the apparition. Is it merely a fantasy, a sign of sinful helplessness, or a trustworthy promise of future bliss?

That all of these allusions are, however, tied to contemporary historical and autobiographical contexts, especially to a peculiarly male sense of guilt over the social and spiritual exemption of men from what women had to endure as a consequence of the physical aspects of married life, has not been fully recognized.[27] As I said, the first two allusions are brought

[25] Some possible answers to the question "why Admetus?" have been offered by Kurt Heinzelman in "'Cold Consolation:' the Art of Milton's Last Sonnet," *Milton Studies* 10 (1977), 111–25; McLoone, "Milton's Twenty-Third Sonnet," 11–14, 17–18; and Sokol, "Euripides' *Alcestis* and the 'Saint,'" 134–6.

[26] Spitzer, "Understanding Milton," 20–2. See also John Spencer Hill, "'Alcestis from the Grave:' Image and Structure in Sonnet XXIII," *Milton Studies* 10 (1977), 127–37; McLoone, "Milton's Twenty-Third Sonnet," and Dixon Fiske, "The Theme of Purification in Milton's Sonnet XXIII," *Milton Studies* 8 (1975), 149–63.

[27] Sokol's reading comes closest, suggesting that the self-denigrating identification with Admetus is expressive of Milton's sense of guilt in relation to Mary. For Sokol, the poem's positive vision of the "Saint" expresses Milton's desire to cleanse his memory of the "taint" of his ongoing anger over the abandonment. The childbed figures into the emotional complexity of the memory and the allusion, but functions primarily as a marker of the poem's reference to Mary ("Euripides' *Alcestis* and the 'Saint,'" 140–3).

to mind by the speaker's present condition, which is not just one of general human sinfulness, but one of a particular kind of bereavement that entails a much more specific kind of guilt. The allusions reflect this condition in all of its dimensions. The Alcestis allusion, in particular, allows the poem to signify a male sense of reproductive guilt in several ways. Most critics have assumed that Milton's reversal of Euripides' comedic ending (the fact that his wife does not come back from the grave as Admetus' does, but only appears to, and then disappears) is meant to signify a critique of the classical myth, which is shown – in contrast to the at once painful and yet hopeful Protestant conclusion of the poem – to be nothing but fantasy. Milton, the Christian widower, unlike Admetus, has to fall back into his state of darkness, bereavement and guilt, but with a trust that this state is temporary and that his desires will be more perfectly fulfilled in the Christian heaven than Admetus' could ever have been on earth. Even had his spouse really come back to him as the story says Alcestis came back to Admetus, his joy would still be imperfect in comparison with the higher joy he expects to have in the afterlife. It would, after all, be only temporal and temporary. Still, that the speaker awakens from his "fancied" vision back into a state of postlapsarian darkness, with only his trust in a future restoration to give him comfort, does offer a compelling and starkly realistic representation of the suspense and the struggle of a suffering believer's continued existence in time, even if it does not wholly subvert the promises of his trust. His problem is not with the trust *per se*, but with how to hold onto it securely while its fulfillment is delayed. Spitzer notes that this is the special emphasis that distinguishes the poem: its insistence on the distance between the Neoplatonic and Christian promise that we can finally be reunited with the ideal, and the difficulty of life in the present world, which for the speaker is one of "irremediable loneliness," at least for an uncertainly long period of future mortal life.[28]

Buried in the classical fantasy that sets the poem's tripartite structure in motion is also a typological signal of what guarantees the truth of this more difficult but also more hopeful state of affairs. As several commentators have noted, Alcestis and Herakles present an overlapping pair of typological images, and these types, like the Mosaic purification ritual alluded to in the second quatrain, themselves suggest the Christian present and future that in the end displace them.[29] The typology helps us answer the question

[28] Spitzer, "Understanding Milton," 19.

[29] Alcestis figures Christ's self-sacrifice on the cross, and Herakles figures both His redemption of mankind and the harrowing of hell. See John J. Colaccio, "'A Death Like Sleep:' the Christology of

"why Alcestis?" enviably well (it also gives us the answer to "why Herakles?"). It does not, however, fully answer the question "why Admetus?" The fact that the poem undermines the hollow and fanciful promises of the myth and gives us instead a strenuously Protestant and Neoplatonic vision of mourning, faith, and hoped for restoration does nothing to disassociate the speaker from the weak-willed and selfish king. According to the logic of the analogy, however, both men ultimately get back their wives (one temporarily on earth, the other permanently in heaven), but neither of them *deserves to*. Typology again can come to our rescue. No matter how pious Admetus was about the laws of hospitality (it is this virtue that inspired Herakles to help him), he is never really absolved in the story of his selfishness, his lack of fortitude in facing his own death, and the fact that he lets Alcestis die for him. As McLoone has observed, to the Christian mind, the rescue of Alcestis by Herakles "rather too neatly let[s] one husband escape guilt over participating in a death-substitution."[30] The fantasy, in other words, is too easy, failing to take Admetus' guilt seriously enough. The story of Christ's sacrifice, to which the double typology of Herakles/Alcestis refers, however, makes a different sort of sense of the "death-substitution," and it is in this sense that Admetus becomes more than just a deeply flawed man who gets rewarded for no good reason. He becomes instead a shadowy type of the Christian redeemed by Christ's grace rather than by his own merits.[31]

For Euripides, Admetus's faithfulness to the memory of his wife because of her self-sacrificial heroism (what she did by her own free choice, what he chose to let her do) is merely an opportunity to display absurd human inconsistency and moral blindness. It then becomes the rather shaky ground for an absurdly tragicomic ending. That happy ending, strictly speaking, makes no sense, and this in fact seems to be the point of the play. "Much that the Gods achieve is surprise," as the Chorus puts it at the end.[32] Sometimes good things happen to people who do not deserve them, and for no particularly good reason other than the capricious whims of certain

Milton's Twenty-Third Sonnet," *Milton Studies* 6 (1974), 181–97; Hill, "'Alcestis from the Grave,'" 127–37; and John C. Ulreich, "Typological Symbolism in Milton's Sonnet XXIII," *Milton Quarterly* 8 (1974), 7–10. Colaccio, J. S. Hill, and others argue that Milton approaches the typology through Neoplatonic sources. On the sonnet's direct allusion to Plato, see Patrick Cheney, "Alcestis and the 'Passion for Immortality': Milton's Sonnet XXIII and Plato's *Symposium*," *Milton Studies* 18 (1983), 63–76. Nardo, *Milton's Sonnets and the Ideal Community*, pp. 41–2 argues for a primarily Christian, rather than Neoplatonic, reading.

30 McLoone, "Milton's Twenty-Third Sonnet," 12.

31 McLoone, "Milton's Twenty-Third Sonnet," 11–14 and 17–18.

32 All quotations from *The Complete Greek Tragedies: Volume III, Euripides*, eds. David Grene and Richmond Lattimore (Chicago, IL: University of Chicago Press, 1959).

forces in the universe. Milton's speaker, however, inhabits a universe flush with meaning and with no room in it at all for caprice. He must maintain faith in a God who has allowed the death to happen for a reason, but who also promises that by virtue of His own self-sacrificial death and resurrection, all will be restored and bettered. And this is also for a reason: to manifest His goodness and grace, the essentially Christian comedic nature of the plot that Milton's speaker imagines he is playing out in contrast to Admetus, whose story, despite its happy ending, cannot be said to have any meaning in this sense at all.

Moreover, the original story was fancifully collapsed by Euripides into the twenty-four hour, present-tense span of the play's action, which covers the final day of Alcestis' life and her resurrection at the end of that day. Milton's speaker must, however, live out (over and over again) one tiny fragment of the dilating time between Christ's resurrection and the final redemption to come, and this is a long, dark day indeed. As McLoone observes, this suspension is furthermore compounded for Milton by his mortalism.[33] The precarious trust that he will be reunited with his beloved in heaven has less power to console because it is deferred not simply to the point of the speaker's death, but until the final judgment. In the meantime, death is a true absence of the whole person, "body, spirit, and soul."[34]

This aspect of the poem, as we will later see, has some importance in terms of genre, allowing the sonnet to project itself forward into the much wider theological and narrative realms of the epic that would follow. It also gives us a much better answer to the question "why Admetus?" than any we have so far explored. However, it still does not fully capture the resonance the allusion has for Milton. In this poem's biographical context, the allusion to Admetus is primarily important as a symbol of something more specific than the general condition of human sinfulness. The figure suggests the bereaved husband's feeling, not only of original sin (the act that "brought death into this world with all our woe"), but his feeling of having been *in a specific sense* responsible for the deaths of his wives. The allusion to Admetus suggests that for Milton, what McLoone calls the "death substitution" had a very specific resonance. The Milton of the sonnet experiences himself as an Admetus whose returned wife is merely a tantalizing image. Her flight at the end leaves him in a state of darkness that not only severely tests the trust of any Christian, but tests it differently for men and for women. Euripides' Alcestis herself, although in a different context, puts that gender difference succinctly:

[33] McLoone, "Milton's Twenty-Third Sonnet," 11.
[34] McLoone, "Milton's Twenty-Third Sonnet," 11.

> O Marriage bed
> it was here that I undressed my maidenhead and gave
> myself up to this husband for whose sake I die.
> Goodbye. I hold no grudge. But you have been my death
> and mine alone. (lines 176–80)

Jonathan Goldberg has noted, in his discussion of the relationship of the poem to the myth of Alcestis, that the play contains a complex set of associations of death, maternity, and espousal.[35] Goldberg notes, for example, that Admetus at line 667 of the play calls Alcestis his "mother" because she gives him life in her dying.[36] This is something his actual mother did not do for him, but it was of course something she risked in giving birth to him. However, it has not to my knowledge been much noted in the criticism that in the play, Alcestis dies after several years of marriage to Admetus. She is a mother of two young children, a son and a daughter, and is greatly concerned in the last hours of her life for their welfare after her death. The reason she asks Admetus not to remarry is not jealousy, but worry that a stepmother will mistreat her children.

One could speculate about the ways in which this play and the myth it draws on helped mediate Hellenic civilization's confrontation with dangerous childbirth. There is no doubt in my mind, however, about the way the words of Alcestis's speech and those of her death scene echoed in Milton's consciousness, what mythic paradigms they suggested, and what anxieties they touched in him. The typology he draws on, in fact, makes this very clear. As we saw in Chapter 3 of this study, seventeenth-century Christianity provided a complex redemptive figuration of childbirth pain and danger, one that was worked out both ritually and textually. In this context, the typological relationship between Alcestis and Christ takes on a richness that is not, I think, fully captured by the treatment offered, for example, by McLoone.[37] A woman in childbirth could and often was thought of as experiencing both the curse of Eve and the grace of Christ, her birth and lying-in suggesting the entire spiritual history of mankind. In addition, she was often thought of as herself Christ-like. This figuration, as we have also

[35] Jonathan Goldberg, *Voice Terminal Echo: Postmodernism and English Renaissance Texts* (New York, NY: Methuen, 1986), pp. 151–8.

[36] Goldberg, *Voice*, p. 151.

[37] McLoone movingly touches on the relationship between reproduction and death at the end of his essay ("Milton's Twenty-Third Sonnet," 17–18), but he focuses on the speaker's sense of his own sexual falleness, not on how that speaker imagines his wives might feel about what killed them. See also Sokol, "Euripides' *Alcestis* and the 'Saint'" for a different approach to the allusion's biographical specificity.

seen, works whether she survives or not. A sense of the Resurrection could attach to either her temporal salvation (her rising up from the childbed to her churching and then, Alcestis-like, her return home to her husband), or it could attach to her redemption in heaven or at the end of time. Should she live, she will – unless she is in, say, her late forties – experience the curse of Eve again, perhaps every fifteen to twenty-eight or so months thereafter until she either dies or enters menopause.[38]

Mary Powell herself, we should note, got pregnant for the first time very shortly after returning to her husband in the summer of 1645, and had all of her four children in a little over six and a half years before dying in the birth of the last one.[39] We do not know what would have happened in Katherine's case, but it is certainly true that she and Milton set about having children right away (she gave birth just eleven months after the wedding). Milton's speaker has experienced a version of the typological figure reserved for those women who died in childbirth, and the sonnet's movement through and then beyond the stories of Alcestis and the Old Testament women is designed to signify in no uncertain terms the experience of a man who has, in the past, had his wife return to him after a birth, and now misses her terribly. Mary had been restored to Milton temporally three times, and as we shall see, in all probability, after being churched. The fourth time, however, she did not return. His story, in its last installment, was not one of Alcestis-like restoration, but of dark bereavement. In Katherine's case, that is all he ever had.

The contemplation, however, of the typological significance of the first two allusions (to Alcestis and Leviticus) yields to a conclusion similar to the one offered by the childbirth discourses, one that parallels in its pained

[38] Roger Finlay, *Population and Metropolis: the Demography of London 1580–1650* (Cambridge University Press, 1981), pp. 133–50. See Chapters 1 and 2.

[39] Milton and Mary were reconciled some time in 1645. We do not know exactly when, but it had to have been sometime before September because we are reasonably certain – particularly given that their first daughter, Anne, was born on July 29, 1646 – that they were living together by then, and they must have moved together into the new house in the Barbican during that month (their reunion may have been the reason for the move). It is, of course, difficult to pin-point when connubial relations started, but if it was in the late summer, as seems likely, Mary got pregnant relatively quickly. The next child (named after her mother) was born on October 25, 1648, about twenty-seven months after her sister, and John Jr. was born on March 16, 1651, between twenty-eight and twenty-nine months after that. These are more or less average birth intervals, slightly on the long side, but Deborah was born after a much shorter interval – barely thirteen and a half months after her brother. Just what the difference in intervals means is hard to say, but the short one before the birth of Deborah does suggest that something had changed in the pattern of the Miltons' reproductive life. We have, of course, no way of knowing whether this was the result of chance or of deliberate design on their part, but it could certainly have lent even greater pathos to Mary's death, coming as it did at the end of a pregnancy that commenced so soon after the birth of the previous child, who was also a first son.

hopefulness the typological readings offered by earlier critics, but with an added complexity of resonance. One side of this conclusion is consoling in ways that draw on the theology of childbed suffering and on Milton's own earlier poetic treatments of it. In the poem, the speaker imagines that his late espoused saints were saved, and that he will be too, even if, for the time being, he has to remain in a trying darkness. His vision of the redeemed state of his wives, not just "washt from spot of child-bed taint" but entirely rescued from it, echoes the apotheoses Milton imagined for Lady Jane Paulet and, through the figure of Psyche's "spotless side," for Lady Alice Egerton's future. In both of those instances, the proper facing of the cycle of reproductive suffering yielded, in the end, to a state bathed in light and characterized by a restored physical integrity – an end to the cycle.[40] Here, the husband's darkness is lightened by this thought, but also by his consideration of his own cycle of suffering. The darkness he remains in at the end of the poem constitutes the masculine trial that accompanies and complements the trials of the birthing women. This is, I believe, in fact the deepest significance of Admetus for Milton. He represents the trial of and the ultimate reward granted to the undeserving husband who has to inhabit the now darkened bedchamber that was once lit by the presence of a wife and mother, had once been the birthing chamber itself, full of the (much dimmer) light and heat and close communal pressure and presence created by the childbed rites. It was also the place to which his first wife had returned to give herself over once again to the embrace that would lead her to another trial. Then, of course, it became the place to which she did not return, and that failure to return was repeated in the case of his second wife.

In other words, the allusions to Alcestis and Leviticus, Luke, and the Churching of Women are designed not simply to make a polemical point about sacred history, but to address the specific pains of Milton's own experience, to offer a specific comfort, the same one he had more abstractly, and with less recognition of the real nature of pain, offered in his imagination to Ladies Jane and Alice. It is also, however, one that he had, somewhat mean-spiritedly, failed to offer in his imagination to John Paulet. At this point, some thirty years later, Milton explored that difficult male position much more fully, and tried to find some way through its darkness back to light. This turns out to be quite difficult. Milton's mourner is left in a starkly vulnerable position both psychologically and spiritually. Men do not give birth. Milton, therefore, finds himself not only

[40] A connection between the "shining" person of the espoused saint and the "radiant sheen" of Lady Jane at the end of the epitaph was noted by Le Comte, "The Veiled Face," 245–6.

helpless in the face of his wives' suffering, but forced to recognize that this suffering was caused by his own desires to express love and to procreate, his need for his wives' cooperation, as well as their probably mutual desire to obey the first commandment. This is an irony we are familiar with from our discussions in Part I: both a man's love and his own and his wife's obedience to God's will can cause painful death, as well as new life. This is most painfully registered by the poem's conclusion, the terrible moment marked by the internal rhyme of "face" and "embrace." The speaker cannot see the woman's face, but he can see the virtues shining forth from her whole "person." As she moves to embrace him, however, a movement that seems to follow along the lines of desire from the way he abstractly apprehends her "person" to the body that her "personhood" suggests, he awakens and the dream is shattered. The dream will not allow the fantasy of *touch*.

It is particularly significant that the final line gives us this painful moment in an unexpected sequence: "I wak'd, she fled, and day brought back my night." It is, of course, common in poems of this kind for the dissolving of the vision to occur as a result of the speaker's being awakened by something, usually an excess of desire, or some external interruption, but Milton's choice to have the lady flee, rather than simply disappear, is of tremendous importance. It suggests that the vision has not simply been ended by his waking, but that, still within the dream, she reacts to the speaker's waking and *flees from him*. As I noted in my earlier discussion of the epitaph on Jane Paulet, Milton almost always used the verb "to flee" and its various forms to denote escape from some confining or otherwise negative condition. In the epitaph, he used it to denote Lady Jane's escape from the earthly conditions that defined her, constrained her, and in which she struggled toward a state of heavenly felicity. In the sonnet, in other words, "she fled" is more than a figure for the shattering of the dream (more like "they flee from me" than "the dream is fled"). It suggests that the condition of the speaker is not only a negative and constraining one from his perspective, but also one from hers. It might be said to suggest the disdain of a redeemed soul for the constraining, earthly condition of the not yet saved, or in McLoone's reading of the speaker's ambivalence, a sense of both the "censorious" rebuke of her purity and his feelings of sexual guilt.[41] But then why the suggestion of fear that comes in the sequence, the fact that Milton's speaker tells us she "fled" just after and, as we are invited to imagine, because of his waking? Why, also, the fudging

[41] McLoone, "Milton's Twenty-Third Sonnet," 17–18.

of the boundary between waking and sleep? Following the convention of this sort of dream-vision, the speaker seems to be "awake" within the dream, though asleep physically. And yet his "waking," which we must assume is *from* the dream, seems to affect her as if it were an awakening *within* the dream.[42]

The key here is the fact that, as the speaker tells us, she was about to *embrace* him. For a confused moment, in anticipation of the embrace (and in the memory of it), the speaker was and remembers himself to have been both prone and passive with sleep. His awakening from that passivity awoke in him an erotic response within the dream, and something about the emotional intensity that surrounded the anticipation of consummation, of touch, was so strong that it woke him, too, from his actual sleep. What was so strong is as clear as it is complex. A part of it is sexual arousal, but along with this comes a spiritual and emotional arousal, as well as a tender memory of a past physical intimacy mixed with the special meaning that touch would have had for any blind man, especially one who had never seen one of his wives and lost sight of, and then completely lost, the other one in the two years that also produced their last two children. Milton probably could see to some extent when he and Mary conceived John Jr., and still to some extent, but not at all well, when they conceived Deborah some time shortly after John was born. When Mary *gave birth* to Deborah nine months later, however, he could no longer see her at all; he could only have touched her. To whatever extent he expected to conceive more children with her (and we have no reason to assume he did not), he would have expected to do so with only touch as a primary way to sense her (along with his hearing and sense of smell). Touch would also have been his primary way of interacting with the new baby, not to mention with his infant son, whom he also could no longer see by the time he died so soon after his mother.

Of course, Milton's sexual relationship with Katherine was always primarily one of touch. The thought of touch was therefore, in relation to his experiences with both wives, fraught enough to wake him and blur the boundaries of the psychological experience and the conventions of its literary representation. For *them*, however, for his fraught imagination of them, his poetic figure of his wife or wives, it was another matter entirely. The lost physical intimacy, in their case, was to Milton's highly empathetic and, in this case, self-lacerating imagination also *the cause of their deaths*. The

[42] I would like to thank William Flesch for first bringing the strangeness of the sequence to my attention in a class discussion many years ago.

speaker imagines his wife as suddenly afraid, betraying a marked ambivalence in his own mind and spirit. He cannot bear to re-experience their nuptial embrace, although he cannot help but fantasize about nearly doing so. All of this is projected onto her. She was willing, it seems, to bend to touch him as long as he remained in the passive state of the vision. We can imagine, perhaps, a rather chaste embrace, one remaining to some extent abstract from the physical aspects of the personal virtues the speaker numbers ("love, sweetness, goodness"). Once he responds to her, however, it is she who cannot abide it, and she runs away from what we must – and the speaker must – remember killed her. That she flees back into what Milton called in "An Epitaph on the Marchioness of Winchester" (hereafter "An Epitaph") "the boosom bright/ Of blazing Majesty and Light," having had the "like fortune" of women like Rachel and Jane Paulet (becoming, like them, a "saint" and, like them, "clad in radiant sheen"), only serves to mark again the tense difficulty of Milton's representation of the male trial (in both cases the women "fled," but in the second case it is because of fear, not just a Christian Neoplatonic disdain for the earth). He imagines that they have passed their trials, but that he is still in the midst of his, a trial that requires he understand his ironic responsibility for theirs, the role he played in their deaths. It is not only Admetus' position he identifies with; it is also, belatedly – and as I suggested before – John Paulet's.[43]

"HER FACE WAS VAIL'D:" MARY POWELL AND THE CHURCHING OF WOMEN

I am unaware of any other poem written by or on behalf of a husband whose wife had died in childbirth that suggests the husband might have been responsible for the death. Milton, however, had not only flirted with such a suggestion before, he resurrects it here with a terrible immediacy. Milton's allusive structure seems designed, in fact, to do even more than simply

[43] After his 1648 release from prison (he had remarried and had four new children by then), Paulet went on to set himself to tasks of which Milton may very well have approved. He published translations from the French of three works of piety and history, including, in 1652 (the year of Mary's death), a translation of *La galerie des femmes fortes* by Pierre Le Moyne, entitled *The Gallery of Heroic Women* (London, 1652). What this had to do with any ideas either Paulet or Milton may have developed about women's heroism will have to wait for a more careful examination of the text than I have been able to do so far (birth is only mentioned in a few places in passing). Paulet's translation, published just a year later, of Nicolas Talon's biblical paraphrase, *Histoire sainte, A Holy History* (London, 1653), does contain an account of Rachel's story. Whether or not Milton knew the work, and if it influenced his own paraphrase of biblical history in *Paradise Lost*, will also have to await further study. That Milton would have known something of Paulet's fate and activities seems likely, given his notoriety and Milton's own earlier interest in the family.

raise the issue. In the process of doing so, it encompasses and comments upon another aspect of seventeenth-century childbirth, and gives us a fascinating glimpse of how conflicts over the value of certain public rituals actually affected individual human relationships at the time.

The churching ceremony, as I have already noted, was the official Anglican rite of thanksgiving for safe passage through childbirth, and a rite of passage for women from the exclusively female world of birth and lying-in, back to the world of public worship and the norms of ordinary domestic life. It was also a social ritual of complex significance and no little controversy. The rite had its origins in early medieval Catholic practices that perhaps, in turn, had their roots in the purification rituals required in Leviticus. The fact that, in Luke 2:22–4, we are told that Mary underwent the Levitical purification rites after the birth of Jesus seems to have been the link that brought the rite over from Hebraic to early Christian practice. Although the medieval Church denied the rite sacramental status and proclaimed it merely a thanksgiving ceremony, in practice it retained, for many women and clergy, the character of a ritual cleansing all the way up to and beyond the Reformation.[44] In Catholic practice, women traditionally attended the ceremony in a white veil; they carried a candle, were met at the church door by a priest who sprinkled them with holy water before they entered, and often had lines from Psalm 51 ("Thou shalt purge me O Lord, with hyssop") said over them.[45] These elements of the ritual, which suggest purification, were muted, however, in Anglican practice, and the 1552 prayer book pointedly changed the name of the rite from "The Order of the Purification of Women," which had been its title in the edition of 1549, to "The Thanksgiving of Women after Childbirth, commonly called the Churching of Women."[46] In addition, the ceremony was moved from the church porch to "some convenient place nigh unto the place where the table standeth," and the sprinkling with holy water was removed. The psalm specified was Psalm 121.[47] Much to the chagrin of Puritan reformers,

[44] Keith Thomas, *Religion and the Decline of Magic* (New York, NY: Scribner's, 1971), pp. 38–9 and David Cressy, "Purification, Thanksgiving, and the Churching of Women in Post-Reformation England," *Past and Present* 141 (November 1993), 106–46, especially 120–1.

[45] Thomas, *Religion and the Decline of Magic*, pp. 38–9; Cressy, "Purification," 117–19.

[46] This title was retained in 1559 and subsequent versions. See *The Book of Common Prayer, 1559: the Elizabethan Prayer Book*, ed. John E. Booty (Charlottesville, VA: University Press of Virginia for the Folger Shakespeare Library, 1976), p. 314. The Anglican position on the ceremony (indeed, a defense of it) was expressed with pointed clarity by Richard Hooker in Book 5 of *The Laws of Ecclesiastical Polity*. See *The Works of that Learned and Judicious Divine, Mr. Richard Hooker*, 3 vols. (London, 1888; facs. New York, NY: Burt Franklin, 1970), vol. II, p. 434.

[47] Booty, *The Book of Common Prayer*, pp. 314–15.

however, popular symbols and practices pointing to purification remained a part of the service – as well as the various celebrations that surrounded it in public and at the home – well into the seventeenth century. Most importantly for our purposes, these included the woman's being escorted to the church (by her gossips and her midwife) wearing a white veil.[48]

Although their opinions differ as to the extent to which the ritual "empowered" women, both Adrian Wilson and David Cressy have demonstrated that churching was a highly popular ritual, whose cultural function for women, as the conclusion of the ritual sequence of birth and lying-in, was probably more important than its theological implications.[49] There is strong evidence, despite the disdain of Puritan divines, that many women wanted the ceremony performed for them (and were willing to pay a fee) largely because it was the one public ritual in which they alone played the central role.[50] The Anglican removal of churching from the church porch to a place near the altar did away with the idea that the woman was being made pure enough to enter the church, but it also had the effect of transforming her, as Cressy argues, "from a petitioner at the margin to the focus of community attention."[51] Even more importantly, the rite celebrated – often augmented by social gatherings over cake and ale at home – the woman's survival of an event that, as we have seen, could be very dangerous.[52] Jeremy Boulton has shown that in one large urban, and significantly Puritan, parish, over 90 percent of the mothers who had their children baptized (76 percent of all mothers) were churched.[53] Wilson reports, from private correspondence with Boulton, that this was also the case in at least one other parish of similar demographic make-up.[54]

However, as the years of Milton's first two marriages took place after the dissolving of the Church, we need to explore to what extent the rite of churching and other Anglican rites survived during the Interregnum. Statistics of the specificity of Wilson's and Boulton's are only available for the years leading up to the first Civil War. Although Boulton reports that

48 See Thomas, *Religion and the Decline of Magic*, p. 39 and Adrian Wilson, "Participant or Patient?: Seventeenth Century Childbirth from the Mother's Point of View," in *Patients and Practitioners: Lay Perceptions of Medicine in Pre-industrial Society*, ed. Roy Porter (Cambridge University Press, 1985), p. 139. Cressy notes that the veil was largely a matter of indifference in discussions of the rite until the 1620s and 1630s, when high ceremonialist bishops began to insist upon it ("Purification," 111, 132–40).

49 Wilson, "Participant or Patient?," p. 139; Cressy, "Purification," 108–17.

50 Cressy, "Purification," 126–7 and Jeremy Boulton, *Neighborhood and Society: a London Suburb in the Seventeenth Century* (Cambridge University Press, 1987), p. 277.

51 Cressy, "Purification," 120.

52 Cressy gives several accounts of typical celebrations ("Purification," 111–17).

53 Boulton, *Neighborhood and Society*, pp. 276–9.

54 Wilson, "Participant or Patient?," pp. 139–40.

there is "a little evidence" that the practice of churching fell off during the Civil War itself, it is unclear just how extensive that falling off was. It is clear, however, that the ceremony did remain in use despite its official suppression. Because they had no sacramental status, churchings were often under-recorded in parish registers, even at the height of the Laudian reforms. It is likely, given the disorder of the war years, that what seems in the already spotty documentary record like a falling off of practice, is simply an even greater falling off of record keeping. Most historians agree that many Anglican rites remained in practice during the 1640s and 1650s, and it is reasonable to assume, given their popularity even in largely Puritan parishes before the war, that churchings were common in the years between the first war and the Restoration, and certainly were available for anyone who sought to have one performed.[55]

The socio-religious make-up of London during the years of the Civil War and the Interregnum was varied and complex, and in no way conformed across the board to the desires of the Presbyterians or Independents in Parliament.[56] Although the Book of Common Prayer, with its churching order, was "officially" outlawed, many parishes continued to use it, and the Directory of Public Worship, which was supposed to replace it in 1645, was poorly distributed.[57] This situation was further complicated by the fact that one of the key innovations of the war years was to get rid of conformity in worship. This made enforcement of a strictly Presbyterian order difficult (as difficult, John Morrill notes, as Anglican conformity had been for the Laudian church to enforce in Puritan districts before the war). The Directory of Public Worship was itself a vague and open-ended document. There was even some debate in the Westminster Assembly as to whether or not a churching service should be included in the Directory. The Assembly, in the end, decided against it, but they did so primarily on the grounds of Scots precedent (it had never been a separate ceremony).[58] In addition, although the Presbyterian discipline was declared with The

[55] This was certainly the case with other popular rituals. Illegal marriage rituals, for example, have been studied extensively in this regard. See Christopher Durston, "'Unhallowed Wedlocks': the Regulation of Marriage during the English Revolution," *The Historical Journal* 31 (1988), 45–59.

[56] See John Morrill, "The Church in England, 1642–9," in *Reactions to the English Civil War 1642–1649*, ed. John Morrill (New York, NY: St. Martin's Press, 1983), pp. 89–114 and Barry Reay, "Popular Religion," in *Popular Culture in Seventeenth-Century England*, ed. Barry Reay (New York, NY: St. Martins Press, 1985), p. 119.

[57] Morrill, "The Church in England," pp. 93–4.

[58] See Thomas Leishman, *The Westminster Directory* (London: William Blackwood and Sons, 1901), pp. 114–15.

Solemn League and Covenant in September 1643, it only gradually made its way into the parish churches that did, in the end, conform. As Morrill has noted, "the office, title and authority of the bishops were not suspended or abolished until October 1646," and it was some time, in any case, before the abolition had an effect on practice in the parishes (the Miltons' reproductive life, of course, began in that year).[59] Of London's 110 parish churches, only about 64 officially became a part of the new Presbyterian structure.[60] Within these churches, practice varied, and in many, the new church government never became fully organized, decaying as time passed and the Puritan zeal of the early days of the revolution faded.[61] In addition, the governing institutions who were supposed to oversee the reorganization were, as Tai Liu observes, "never given any coercive superior jurisdiction," and, as Christopher Durston notes in regard to the government's failure to fully enforce the Marriage Act of 1653, which outlawed church weddings, the limited bureaucracy typical of early-modern England was simply no match for widespread popular resistance in matters of church ritual.[62]

There is therefore strong reason to believe that a woman who wanted to have a churching performed could easily have found a clergyman in London who would have performed one for her, particularly in the early years of the Civil War period. It is also possible that Mary Powell was one such woman. In 1945, when Parker made biography central to the debate over Milton's sonnet by suggesting that, for various reasons, it did not refer to Katherine Woodcock, among the pieces of evidence he brought to bear was the possibility that the veil in the poem was a reference, not just to Euripides, and not just to the fact that Milton was blind by the time he met and married Katherine Woodcock, but to this popular Anglican service.[63] The possibility is a controversial one. Anthony Low, for example, in his *Milton Quarterly* note in 1975, dismissed the notion that Milton could have been referring to this ceremony on the basis of what we know about his attitude toward it.[64] The ceremony was supported by conservative clergy and was often singled out in the anti-episcopal tracts of the 1640s as a superstitious Jewish or papist hold-over. The right of the clergy to require

59 Morrill, "The Church in England," pp. 92–3.

60 Tai Liu, *Puritan London: a Study of Religion and Society in the City Parishes* (Newark, NJ: University of Delaware Press, 1986), p. 55.

61 Liu, *Puritan London*, p. 55.

62 Liu, *Puritan London*, pp. 52–4; Durston, "'Unhallowed Wedlocks,'" 54.

63 Parker, "Milton's Last Sonnet," and "Milton's Last Sonnet Again." See also Le Comte, "The Veiled Face," 245–6.

64 Low, "Milton's Last Sonnet," 80–2.

that women wear a veil during the ceremony had been a matter of active contestation, and was upheld in ecclesiastical court on a number of occasions during the reigns of James and Charles.[65] Milton himself made a very snide remark about the use of Psalm 121 during the service in *An Apology* (published in April 1642, a month or so before he married Mary).[66] This, and just about everything else we know about Milton's theology and politics, supports Low's assertion that "Milton would never have approved of his wives' undergoing the ceremony, nor if they did would he have spoken about it as he has been thought to do in this sonnet" (that is to say, with affectionate longing and approval).[67]

Such a position fails, however, to take the ideas and desires of Mary (and perhaps, though less probably, Katherine) into consideration. It is also too quick to jump to conclusions about the psychology of Milton's grief and how his poetry might have expressed it. Mary came from a conservative, Royalist family.[68] She spent the first three years of her marriage near the king at Oxford – probably a willing prisoner at her parents' house in the very heart of Royalist territory. She returned to Milton's household in largely Puritan London only after the king's forces had been defeated. There is

[65] See Boulton, *Neighborhood and Society*, p. 276 and Thomas, *Religion and the Decline of Magic*, pp. 59–60. Cressy gives several accounts of cases of this kind ("Purification," 136–40).

[66] He refers to such "errors, *tautologies*, [and] impertinences, as those thanks in the womans Churching for her delivery from Sunburning and Moonblasting, as if she had bin travailing not in her bed, but in the deserts of *Arabia*" (*CP*, 1.939). The reference is to Psalm 121:6, which reads, in the version used in the 1559 Book of Common Prayer: "So that the sun shall not burn thee by day: neither the moon by night" (Booty, *The Book of Common Prayer*, p. 314). Low also notes a passage in *The Doctrine and Discipline of Divorce* that suggests Milton believed churching was at best superfluous and at worst superstitious (*CP*, 2.225).

[67] Low, "Milton's Last Sonnet," 80. McLoone later suggested that the reference to churching expresses the mourner's spiritual ambivalence ("Milton's Twenty-Third Sonnet," 14–15).

[68] Katherine Woodcock came from a family in some ways oddly like the Powells. Their fathers, in particular, resembled one another in temperament and behavior. However, the Woodcocks had a much more politically and religiously mixed heritage, with a strong Parliamentarian side. Details about the two families can be found in Parker, pp. 866–70, 1053–5. Further details about the Woodcocks, not all of them accurate, can be found in John S. Smart, *Sonnets of Milton* (Glasgow: Maclehose, Jackson and Co., 1921; rpt. Oxford: Clarendon Press, 1966), pp. 107–10. Katherine and Milton were members of the parish of St. Mary Aldermanbury. According to Liu, this was "one of the most important parishes in Puritan London," whose minister was the well-known and influential Presbyterian divine, Edmund Calamy, the "EC" of the "SMECTYMNUUS" group whom Milton had defended in *An Apology* (Liu, *Puritan London*, pp. 29, 73–6). They had the wedding banns published in the church, but they were married by a justice of the peace, not a clergyman, as the law at the time required (see below). The more Puritan context of the marriage makes it seem less likely that Katherine would have undergone a churching, despite the fact that she lived long enough to have done so (whether or not she would have had the strength is a matter of conjecture). The birth of her daughter is registered in the parish of St. Mary's, but there is no record that the child was baptized. Unfortunately, we have no record of Milton's wedding to Mary Powell, which, like the records of her death and burial, are not where they ought to be (Parker, p. 1009).

every reason to assume that, whatever her husband might have thought of it, she would have wished and expected to undergo the thanksgiving ceremony. We do know, for example, that she had at least one of her first three children baptized, despite the fact that Milton's feelings about infant baptism were similar to those he had about churching.[69] Low himself, in the nuanced account of Milton's ideas about marriage he later provided in *The Reinvention of Love*, notes that Milton was more flexible in matters of religious ritual than we might be tempted to assume.[70] Milton married Mary in Oxfordshire, and we can imagine that the wedding was arranged by her family in their parish church. He married Katherine in a civil ceremony, which was the only way to *legally* marry after the Marriage Act of August 24, 1653 outlawed church ceremonies. This did not, of course, stop people from marrying in church clandestinely, but Milton would have, presumably, been in agreement with the new rules. In the divorce tracts, he had already gone some distance in arguing for the separation of marriage from the church. In addition, in *Considerations Touching the Likeliest Means to Remove Hirelings*, published in 1659, but probably written for the most part in 1653, he put his position in no uncertain terms, praising Parliament for "prudently" recovering "the civil liberty of marriage" from the encroachment of a clergy that still wanted to control its celebration, even in the wake of the changes wrought by the revolution, and even though they had already declared that it was not a sacrament. He was glad that Parliament had "transferrd the ratifying and registring therof from the canonical shop to the proper cognisance of civil magistrates" (*CP*, 7rev. 300).[71] However, Milton did, as John Shawcross has recently noted, have the banns for the wedding published in his parish church.[72] This is significant because he did not have to do so. The new law had made it possible to completely divorce the ceremony from the church's authority by allowing a couple to publish their banns in the marketplace rather than the church. That Milton either decided to publish – or decided to allow his banns to be published – in

69 On the baptism of Mary's children, see Parker, p. 340.

70 Anthony Low, *The Reinvention of Love: Poetry, Politics and Culture from Sidney to Milton* (Cambridge University Press, 1993), pp. 158–201.

71 William Hunter briefly sets out the evidence for the earlier date of composition in his introductions to the treatise in *The Prose of John Milton*, ed. J. Max Patrick (New York University Press, 1968), pp. 475–8 (see also *CP*, 7rev. 229–37; especially p. 230, n. 6). Shawcross offers a vigorous defense of Hunter's suggestion in *Rethinking Milton Studies: Time Present and Time Past* (Newark, NJ: University of Delaware Press, 2005), pp. 69–74. If Hunter and Shawcross are correct, the statements about the Marriage Act, which would have just recently been passed, decisively predated Milton's marriage to Katherine. The remarks therefore probably reflect relatively long-standing opinions, making the flexibility I go on to discuss all the more noteworthy.

72 Shawcross, *Arms*, p. 206.

church suggests a flexible willingness to abide by religious custom. The fact that in 1663, Milton married Elizabeth Minshul, his third wife, in a church also suggests such flexibility, or at least a sense of pragmatism in the face of a particular legal climate.[73] It is very difficult to know what all of this means about Milton, to what extent his actions were determined by simple practicality, the legal situation, or the desires of his brides or the families involved. It does not, however, look like the record of a man with a particularly dogmatic approach to matters of church ritual.

Milton might therefore have also been less dogmatic about churching than his remarks in a piece of polemical prose might suggest in isolation. We cannot know for certain that Mary was churched, but we cannot dismiss the intriguing possibility that it happened perhaps three times while Milton could still see. Although there is nothing to rule out a churching after the birth of each of Mary's first three children (she died, of course, too soon after the birth of Deborah), the evidence is particularly strong for the birth of Anne, the Miltons' first child. Mary's family, made homeless by both the war and her father's financial irresponsibility, followed her to London some time after June 27, 1646. Milton housed them from early July until the death of Mary's father in December. Since Anne was born on July 29th, about a month after the Powells arrived, it is reasonable to assume that her mother was chief gossip at the birth. This was also about two months before the abolition of the bishops, and well within the period of greatest confusion in matters of church discipline in London. It is therefore highly likely, given what we know of the family background, of church organization at the time, and of the role that gossips generally played in the rites of childbirth,[74] that

[73] See Low, *Reinvention*, pp. 183–4, and Parker, pp. 1053, 1095. I thank Professor Low for pointing this out to me in correspondence. The "Act for Confirming Marriages" of 1661 had declared all marriages performed during the Interregnum – no matter how they were performed, by whom, or where – valid, but it also outlawed civil ceremonies from that point on. It is therefore very unlikely that Milton and Elizabeth Minshull would have been married by a Justice in 1663. Some people, as Outhwaite shows in detail in his study of clandestine marriage, certainly defied canon law after the Restoration (just as they had defied it before the Interregnum, and just as, for that matter, they defied the 1653 Act *during* the Interregnum), but I doubt very much that Milton would have been tempted to do so given his precarious legal situation in those years. See R. B. Outhwaite, *Clandestine Marriage in England, 1500–1850* (Rio Grande, OH: Hambledon Press, 1995). I suppose that John and Elizabeth might have simply made vows in front of witnesses (this was still allowed under the restored canon law) but this also might not have been an attractive option for them. Another aspect of the documentary evidence suggests that they did not want to invite any undue scrutiny. No banns were published for the wedding, but an ecclesiastical license was issued about two weeks prior to the ceremony. Such a practice was common among couples who desired to get things taken care of as quickly and with as little fuss and public attention as possible. The fact that John was fifty-five years old and on his third marriage, and that Elizabeth was twenty-four, might have had something to do with this. I am grateful to John Shawcross for his comments and suggestions in correspondence on this issue.

[74] Wilson, "Participant or Patient?," pp. 133–41.

Mary could have been churched sometime in late August. It could have happened again after each of the next two births, although the chances of our finding a record of this are slim at best. It is unlikely that churches would have kept records about such ceremonies.

The possibility is particularly tantalizing in the case of John Jr.'s birth. The interval between the birth of John and the birth of Deborah was a good deal shorter than those between the births of Anne, Mary, and John Jr. Mary Powell did not get pregnant again for about two years after the births of Anne and Mary, but she became pregnant with Deborah only thirteen months after John's birth. This suggests that she and Milton resumed sexual relations shortly after her lying-in was over. It is possible that they had resumed just after the lying-in in all three cases, and that the quick pregnancy in the last case was the result of a decision on Mary's part not to nurse John Jr. herself, or it may have simply been a matter of chance. We have no way of knowing whether or not the Miltons ever employed a wet nurse other than the one Phillips thought killed his cousin. However, the possibility that the Miltons were either in the habit of resuming relations shortly after lying-in, or that they were, for whatever reason, anxious to have another child very soon after the birth of their first son is intriguing. It was common for the churching ceremony to not only provide an occasion for giving thanks for safe passage, marking the resumption of public worship (indeed, of public existence), but also to mark the resumption of ordinary domestic life, including conjugal relations.[75] The period immediately surrounding the birth, including the lying-in period, could have meant complete separation of man and wife for almost a month, and their reunion in the marriage bed could often have had powerful emotional and symbolic significance. Were the Miltons especially amorous or happy about family life in the wake of the birth of a boy, and did this make them resume sexual relations early or with particular intensity? Were they trying to affirm their bonds in the context of the legal battle with Mary's mother? Had their marriage bonds simply deepened over the years? Did it have something to do with Milton's depressed mental state over his blindness? We have no way of knowing. The pregnancy might very well have been the result, as I said, of chance on one not particularly warm or even pleasant occasion (one thinks of the "mill of an undelighted and servil copulation" that Milton famously evoked in *The Doctrine and Discipline of Divorce* [*CP*, 2.258]), but the fact remains that the year or so prior to the death of both the boy and his mother (indeed, the two years before) were heavy with birth and infant care, and

[75] Wilson, "Participant or Patient?," p. 138; Cressy, "Purification," 115–17; and Chapter 1.

probably with at least periods of the kind of sexual activity that makes for rapid pregnancies, one following upon another. This suggests a period full of the joys, hopes, and the stresses that come with a rapidly growing family life, and of course the anxieties as well. Within a matter of weeks, it was all over. Not only did Milton lose his partner in the marriage, but also one of the union's most precious fruits.

The possibility that Mary was churched on possibly three occasions during such a period, along with the attendant possibility that the ceremony was a bone of contention in the marriage, as well as, in practice, a prelude to the resumption of love-making during a period of rather high fertility in that marriage, reinforces and complicates our understanding of the guilt that drives the sonnet as palpably as its grief. It is possible that Milton was remembering Mary in her white robe and veil, and thus that the allusion to Alcestis is determined by the memory of Mary in particular, and not simply by typological and literary considerations, and not simply by memories of his unseen Katherine.

While Milton may have disapproved of churching on purely theological grounds, he may not have wished to forbid his wife her desires. Whatever dubious theological implications the rite had for him, its social implications – and the fact that each time it occurred, it tangibly marked the fact that his wife had not died to give him another child – may well have combined to lend it considerable affective power each time it occurred, even more so in retrospect after her death. In addition, as we have seen, the emotional circumstances following Mary's death were very difficult. The image of that veiled woman, who did not return from her last lying-in to unveil herself and help him care for the children, who had, in fact, barely begun her month of lying-in when she died, and who had left him with not only a fourth child, but a third child vulnerable to the neglect of a woman not his mother, must have tapped deep currents of ambivalence, loss, and helplessness for Milton, whether or not he gave expression to these emotions in verse at the time.

We must also remember that Mary had earlier returned to her husband after a three-year separation. He had taken her back, and it stands to reason that some kind of compromise had to have been reached about just how life in the household was to be managed. He may have conceded something to Mary on the issue of churching. In fact, it is likely he had no say in the matter. Childbirth was an area of life that the historical literature tells us was conspicuous for the absence of men altogether, let alone of male authority.[76]

[76] Wilson, "Participant or Patient?," p. 134.

Cressy, for example, cites several cases of women before the war who crossed both the authority of their husbands and that of reform-minded clerics in order to be churched.[77] Finally, the early biographers' silence about any warmth in the marriage does not prove the absence of that warmth,[78] and even if it did, it does not obviously follow that Milton would not have written affectingly about Mary after her death. A quick reading of Thomas Hardy's 1912–1913 poems should serve as a reminder of the complex relationship between grief, guilt, dreams, poetry, and affection.[79]

THE POEM AND ITS TRADITION

A reading of the sonnet in the context of contemporary conditions and biographical events need not contradict readings that place it in the context of a more purely "literary" history. In fact, attention to biographical and historical reference can help us to understand more fully what motivated the rather aggressive approach to genre that Milton took in this case. The sonnet, as we have already seen, ends in an isolated darkness. In this, it is unique in Milton's canon, and all the more remarkable given that, as published in the *Poems* of 1673, it concludes a sequence of sonnets and therefore constitutes not just an imitation of the Petrarchan and Dantesque use of the dream vision, but an extreme and in some ways terrifying revision of them. The English poets of the preceding century, as we know, tended to literalize the conventions of the Petrarchan tradition, rendering them in tense political and social situations that were often referentially specific, or at least designed – somewhat polemically – to assert their own realism against the general idealism of the genre.[80] Milton's collection of sonnets is far shorter and far more heterogeneous than most of those that preceeded it, and it looks back at the heyday of English sonneteering with a pathos of distance generated by a decades-long gap in time. He wrote the individual poems in response to particular occasions and intentions over a period of almost thirty years. Only the first seven, which constitute a Petrarchan

77 Cressy, "Purification," 130–1. 78 Low, "Milton's Last Sonnet," 80.

79 See Hill's sensitive treatment of this matter ("A Dream in the Long Valley," 10–12).

80 The keynote of the trend was struck by Wyatt in "They fle from me that sometime did me seke." See Thomas Greene, *The Light in Troy* (New Haven, CT: Yale University Press, 1982); Steven Greenblatt, *Renaissance Self-Fashioning from More to Shakespeare* (University of Chicago Press, 1980), pp. 115–56; and Louis Schwartz, "'But as for me, helas, I may no more': Petrarchan Imitation and Courtly Sociability in Wyatt's 'Who so list to hounte,'" *The Comparatist* 18 (1994), 1–22. See also Gerald Hammond, *Fleeting Things: English Poets and Poems 1616–1660* (Cambridge, MA: Harvard University Press, 1990), pp. 213–14.

mini-sequence, seem clearly to have been directly concerned with the genre of the sonnet sequence at the time of their composition. Still, Milton retroactively structured and published the whole set (the first ten and one canzone in 1645, a further nine in 1673) in a way that suggests that they should be read as a sequence, not simply as a chronologically arranged set.[81] If we take this cue and approach the set as a sequence, the final sonnet bears a particularly heavy burden, drawing the sequence back to the set of generic expectations it began with and then strayed from. In line with general English practice, the sonnet also literalizes some of the most central conventions of the genre, but it does so in a strikingly original way.

Milton's sequence, in the opening set of eight lyrics (seven sonnets and the canzone), begins by using all of the generic commonplaces of a more-or-less conventional love sequence, although it does unconventionally mix English and Italian. The speaker self-consciously makes the mixture of languages thematic, however, accommodating it to various conventional themes (inexpressibility, the announcement of a poetic vocation, the social isolation that love foists upon the speaker, etc.). The speaker seems particularly concerned with questions about his vocational choices (shall he become a lover or a poet? can he be both? shall he write in English or Italian? will he write verse good enough to ensure that we will be remembered after he dies?). His attention to these concerns tends to overwhelm the more conventional task of idealizing his beloved, dark-haired Italian lady. But this is itself hardly unconventional, even if Milton emphasizes it more than some of his predecessors. After Sonnet 7, however, the sequence drops the theme of love altogether, taking on, in imitation of Tasso and others, matters of politics, satire, and praise, as well as Horatian poems of invitation and advice to friends. Toward the end, the sequence also presents personal

[81] The sonnets addressed to Fairfax, Cromwell, Vane, and one of two addressed to Skinner were left out in 1673, but the Trinity Manuscript indicates that Milton intended to include them in what would have been a sequence of twenty-three sonnets: five in Italian, eighteen in English, plus one Italian canzone. The manuscript also indicates that Milton considered placing the tailed sonnet "On the New Forcers of Conscience" in the sequence just before the poem to Fairfax, but it is separated out in 1673. Political considerations probably affected these decisions. The manuscript sequencing differs somewhat from the published version, and there has been disagreement about Milton's intentions. "Mee thougt I saw my late espoused saint" is, however, the final sonnet in both arrangements. See William McCarthy, "The Continuity of Milton's Sonnets," *PMLA* 92 (1977), 96–109; Nardo, *Milton's Sonnets and the Ideal Community*; Mary Anne Radzinowicz, *Toward Samson Agonistes* (Princeton University Press, 1978), pp. 129–42; Adrianne Baytop, "Milton's Sonnet Sequence: Strictest Measure," *The Language Quarterly* 26 (1987), 20–2; and Annabel Patterson, "That Old Man Eloquent," pp. 22–44.

religious mediations. Only in the last sonnet does it return to the theme of love. More precisely, love reappears only to give way to loss. The dark Italian beauty of Sonnets 2 through 6 has been forgotten, and we are suddenly confronted by what must also seem a forgotten – perhaps repressed – matter of the poet's life. Somewhere along the way, through the sometimes dark wood of a public life, he had, it seems, married, and now his wife has died. It is hard not to see the sudden reappearance of the love theme – and its reappearance in a dream vision, the classic figure of reappearance in the genre – as a deliberate comment on the long thematic detour the poet has taken away from love, as well as on the larger significance of the theme itself.

That the dream conceit is here used in the service of a widower's pain, rather than a young man's choices, hopes, and desires, can, in addition, be read as a deliberate comment on the earlier English tendency to literalize the Petrarchan situation and, in particular, on Spenser's decision to make it apply to marriage in his narrative coupling of the *Amoretti* with his "Epithalamion." The poem seems designed – along with the web of associations produced by the fact that, as we shall see, Milton echoes it at a crucial moment in *Paradise Lost* – to make the conceits of the Petrarchan tradition, within the larger theological context suggested by his epic, bear representation of the tragic, literal realities of postlapsarian procreation as experienced by a married, Protestant Londoner. Milton, like all of his predecessors, ends his sequence in a state of profound suspension. Even Spenser ends his *sequence* that way, providing consummation only in the appended marriage song (which, of course, includes a prayer for fertility). Dante, of course, famously ended *La Vita Nuova* with a promise, in the wake of Beatrice's death, to write something of her that had never before been written of a woman. He makes her his psychopomp in the *Commedia*, fulfilling in his epic narrative the suspended promise of his sequence. Milton, in imitation of both Dante and Spenser, also projects the consummation of his own suspended ending forward beyond the text of the sequence proper, in this case into *Paradise Lost*, which will detail not only how the bereaved mourner got into his situation (how all human beings became subject to grief), but also how he, and all other human beings, can and must live with grief and, finally (hopefully) transcend it. The trajectory is aimed textually forward, but historically backward, to the marriage of Adam and Eve, and only then forward again to the painfully literal context of Milton's own wrecked, mortal marriages and the lonely bed in which he also claimed to dream – and may have in part dictated – the epic itself.

This progression suggests that a complex reading can be made of the sonnet's allusions both back through the Petrarchan tradition and forward into the epic. And we are helped in this task by a pair of echoes so close and so pointed in their suggestiveness that it is impossible to see them as accidents. As several critics and editors have noted over the years, the sonnet not only echoes the dream-vision conceit itself, but also the first line of a well-known example: Ralegh's dedicatory poem to *The Faerie Queene*, "Methought I saw the grave where Laura lay." Ralegh's poem is like a signpost pointing down the road of the poem's generic history, and our entrance forward into *Paradise Lost* is similarly guided by an echo: the echo of the first and last lines of the sonnet in the framing lines of Milton's description of the creation of Eve at 8.462–3 and 478, which we will discuss in detail in the last section of this chapter.

Milton's echo of Ralegh's opening line brings the Petrarchan legacy of his poem full-circle, back to "the grave where Laura lay," only to have the poet discover not only his own precedence over the achievement of Petrarch, but to discover that that precedence is now in a terrible way signified by the body of his own dead wife, the cost, as it were, of literalizing Petrarchan ideals in the representation of an actual, and, of course, *earthly*, marriage. Petrarchan suspension, as in Spenser's "Epithalamion," is here consummated in marriage, or it was at some unrecorded narrative point between the time of the sixth and the twenty-third sonnet. In Milton's poem, however, the suspension is then reinstated. It is now associated with the span of time that unfolds before the speaker as he faces the burden of continued life in darkness (with only his trust in a future reunion to uphold him). What we see here is also a reworking of the topos of the funereal wedding he made use of in the epitaph for Jane Paulet, although in this case it has become a funereal *marriage*, in fact *two* marriages, both of which have ended the way the Paulets' did. In this case, again, it will be necessary (though far more difficult) to frame the deaths in a redemptive, consoling way. The death that is exiled from epithalamic discourse in its conventional functioning – and that Milton had represented in its consoling, redeemed aspect almost thirty years earlier – returns here in the ghostly figure of the veiled woman who is not only a visionary figure, but an earthly spouse who also was – or in the vision resembles – a churched mother.

As Jonathan Goldberg, and more recently Elizabeth Harvey, have noted, the allusion to Ralegh suggests that the intertextual relationship be read as an instance of poetic rivalry.[82] There is clearly even more at work here, however, than is suggested by either Goldberg's rather abstract Derridian and Bloomian meditation, or by Harvey's more historically and psychologically complex contention that the body of the dead wife is here being made the ground

[82] Sokol also notes the allusion ("Euripides' *Alcestis* and the Saint," 141).

upon which Milton converts his wives' capacities "for giving birth into a capacity for poetic renewal, a transposition from female procreation to male creativity."[83] Harvey has her finger on an important dynamic, but it should be noted that the appropriation of female procreative power could not have seemed to Milton unambiguously empowering in this context. Both of his wives had died in the process of enacting that power, and it seems clear that Milton, in using the figure of birth in the sonnet, expresses anxiety over whether or not he can in fact wield such power safely and successfully himself. The worry is similar to the one that governed "On Shakespear," but here his relationship to and understanding of female experience has changed and deepened. He approaches the fact that he is not a woman, and can reproduce as females do only by means of poetic representation, as less an occasion for appropriation of their power than an occasion for both lamentation and guilt-laden relief over his own lack.

Goldberg's association of Milton's anxiety in both poems with the effacing power of the sign is, I think, also compelling. However, it is weakened by his failure to see the poem as referring to something other than the act of writing. In "An Epitaph," by tying Lady Jane's experience to the death of Rachel and the apotheosis of Beatrice, Milton too explicitly tied his aggressive generic revision, his youthful ambitions and anxieties, with his praise of Lady Jane. The invocation of Dante's potent achievement in Christian epic did offer him a way of asserting poetic value in the face of the death, but it could also be argued that he too easily and too quickly appropriated female reproductive heroism to his own vocational concerns, and that, as a young poet, he had not yet earned the right to such an appropriation. He also, as we have seen, dwelled too confidently in that early poem on the power of poetry to console in the face of childbed loss. He had even, if Frost is right about his approach to John Paulet, blamed the husband and his family's dynastic ambitions for the death, while implicitly identifying himself with the power of Jane's religious self-sacrifice. In the face of her mortal suffering and that of her infant and her family, he asserted that they both had produced a perfect, immortal child: she in her deed, he in his representation of it. The sonnet, however, is quite different in a number of ways. It is not only far more disruptive of the generic conventions in which it participates, but, in effect, it calls upon childbed experience in order to offer the reality of a catastrophic birth as a way of adding a new chapter to the development of (and the proper passing on of) Petrarchism within the English tradition.

83 Elizabeth D. Harvey, *Ventriloquized Voices: Feminist Theory and English Renaissance Texts* (London: Routledge, 1992), p. 101.

The sonnet also makes personal bereavement a sign of a new-found but more ambivalently embraced form of poetic power. Poised between Petrarchan sequence and epic, the poem concentrates in a new way upon the problem of how to assert a proper Christian consolation in the face of childbed suffering.[84] The sonnet's answer to that problem, as it projects itself forward into *Paradise Lost*, is far more equivocal than the ones Milton offered his readers in the 1630s.

"WIDE WAS THE WOUND"

While images of reproduction have long been recognized as centrally important to *Paradise Lost*, there are two episodes whose images stand out as particularly direct evocations of human birth itself. These are the allegory of Sin and Death (2.648–870) and Adam's description of the creation of Eve (8.452–85). The allegory, as we will see in Chapter 8, is the most important of a handful of passages in the epic that evoke the pains and dangers of fallen childbirth, and it does so in terms deliberately and specifically evocative of seventeenth-century obstetric conditions, setting off a dark chain of associations in the epic. Adam's account of Eve's creation, on the other hand, might be called that passage's bright twin. It beautifully and evocatively describes an act of creation whose only witness experiences it as the summation of all that God, in His goodness, has planned for His universe. However, the passage is also seeded with allusions and images that associate it with fallen childbirth, and this gives the episode a curiously mixed, affective quality. The echoes of the sonnet (the primary ones at 462–3 and 478 and the secondary ones at 461, 482, and 484–5) are, in particular, alive to the implications of a powerful ambivalence, bringing the allusive structure and occasion of the sonnet to mind, and forcing a number of points in scriptural history, literary history, and biography to stand together tensely.[85]

[84] My reading differs to some extent from one offered by John Rumrich, who suggests that the connection between the epic and the sonnet is one of "heroic resistance" to death and oblivion as figured in the maternal woman, "a resolution to go on living in the darkness of this world" and to "deliver an epic conceived in the realm of dreams" (Rumrich, *Milton Unbound*, p. 89, drawing on Hammond, *Fleeting Things*, p. 216). There is certainly something heroic in the sonnet's frank embrace of loss. What this embrace sets the stage for, however, is a confrontation with the question of whether or not a full recognition of such a loss is at all compatible with consolation. See below.

[85] The echoes have been noted, but little discussed. Edward Le Comte is one of the few critics who deals with them at any length, but he was uncertain about their significance: see Edward Le Comte *Yet Once More: Verbal and Psychological Pattern in Milton* (New York, NY: AMS, 1969), pp. 16–17. The Richardsons noticed the similarity in motif, but said nothing about the verbal echoes: see J. Richardson, Father and Son, *Explanatory Notes and Remarks on Milton's* Paradise Lost (London, 1734), p. 376.

John Shawcross has noted that the central lines of Adam's account mark the epic's golden section, suggesting that Milton considered it crucial to its structure.[86] John Rumrich goes so far as to call the nativity of Eve "a mythopoeic axis upon which the epic, and the encyclopedic knowledge it deploys, turns." He notes that various and "sometimes irreconcilable" spheres of association revolve uneasily around the episode, especially those concerning generation in its various forms, from sexual reproduction to the "*poesis* of creation" itself.[87] In the following pages, I will argue that among these "spheres of association" is that of the childbirth consolations and conditions we explored in Part I of this study. Milton evokes the childbirth discourses not only by echoing the sonnet, but by making the episode uncannily suggestive of both what birth could have been and what it became. Susan McDonald, for example, has suggested that the passage is as close as we get in the epic to a depiction of a prelapsarian birth, a fantastic vision of what birth might have been like had the Fall not occurred.[88] The fact, however, that it is a man who "gives birth" in the episode, rather than a woman, also associates the passage with Milton's early conflation of platonic reproduction and maternal mortality in "On Shakespear," as well as his revisions of that figuration in "An Epitaph" and the final scene of *A Mask*. Even more strikingly, as we will see, Adam's description of Eve's creation suggests some of the most painful and frightening aspects of seventeenth-century obstetrical surgery. Coming at such a crucial point in the epic, these echoes and allusions have wide-ranging implications for our understanding of the epic's theological and psychological dynamics.

Here is the passage itself:

> Hee ended, or I heard no more, for now
> My earthly by his Heav'nly overpowerd,
> Which it had long stood under, streind to th'highth
> In that celestial Colloquie sublime,
> As with an object that excels the sense,
> Dazl'd and spent, sunk down, and sought repair
> Of sleep, which instantly fell on me, call'd
> By Nature as in aid, and clos'd mine eyes.
> Mine eyes he clos'd, but op'n left the Cell

86 Shawcross, "The Centrality of Book 8."

87 Rumrich, *Milton Unbound*, p. 117. See also Gordon Teskey, *Delirious Milton: the Fate of the Poet in Modernity* (Cambridge, MA: Harvard University Press, 2006), pp. 107–28.

88 Susan McDonald, "'Wide Was the Wound': Cesarean Section and the Birth of Eve," in *Living Texts: Interpreting Milton*, eds. Kristin A. Pruitt and Charles W. Durham (Selinsgrove, PA: Susquehanna University Press, 2000), pp. 80–98. McDonald expands on remarks I made about the passage in 1993, providing more evidence that Milton drew on childbirth lore and practice. See also Rumrich, *Milton Unbound*, pp. 109–17.

Of Fancie my internal sight, by which
Abstract as in a transe methought I saw,
Though sleeping, where I lay, and saw the shape
Still glorious before whom awake I stood;
Who stooping op'n'd my left side, and took
From thence a Rib, with cordial spirits warm,
And Life-blood streaming fresh; wide was the wound,
But suddenly with flesh fill'd up and heal'd:
The Rib he formd and fashiond with his hands;
Under his forming hands a Creature grew,
Manlike, but different sex, so lovely fair,
That what seemd fair in all the World, seemd now
Mean, or in her summ'd up, in her containd
And in her looks, which from that time infus'd
Sweetness into my heart, unfelt before,
And into all things from her Air inspir'd
The spirit of love and amorous delight.
Shee disappeerd, and left me dark, I wak'd
To find her, or for ever to deplore
Her loss, and other pleasures all abjure:
When out of hope, behold her, not farr off,
Such as I saw her in my dream, adornd
With what all Earth or Heaven could bestow
To make her amiable: On she came,
Led by her Heav'nly Maker (*PL*, 8.452–85)

Perhaps the first thing worth noting here, in addition to the direct verbal echoes, is that Milton chose to frame the episode as another version of the motif that he used to frame his sonnet. The passage therefore not only alludes to the sonnet itself, but also to the same long line of stories about the appearance and disappearance of a beloved woman that forms the primary literary backdrop of that poem. Here, however, the motif is structured comedically. What is traditionally (in poems like Sonnet 23) depicted by a speaker as tragic, or at best as an uncertain fantasy that arises from the speaker's unfulfilled longing, here ends happily. Unlike Aeneas's encounter with Creusa's ghost,[89] for example, or any number of appearances and disappearances in the Petrarchan tradition (including, of course, the one depicted in the sonnet), Eve appears before Adam not as an image of a lost and now painfully remembered woman, but as an answer to his desire for partnership. And she turns out to be very real, present, and available.

[89] Thomas B. Stroup, "Aeneas' Vision of Creusa and Milton's Twenty-Third Sonnet," *Philological Quarterly* 39 (1960), 125–6.

Even more striking, however, are some of the details Milton includes along the way to this happy ending. Adam falls asleep and is given visions twice in the course of the narrative he recounts for Raphael. The first time comes after he falls asleep exhausted by his first experiences of "lively vigour" (8.267–92). God appears to Adam as an "inward apparition," and he is then flown to Eden, a place even more beautiful than where he was first created. He is allowed to see the entire flight as if it were happening in a dream, but when he awakens he finds it all "real, as the dream/ Had lively shadowed," a perfect fulfillment of his earlier sense that he was happier than he knew (8.282, 292–311). In the case of Eve's creation, he again falls asleep in exhaustion (this time due to the strain of his colloquy with God). And, again, he is allowed to witness, while asleep, what happens next: another indication of even greater happiness, the creation of the very "likeness" and "fit help" he had described to God just a few minutes earlier. He falls in love, of course, with the creature who emerges, but then God does something surprising. He takes her away. In an astonishing echo of the motif as it is found in the sonnet, Eve disappears, leaving Adam briefly in darkness. Even more striking is the fact that when he awakens, he finds her not there, but still gone, and the horrible moment lasts long enough for him to actually begin despairing of ever seeing her again. Only then does she finally reappear, "such as [he] saw her," in the dream (8.478–85), and only then does the narrative steer seamlessly into its joyful epithalamic conclusion, bringing us to the marriage bower and to Adam's praise of sexual intimacy, which he describes as "the sum" of his "earthly bliss" (8.522).

There are a number of reasons why Milton decided to have God include a heart-stopping loss (which is then quickly restored) in the middle of Adam's first blissful experience of Eve. Part of its function is proleptic. It adds a painful, dramatic tension to the narrative by foreshadowing what we know will come later. Adam's subsequent description of the power of passion, as many critics have noted, reveals an instability in the consummated ending of this episode. It is not, however, simply passion itself, but Adam's passionate *attachment* to Eve that will leave him vulnerable in his later trial. God has deliberately vexed Adam's first experience of desire and fulfillment with an urgent fear of what we would today call "object loss," and it is this fear in particular that will later lead him to choose hastily to fall with Eve rather than face the possibility of losing her again (he already knows, after all, how it feels to lose a beloved – and, to put it simply, he didn't like it).[90]

[90] This sense probably also affects Adam's desire to keep Eve by his side on the morning of the Fall, and so his subsequent encounter with her would have seemed a fulfillment of his worst apprehensions. This, in turn, we can imagine, increased the sense of urgency that led him to make his fatal choice.

The proleptic loss also links the passage even more closely to the sonnet, and therefore to Milton's own experiences, as well as to his earlier treatments of the childbed discourses, and it does so as part of an elaborate allusive scheme. The passage is actually one of a number of passages in *Paradise Lost* that allude to precursor texts in a way designed to assert Milton's prior authority.[91] In this case, Milton's purpose is to establish the priority of his epic's account of human love over those of the traditions of love lyric and love narrative that he has inherited. He is recounting, after all, what he would have us believe was the moment at which the whole dynamic of desire, loss, and either longed-for or fulfilled reunion was not only first experienced, but first represented in language by a male human being. Adam's account is the first love story told by a man, and it ends with the first epithalamion.[92] Milton's use of the motif of appearance and disappearance for the depiction of such an inaugural moment suggests that all "later" versions of the motif, including that of Sonnet 23, as well as the comedic versions found in intertexts like those of *La Vita Nuova* and the *Commedia* and Spenser's *Amoretti* and "Epithalmion," are merely imperfect echoes of what Adam was actually the first to experience and depict.

Milton's inclusion of the moment of loss in this important etiological passage suggests that for him the experience of male heterosexual desire included both loss and gain in some irreducible way. The structure and verbal texture of the account also suggests that, for him, the experience was irreducibly concerned with reproduction. As I said before, the passage contains a number of allusions to childbirth trauma in addition to its complex echo of the sonnet, and together these serve to heighten the trepidation the episode expresses, making its positive valences affectively unstable. Most importantly, they ultimately suggest that the ensuing narrative is going to be more difficult than its protagonists can yet imagine, not just for them but for their progeny (among whom, of course, is the narrator/poet himself). Even if the possibility of a final glory will ultimately be offered to humankind, that glory will only come in the wake of very difficult trials, and the shape of those trials – their close relationship to the outcomes of the bliss that Adam feels at the beginning of his relationship with Eve – is signaled to us in the way Adam's "prior," comedic episode is seeded with an incipient awareness of later pains and losses. In other words, Adam, as both

[91] On this dynamic, see Harold Bloom, *A Map of Misreading* (Oxford University Press, 1975), pp. 125–43.

[92] Eve's earlier account of her own awakening, delivered to Adam the day before, is interestingly devoid of this dynamic of desire and loss, although the love lyric she recites for him before they go to bed that night does register her sense of what the world would be like for her without him (*PL*, 4.449–91, 641–56).

the first man and as a metonymy for all later men, is happier, but also more unfortunate, than he knows. Milton imagines the first man's fragile condition from a dark and uncertain point in a difficult future – a point after which the wide wound that God opened and closed so miraculously in Adam's side will be opened again in a different way, and well before it is filled-up again and healed.

"METHOUGHT I SAW..."

The echoes of the sonnet themselves are central to the larger implications of this dynamic, so they are worth examining in some detail. The first, the echo of the sonnet's first line at lines 462–3 ("methought I saw,/ Though sleeping, where I lay"), is very close, although there are some important differences. The first four syllables are, of course, the same, although the syntax of the whole differs, and the rest of the syllables, which are displaced over a line break, only echo their counterparts in terms of rhythm, number, and an array of repeated consonants and vowels. The placement of the line-break is itself significant, marking the point at which exact repetition gives way to a subtle play of pararhymes. Also, the last six syllables of the sonnet's first line provide a clear object for the opening main clause ("I thought I saw my saint"), and the object is then modified by the prepositional phrase and comparison offered in line 2 ("I thought I saw her brought to me like Alcestis"). The syntax of Adam's speech is less clear. Depending on how you read the comma before "where I lay," the "methought I saw" of line 462 may or may not have a direct object. Adam is either saying simply that, lying there, he could see, despite being asleep, or he is saying that, despite being asleep, he could see the *place* where he was lying.[93]

The differences are suggestive. In his speech, Adam is telling Raphael about what to him seemed a paradox: the fact that he could see while (or where) he was lying "as in a transe." His eyes were shut, only his internal "Cell/ Of Fancie" was open, and through it he seemed able either to perceive external events he could not see physically, or to receive dream-like impressions of them provided by God. In the sonnet, the speaker is not remarking explicitly on a strange experience, but recounting what is for him (and us) the familiar human experience of ordinary dreaming – something with which Adam is not yet all that familiar. Even if we are aware of the poet's blindness, and attribute that to the speaker, therefore adding stress to "saw" in order to register that fact that this speaker could see in his dream,

93 Hollander briefly notes the ambiguity (*The Work of Poetry*, p. 84).

even though he could not see while awake, we would still have to distinguish his painful experience from Adam's. Blindness would no doubt have made the sonnet speaker's dreaming different from the dreaming of the sighted in an important and especially poignant way, but in others it would still be very much like the dreams most of us have all the time. The primary purpose of the sonnet's first line is therefore to present, simply (if dramatically), the object of this particular instance of dreamed sight (the "espoused saint"). When Adam had his dream, on the other hand, he had had only one before. Both of these first two dreams also immediately come true, and neither have any of the abiding uncertainty that characterizes ordinary human dreaming. The night before the events of Books 5 through 8, Eve had certainly had a more conventional-seeming dream (*PL*, 4.799–809, 5.28–94), and she and Adam had puzzled over its nature and implications just that morning – neither she nor Adam ever discover that her dream was created by Satan. It is possible that Adam also had a few other dreams since his first day of existence, but no others are mentioned. The experience is, in any case, still rather new at the end of Book 8, and is still the source, it seems, of not a little wonder.

The experience is familiar to us, of course, not only from our own dreams, but from the literary traditions of the representation of dreaming, and a knowledge of both experience and tradition informs the sonnet-speaker's narrative as well as that of the narrator/poet who tells us what the first man said to the angel. Indeed, part of the narrator/poet's purpose here is to suggest that this moment is not only the original of both a certain kind of male desire and a certain kind of dream about desire, but also of what would later become a time-worn literary motif. In the sonnet, we are invited immediately to identify with the speaker and his experience (it is like ours, even if we have not had a dream quite like this particular one). Our relationship to Adam's narrative, however, is a good deal more complex. In so far as we associate the narrator of *Paradise Lost* with Milton, we are invited to distinguish between Adam's naive telling, which is infused with wonder both at the event and at the language he is coming up with at that moment to describe it, and the narrator/poet's different and very painful investment in the very same things. Such a distinction still holds if we read the sonnet, following Spitzer,[94] as having no specific biographical reference (the speaker remains a fallen man). Such distinctions allow us also to register the distance between the freshness of all of Adam's experiences (what he saw, what he felt, what he said, and even what it felt like to say it) and those

[94] Spitzer, "Understanding Milton."

of Milton and ourselves generations and generations later, subject, as we all are, to severe physical limitations and frailties and operating within a history not only of loss, but also the representation of loss.

The later echo of the sonnet at line 478, "She disappeerd, and left me dark, I wak'd," intensifies this aspect of the intertext. It is less close than the first echo to its corresponding line in the sonnet, "I wak'd, she fled, and day brought back my night." However, it still tellingly echoes, in its last six syllables, the monosyllabics of the poem's final line, and it neatly reverses the painful sequence suggested by the sonnet's conclusion (she disappeared first, then he awoke). Furthermore, the final verb of Adam's line is tied to a syntactic sequence that extends through his few despairing moments to this final happy exclamation of "behold her," which then leads us right to another echo of the sonnet: "Behold her, not farr off,/ *Such as I saw her* in my dream" (my italics) (lines 481–2). These lines provide the fulfillment, albeit temporarily, of the desire that Milton's sonnet speaker expresses so hopefully in lines 7–8 ("And such, as yet once more I trust to have/ Full sight of her in heav'n without restraint"). It is also significant that the first thing that Adam sees Eve do after her reappearance is come toward him. This also echoes important details of the sonnet. Lines 484–5 ("On she came,/ Led by her Heav'nly Maker...") echo two important verbs in the sonnet's opening descriptions of the late espoused saint (that, at line 2, she is described as having been "brought" – and later given – by Herakles, and that, at line 5, we are told she "*came* vested all in white" [my italics]). In addition, both poem and passage are structured around the juxtaposition of temporary or illusory arrivals with permanent (or at least more permanent) ones. In the sonnet, the active verb "came" implies something better and higher than the passive "brought," associating the saint's purity and personal virtues, which are described after the verb itself arrives, with the salvation and reunion in the afterlife that are described just before the verb. The passive and even objectifying verbs, which make her seem a gift or object of exchange between two men, adhere only to the mythic and, for Milton illusory, allusion. The higher apprehension does give way to loss after the failed embrace reveals the dream's ephemeral nature, but the future is still something that inspires the speaker's hopeful trust. In Adam's account, on the other hand, the re-arrival of Eve is a true and present restoration (at least for the time being), and it includes both the self-possessed and active sense of "came," along with a clarified version of the passive sense of "brought." In Adam's case, it is God, not the mythical, if typological, Herakles who is the agent, and his action has become a leading, rather than a bringing and giving, suggesting guidance of Eve rather than her objectification as a gift for Adam.

It is striking how closely plotted these echoes are. Even the syntax reinforces the ways in which Milton has adapted the motif to two distinct but closely related purposes. In the sonnet, lines 7–8 constitute the second of two dependent clauses that delay the arrival of the verb at the heart of the long sentence that winds from the beginning of line 5 to the end of line 9, overrunning the octave/sestet break. The conventional turning-point of the sonnet is therefore unconventionally marked by the punningly delayed arrival of the verb "came," which only comes, as it were, finally fulfilling our syntactic expectations, at the start of line 9, exactly where sonnet form would lead us to instead expect a turn of the conclusion of the second quatrain's attenuated main clause ("Mine…Came"). The actual turn does not occur, if it is a turn at all, until line 10, with the slightly unexpected "Her face was vail'd," which almost sounds like a response to an "off-stage" biographical query ("so, which spouse was it?" "I don't know, her face was veiled"). Or perhaps no turn occurs until line 12, where the speaker's exclamation brings us to the final painful twist of the narrative.

This is more than just a subversion of the expectations of sonnet structure. The extension of the second period of the poem beyond the end of its second quatrain delays the completion of the sonnet's account of the saint's first action within the dream. Her arrival is presented to us, as I said, at first passively (she is "*brought*…like Alcestis" [my italics]). Then, at line 5, the speaker returns from his first extended comparison to emphasize certain ways in which *his* envisioned wife actually differed from Alcestis ("mine" asserts both *whose* she is and *that* she is therefore different – she is real, for one thing, although no longer alive, and even more importantly, she is Christian). In the lines that follow, he maintains the syntactic suspension I have just described all the way through his Old Testament comparison and his expression of trust that he will see her again in the future, when she will actually look just as she only seems to look now. We are given the emphatically possessive pronoun, but no verb (that is, until we have gone by way of analogy and faithful imagination first back to the Old Law and then forward into Christian salvation). Only at that point is her arrival presented actively rather than passively.

As I said before, the active voice is designed perhaps to mark the higher, freer nature of the redeemed state to come, but the fact that the vision and its climactic, active verb takes up the *middle*, rather than the end, of the sonnet serves to emphasize for us the fact that the speaker knows he has not really seen his saint at all, only that he has imagined her. This is, in part, what makes the sudden, uncertain disclaimer, "Her face was vail'd," so poignant. He has not seen her "face to face" in the dream. True sight, true presence, even knowledge of who she was, will only come later, in the future that he hopes will conclude his larger story. At this moment, however, he knows that his sonnet, with perfect generic propriety, is a representation of his ongoing, mortal condition, and cannot end with such a consummation. In a sense, the expectations of the genre, despite the internal subversions of its structural expectations, which run ahead of and gesture beyond the generic frame, ultimately mark the limits of what the speaker believes we can expect in his mortal life.

In the epic's etiological account, however, the sonnet speaker's hoped for conclusion has been displaced from the middle of the narrative and moved to its consummated end. It is not part of the description of Eve's appearance, but of her later reappearance, and this is part of what makes the episode not just comedic in comparison with the sonnet, but in some sense directly redemptive of its darkness and pain. It is as if we were meant to read this after the sonnet and feel the speaker's pain ameliorated by the revision (that is, until we are forced to contemplate the historical relationship between the two texts). At that point, aspects of the sonnet's version of the motif, which still echo in the darkness at the middle of Adam's account, assert themselves. "Left me dark" (line 478), for example, is a reminder of the sonnet speaker's "night," the later mortal darkness that was only momentarily enlightened by the dream (and perhaps also of Milton's blindness). For Adam, of course, this darkness describes a brief and temporary state of loss, not a physical state briefly alleviated only to return to last prospectively until the trusted ressurrection. Still, the feeling of the dark moment – and later its memory – troubles Adam's state of happiness, reminding us that his short moment of loss foreshadows the greater mortal losses to which he, in his panicked weakness, will later consign both himself and all later human beings (Milton in particular). And, of course, it matters that Eve's own fall, which Adam chooses to share, will make her mortal in a way that will later painfully affect what it would be like to be married.

The passage in Book 8 also includes another ambiguous revision of another important element of the sonnet's conclusion, one even more closely related to childbed anxiety and guilt. Although Milton repeats the vanishing here, it is significant that he does not repeat the word "fled," which had carried so much of the burden of masculine guilt in the sonnet. He uses instead the more neutral "disappeerd," which can refer to either Adam's or Eve's perspective, and has none of the connotations of projected fear that haunt the sonnet's final lines.[95] The word also obscures God's

[95] My thanks to John Shawcross for his comments on the distinction.

agency. We can assume that God is the one who made Eve disappear from Adam, but such a thought does not seem to have occurred to Adam himself in any conscious or clear way. He simply reports what he "saw," then did not see, then saw again, and the disappearance is described as a thing that happened *to him*, rather than as something *done* to him *by someone*. The obscuring of agency (either she chose to do it at that moment for some reason, or God simply made it happen for reasons of His own) lightens the emotional weight of the moment. It also, however, burdens it with suggestions of later actions that are just as, if not more, painful. Not only does it suggest the active flight of Milton's dreamed-of wife or wives, but Eve's later leaving on the morning of the Fall, her choice to fall itself, his angry repelling of her first attempt at reconciliation with an exclamation of "out of my sight" (*PL*, 10.867), and even her possible death before his at some future point.

The fact that Eve says nothing about this disappearance in her own account of her creation (*PL*, 4.449–91) is also interesting. According to that account, she was not, apparently, aware of anything prior to her own awakening on a bank of flowers after being removed (presumably unconsciously) from Adam's presence. The disappearance, therefore, seems wholly an experience that God has designed for Adam. This suggests, I believe, that Milton has created the episode to correspond to, and in part explain, something that he felt was at the heart of the male experience of heterosexual desire, something drawn from his own experience and psychology and extrapolated into a general condition. Both Eve's and Adam's accounts combine desire and reproduction, although the sequence and some of the terms are significantly different. In Book 4, upon awakening and after being allowed to view and fall in love with her own image, Eve is told that she must encounter a different kind of image (in a partner both like and unlike herself). However, she at first famously rejects Adam, preferring her own image, and it is only when he seizes her hand and she yields to him (*PL*, 4.488–9) that she comes to desire him as he desires her right from the start. At that point, she also implicitly accepts her identity as a mother of "Multitudes" who will be both like herself and more real than the watery reflection she at first found so compelling. In other words, in her account, a desire for sameness gives way – at first unstably – to a desire for sameness in difference, which then leads to motherhood, which is ambiguously marked by an experience of both desire and submission. Although they are presented here in a positive and erotically charged manner, it is no coincidence that all three of these things will appear again in negative terms in the curse to which she and all women will later become subject.

Adam, however, experiences a desire for a corresponding other first, and this desire is furthermore awakened by a sense of lack that he is given plenty of time to discover for himself. He is then allowed, after articulating his desires clearly to God, to witness the creation of his same but different partner ("Manlike, but different sex," as he puts it at 8.471) in a way that suggests both a birth (a figurative maternal experience) and Milton's own later childbed losses. He then loses her himself before gaining her back again.[96] In other words, reproduction is central to both narratives, and both bear signs of later childbed trauma. Only Adam's, however, is marked by signs of traumatic object loss.

READING ADAM'S DREAM AS A BIRTH-NARRATIVE

As I mentioned earlier, Susan McDonald has pointedly observed that, although the birth is clearly not "normal" by any stretch of the imagination, Adam's dream narration describes the only human birth in the epic.[97] The "abnormalities" are uncanny, although presented positively, and they have important thematic and emotional resonances. Not only does a man, not a woman, give birth in the passage, but that man, while he is attended in the process by a midwife figure (as most women were in the seventeenth century), the midwife is no mortal woman, no pagan or literary Lucina, nor, of course, Atropos with a pair of shears, but God Himself. The man also experiences no pain, and he is spared (or deprived of) the experience of having another human being gestate inside his body. In a physically concrete version of the process of imagination that Milton explored years earlier in "On Shakespear," Adam conceives of and gestates, in colloquy with God, an idea of the creature to whom he finally gives birth. The language that Adam uses in lines 452–9 is even interestingly suggestive of the exhausted aftermath of an overwhelming sexual act, and it is important that the material from which Eve is made actually emerges from within his own body. Her physical development, however, takes place outside that body, while he lies on the ground in a trance, a passive witness. The process is also

96 My approach to these passages and their discrepancies has been deeply influenced by W. Gardner Campbell, "Hierarchy, Alterity, and Freedom in *Paradise Lost*," in *Milton's Legacy*, eds. Kristin A. Pruitt and Charles W. Durham (Selinsgrove, PA: Susquehanna University Press, 2005), pp. 50–69, and Ronald Levao, "'Among Unequals What Society': *Paradise Lost* and the Forms of Intimacy," *Modern Language Quarterly* 61 (2000), 79–107. However, see also Peter Herman, *Destabilizing Milton*: Paradise Lost *and the Poetics of Incertitude* (New York, NY: Palgrave, 2005), pp. 53–4 and Elizabeth Sauer's extensive discussion of both narratives in *Barbarous Dissonance and Images of Voice in Milton's Epics* (Montreal, QB: McGill-Queen's University Press, 1996), pp. 97–110.

97 McDonald, "'Wide Was the Wound,'" pp. 84–5, 94–5.

rapid, taking no more, it seems, than a few moments. McDonald is surely correct that – distant though it is from the physical conditions of normal human birth (in fact, in part *because of* that distance) – the episode gives us our only glimpse of what Milton imagined was the lost perfection that birth was to have had in Eden. In other words, it reflects aspects, although not all aspects, of what might have been Eve's experience had the Fall not taken place.

As McDonald observes, Milton was constrained by his biblical source. He could not show Eve giving birth before the Fall, and was perhaps therefore inspired to use this episode to suggest what was lost with the institution of her curse.[98] In presenting such a birth, however, Milton also chose not only details designed to evoke his own personal losses in the childbed, but general contemporary obstetric conditions as well. The language of the passage suggests, in particular, surgical procedures (caesarian-section and the removal of a dead infant by crochet) that almost always had tragic associations in contemporary contexts. As we saw in Chapter 2, having to undergo either procedure was among the key nightmares for any laboring woman. Caesarian section was performed only when a mother had actually died or, in rare cases, was dying. Extraction by crochet, on the other hand, involved surgical dismemberment and removal of the dead infant's body through the vagina of a woman who was herself still alive. An announcement that such a procedure was necessary not only announced that the child had died, but almost always also meant the eventual death of the mother, often due to lacerations leading to infection or hemorrhage. The emotional impact of having to undergo such a procedure can be easily imagined. It is also worth remembering that the physical dangers were often exacerbated by the pressures that caused midwives to delay calling on a male surgeon (a desire to keep the female exclusivity of the rites intact, concerns over the psychological and spiritual state of the mother, etc.), and that such delays often meant that the woman was in a severely weakened condition by the time a surgeon would have begun working.[99]

Milton could very well have had descriptions of such procedures and cases in mind as he imagined Adam's experience of God's "surgical" removal of the rib. McDonald notes, in particular, that Milton's decision to have

[98] McDonald, "'Wide Was the Wound,'" pp. 94–5.

[99] For more details, see McDonald, "Wide Was the Wound," pp. 87–90; Schwartz, "Spot of child-bed taint"; Renate Blumenfeld-Kosinski, *Not of Woman Born: Representations of Caesarean Birth in Medieval and Renaissance Culture* (Ithaca, NY: Cornell University Press, 1990), pp. 61–91, and Chapter 2, above.

Adam specify the side from which God extracted the rib (the left) was likely determined by *both* a set of traditional symbolic significances and a specific medical reference. The left side is nearest Adam's heart and has traditionally "sinister" associations, but it is also the side that most surgical manuals said was the best for a caesarian-section incision.[100] In other words, Milton's portrayal of Eve's creation, particularly the portrayal of God's opening a "wide wound" in Adam's side and then removing a rib, "with life-blood streaming fresh," would have suggested to contemporary readers not so much the activities of a midwife, but a strangely idealized version of an obstetric surgeon, a man whose activities would have been in actuality physically terrifying, emotionally overwhelming, and an intrusion into the female world of the lying-in chamber. All of this would have brought to mind some of the most powerful tensions and anxieties at work in the contemporary experience of childbirth.[101]

Milton's choice of reproductive resonances may also have been affected by the general exclusion of men from the birthing chamber. The figure of a male birth in the passage has struck some as an example of a male poet's fantasy of appropriating female creative power, or as part of a Miltonic impulse to idealize a purely masculine Eden before the creation of what Adam later calls the "fair defect" of Eve (a prolepsis, in other words, of Adam's later misogynistic regret that Eve had ever been created [*PL*, 10.888–908]). These may very well have been significant factors in Milton's conception of the passage. I do not, however, agree with the notion expressed in Elizabeth Harvey's very brief remark about the passage in *Ventriloquized Voices*: that the displacement of woman from the subject position of the caesarian birth offers "a metaphoric fantasy ... of a birth that bypasse[s] nature and the female body."[102] McDonald suggests, I think more plausibly, that the figure of male birth in the passage allows men the fantasy of being both witness to and the subject of a birth, not so that they can appropriate the powers it represents, but to intensify the reader's sense that pain in birth *included* men, especially given the "self-conscious anxiety" with which, she reminds us, they witnessed such events from afar under contemporary conditions.[103] The fact that the male "mother" here experiences no pain might also reflect directly on

100 McDonald, "'Wide Was the Wound,'" pp. 90–3.

101 Milton may also have been aware of a connection between iconographic renderings of the Genesis story and manuscript illuminations of the birth of Caesar, as well as certain literary and theological implications commonly attached to caesarian-section, including Christological and hagiographic lore concerning miraculous caesarians performed by saints and traditions that claimed that the Anti-Christ would come into the world in this way. On these, see Blumenfeld-Kosinski, *Not of Woman Born*, pp. 73, 120–42, 172.

102 Harvey, *Ventriloquized Voices*, p. 150, n. 9.

103 McDonald, "'Wide Was the Wound,'" pp. 93–4.

Milton's acute sense of the exemption of men from such pain. It is perhaps a guilty reflection on the fact that, later in the story, only women will become subject to such suffering (although, men, of course, will still be subject to loss). It is for all these reasons that the depiction of a fantastic, idealized male birth in the Edenic past is shot through with trapdoor allusions to a nightmarish present reality.

In any case, the passage is clearly fraught with a complex psychological burden that resonates not only with Milton's biography, but with the wider material and literary context he inhabited. It is also aimed at a key aspect of its author's larger intention: to force older epic conventions to the new task of expressing a Prostestant theodicy, including a subtext designed to ameliorate childbed suffering. In this passage, Milton intends nothing less than a description of the inauguration of human sexual life from the male perspective. This key etiological passage, in presenting a nostalgic fantasy as a prolepsis of its own loss, is designed not just to recall lost happiness, but also to enable the epic to recall and then hopefully dissolve or ameliorate some of what Milton would have considered the worst consequences of fallen heterosexual union. Most readers of *Paradise Lost* have long taken for granted that, for Milton, married sexuality – or at least sexual intercourse in what Milton would have thought of as a *good* marriage – was meant to recall Eden. That his poetic recollection of Edenic experience should, at this key moment, also recall us to the surgeon's knife is strange, but it makes sense in light of what the intertext of the sonnet and the passage suggests about the more difficult side of married sexuality – something that, at this point, Milton felt a need to confront more fully than he did in the 1630s.

The intertext is congruous with the approach he had taken earlier to childbirth trauma, but it is far more emotionally complex and self-aware. Note, for example, that the passage recalls not only the dreaming, widowed poet, prone and alone in his bed, but the suggestions of obstetric surgery that Milton earlier wove into his account of Lady Jane's death. The opening and healing of the wound, furthermore, suggests the passage from Dante that concluded the epitaph. The image of "Life-blood streaming fresh" also gives Adam's experience a Christological element that has powerful resonances in the context of the typology we explored in Chapter 3. The prone Adam and the prone widower even suggest the prone and wounded Adonis in the tableau that ends *A Mask*. There, secreted away by Venus, Adonis represented the realm of natural desire and fertility both within and outside of marriage, while Cupid and Psyche represented what might be possible in both a chaste earthly marriage and in salvation (especially after the trial of earthly reproductive suffering). The masque's allusion to Spenser makes us imagine Adonis locked forever in a cycle of "eterne in mutability." In Book 8 of *Paradise Lost*, however, the wound of the prone male figure is "suddenly…fill'd up and heal'd," and he feels no pain, suggesting in an uncanny way the collapse of the entire cycle of future married reproduction, with all of its negative *and* positive implications and experiences, into this one instituting moment. The moment is not itself eternal, but it holds in itself signs of all that is to come, including the prone widower, the suffering of mortal mothers, and the final amelioration of all of that suffering, which is not only displaced to the final, future redemption, but figured by an aspect of the lost Edenic past that is restored by the poem to the human imagination.

Milton went out of his way to freight this moment with details so suggestive of both negative and positive experiences (both his own and those of others), not just to project his personal pain into the epic in an idealizing and perhaps psychologically comforting fashion, but also to bring his epic machinery to bear in a way that might ultimately meet the general condition of childbed suffering head-on, offering the kind of conclusion that the sonnet could not fully express or uphold. The birth of Eve therefore constitutes an ambivalent nostalgic fantasy, a dream of perfection as it might be imagined by a man who had suffered deeply the consequences of what the passage makes clear are imperfections that will come by the end of the epic's narrative to define his own (and our) present state. Like the bright vision of the sonnet-dream while it lasted, but projected toward the past rather than the future, the passage provides an idyll that dissolves grief by allowing contemplation of an event that was never allowed actually to happen. In the idealized imagination of the creation of the first man's first sexual partner, it becomes possible for the suffering male reader and/or poet to contemplate what was originally to have been the result of the first human sexual partnership: the perfect, painless birth of a human child to a human mother untainted by a curse. At the same time, it suggests the whole nightmare of the present. Adam's temporary bliss in paradise is therefore at once an idealizing projection back to a time of perfect hopefulness, as well as a sign of losses to come. The episode provides a proleptic reversal of some of the most painful aspects of human love and procreation, as though the pains to come could be somehow already dissolved in the joy that preceded them (a version of which will be restored to humankind eventually), and it does so while still insisting on the abiding force of those pains in the meantime.

The episode is not allowed to be entirely consoling, because the attainment of a perfect consolation will, as far as Milton is concerned, turn out to be far more difficult than the hopeful valences of this episode or the poems of the 1630s to which it alludes might suggest. As Chapter 8 will show, in the etiological and eschatological schemes of the epic, birth will become both the transmitter of sin to later generations, and the mechanism by which that sin will be reversed. However, the pivotal experience that stands between the two functions, and, for that matter, the pivotal figure of the whole poem, will remain that of trial. In order to represent human trial in the form it took in the childbed, Milton will have to turn away from the sorts of personal allusions we have been exploring here, and toward allegory instead. As he approached childbed suffering even more immediately and fully than he does in either the sonnet or Book 8, and without the aid of nostalgic fantasy, I believe he found the material too difficult to handle, either naturalistically or by way of direct allusion to his own life. In Book 2, however, allegory – especially given the hybridized and open-ended ways in which it was practiced in the mid and later seventeenth century – provided him with a method for suggesting the extremity of seventeenth-century birth experience, while at the same time applying a rigorous theological framework to its interpretation. Later, in the epic's final books, he will set himself the even more difficult task of seeing that theological interpretation all the way through to its consoling conclusion, a task not fully completed in the poem. That incompletion, indeed, turns out to be a major element in the final books' peculiar blend of hopefulness and sorrow.

CHAPTER 8

"Conscious terrours" and "the Promis'd Seed": seventeenth-century obstetrics and the allegory of Sin and Death in Paradise Lost

The nature and function of the allegory of Sin and Death has been a bone of contention in Milton criticism as far back as the eighteenth century, when Addison and Johnson criticized it as a failure of decorum. Most critics today accept the allegory, along with the other allegorical episodes in the poem, as appropriate and significant parts of its structure. However, there is still a good deal of argument about what the allegory signifies, and why Milton used the mode at all in an otherwise naturalistic epic. As a result of these debates, a rich critical literature has accumulated. The various permutations of the relationships between Milton's figures have been worked out, and a large number of sources, analogues, and allusions have been uncovered and interpreted.[1] My purpose in this chapter, however, is to suggest that, because few critics have paid much attention to the naturalistic elements of Milton's

[1] Some have argued that Milton meant us to understand Sin and Death as having actual being in the universe of the poem, others that they are figures of Satan's inner life, or instances of the convention of the "*credibile maraviglioso,*" or that Milton used allegory deliberately, allowing its obsolescence as a mode to suggest that figures like Sin and Death were of lower ontological status than fully "real" characters like Adam and Eve. On Milton's practice with allegory, generally, see Catherine Gimelli Martin, *The Ruins of Allegory:* Paradise Lost *and the Metamorphosis of Epic Convention* (Durham: Duke University Press, 1998); Mindele Teip, *Allegorical Poetics and the Epic: the Renaissance Tradition to* Paradise Lost (Lexington, KY: University of Kentucky Press, 1994); Sarah R. Morrison, "When Worlds Collide: the Central Naturalistic Narrative and the Allegorical Dimension to *Paradise Lost,*" in *Living Texts: Interpreting Milton*, eds. Kristin A. Pruitt and Charles W. Durham (Selinsgrove, PA: Susquehanna University Press, 2000), pp. 178–97; and John Shawcross, "Allegory, Typology, and Didacticism: *Paradise Lost* in the Eighteenth Century," in *Enlightening Allegory: Theory, Practice and Contexts of Allegory in the Late Seventeenth and Eighteenth Centuries*, ed. Kevin L. Cope (New York, NY: AMS Press, 1993), pp. 41–74. On Sin and Death in particular, see Stephen Fallon, "Milton's Sin and Death: the Ontology of Allegory in *Paradise Lost,*" *ELR* 17 (1987), 329–50; John M. Steadman, "Tradition and Innovation in Milton's 'Sin': the Problem of Literary Indebtedness," *Philological Quarterly* XXXIX, I (January 1960), 93–103 and "Allegory and Verisimilitude in *Paradise Lost*: the Problem of the 'Impossible Credible,'" *PMLA* 78 (1963), 36–9; Michael Lieb, *The Dialectics of Creation: Patterns of Birth and Regeneration in* Paradise Lost (Amherst, MA: University of Massachusetts Press, 1970), pp. 142–83; Philip J. Gallagher, "'Real or Allegoric': the Ontology of Sin and Death in *Paradise Lost,*" *ELR* 6 (1976), 317–35; Maureen Quilligan, *Milton's Spenser: the Politics of Reading* (Ithaca, NY: Cornell University Press, 1983), pp. 79–128; and Mary Adams, "Fallen Wombs: the Origins of Death in Miltonic Sexuality," *Milton Studies* 29 (1992), 165–79. See also Margaret

allegory, an allegory that deftly and somewhat strangely mixes modes, an important aspect of the way it presents itself to readers, has been ignored.

Few critics have noted, for example, that Milton not only goes out of his way to present us with terrifying and grotesque figures of childbirth, going well beyond the suggestions of birth he found in his sources, but that in constructing these figures, he drew on contemporary obstetric experience and practice.[2] The birth imagery has, of course, been considered, but usually only as part of a discussion of the ways in which the natures of Sin and Death suggest fallen human sexuality (usually confined to lust), the negative side of a dialectic of creation and destruction, or patriarchal anxieties over "the maternal" and/or about women in general. The contemporary experience of childbirth, however, provided Milton with painful and powerful referents that would have suggested to contemporary readers a very different axis of engagement, significantly complicating the allegory and allowing the epic's theodicy to confront, in a strikingly direct way, the vexed theological and psychological questions we have been exploring in this study.

Attention to the obstetric content of the naturalistic referents of the episode in Book 2, which most critics have not wanted to take too literally, complicates the referentiality of its allegory, drawing the reader into an elaborate network of identifications with Milton's dramatically rendered personifications. Failure to notice this dynamic has limited both traditional theological approaches to the allegory as well as those that have attempted to read it against the backdrop of other contemporary concerns. The allegorical reference of Sin should not be confined – as most traditional readings would have it – to the experience of temptation to what Milton calls in *De Doctrina Christiana* "individual sin" (*CP*, 6.382–92).[3] Readings that make this assumption necessarily construct a temptation narrative whose subject

Olofson Thickstun, *Fictions of the Feminine: Puritan Doctrine and the Representation of Women* (Ithaca, NY: Cornell University Press, 1988), pp. 63–70, who looks at the allegory against the backdrop of contemporary ideas about women's domestic duties, and Elizabeth Sauer, *Barbarous Dissonance and Images of Voice in Milton's Epics* (Montreal, QB: McGill-Queen's University Press, 1996), pp. 88–97, which discusses the passages' debt to political imagery derived from accounts of monstrous birth.

[2] See the earlier version of this argument in Louis Schwartz, "'Conscious Terrors' and 'the Promised Seed': Seventeenth-Century Obstetrics and the Allegory of Sin and Death in *Paradise Lost*," *Milton Studies* 32 (1995), 63–89. See also John Rumrich, *Milton Unbound: Controversy and Reinterpretation* (Cambridge University Press, 1996), pp. 99–100 and "Milton's Poetics of Generation," *TSLL* 38 (1996), 191–208.

[3] Controversy still hovers over the authorship of *De Doctrina Christiana*, but I agree with Rumrich that the text is more or less finished, and that the stylometric analysis that has been used to call Milton's authorship of sections of it into question is inconclusive: John Rumrich, "The Provenance of *De Doctrina Christiana*: a View of the Present State of the Controversy," in *Milton and the Grounds of Contention* eds. Mark R. Kelley, Michael Lieb, and John T. Shawcross (Pittsburgh, PA: Duquesne University Press, 2003), pp. 214–33. In any case, the particular distinction to which I am referring is widespread enough in Christian thought as to be uncontroversial.

is male. In such readings, Satan or the reader is enticed by Sin's original "beauty," only to see her transformed into something manifestly terrible (or, after her Fall, by the alluring upper half of her body, only to discover her scaly lower half and stinging tail). I would instead suggest that the allegory, while still making use of the more traditional narrative, complicates that narrative with reference to "general sin," the sin that, again, according to Milton in *De Doctrina Christiana*, is common to all human beings after the Fall, and that to a large extent limits and challenges the individual's exercise of free will. "General sin," as Milton defines it, is best understood as the context in which the temptation to "individual sin" is acted out. The obstetric focus that Milton's unconventional manipulation of his literary and theological sources gives the episode places birth at the center of this complex allegorical tableau. This not only makes birth a central figure for the fallen condition itself (a condition that is "general" in more than one way), but also ties birth to the negative side of the poem's dynamic of fall and redemption, while at the same time suggesting how, via trial, it can lead us to the positive side. In other words, the allegory connects the dramatic trials of the sinful condition to the positive and negative aspects of human reproductive experience we explored in the last chapter. Most importantly, and unlike Adam's dream of Eve's nativity, the allegory does so in a way that provides subject positions that are gendered both male and female.

Even readings that have attempted to understand the allegory in wider psychological and ideological terms have tended to remain committed to readings that either place the male reader in the primary subject position (confronting, for example, female unruliness), or that confine Sin's referentiality to aspects of a wider figure of "the Satanic," offered to the reader satirically.[4] Few readers, however, have paid enough attention to the function of the episode's pathos, the way it seems to be inviting us, to some extent, to respond to Sin as a subject, and how this profoundly affects the scope of the allegory.[5] In setting out my argument, I will first closely examine the ways in which Milton's descriptive choices suggest specific obstetric conditions, techniques, and assumptions. I will then turn to the literary context of the passage in order to analyze Milton's manipulation of his models, and to discuss the rhetorical force that the obstetric imagery ultimately develops, especially in so far as it helps to create the passage's

[4] Sauer, *Barbarous Dissonance*, pp. 88–97 offers a compelling example.

[5] One important exception is Thickstun, who insists that Sin be approached not just as an abstraction but as a character "who has been given an inner life" (see *Fictions*, p. 65 and *Milton's* Paradise Lost: *Moral Education* [New York, NY: Palgrave, 2007], pp. 45–52).

pathos. The last section of the chapter will then show how the obstetric referents, in so far as they represent what fallen women will become heir to, complicate the Christian consolation offered in the epic's final books, a consolation constructed around prophesies of the Nativity – a birth that can only come to pass if Eve submits herself in faith to the conditions of the curse this episode so unflinchingly examines.

"CONSCIOUS TERROURS": READING CONTEMPORARY OBSTETRICS IN SIN'S NARRATIVE

To a reader familiar with the suffering experienced by many women in childbed during the seventeenth century, Sin's pitiable and extravagant account of her own experiences has a referential concreteness not wholly accounted for in the interpretive contexts offered by the available criticism. Her narrative, in fact, reflects several specific ideas about birth held by most educated Londoners of the age, and suggests some of the consequences of seventeenth-century surgical solutions to various forms of abnormal childbirth. Reference to these matters, once we become as aware of them as Milton and his original readers were, has the power to distract us from the rather stark abstractions we usually think of as the primary referents of the allegory. For example, the account concerning Death's tearing through his mother's entrails, effecting his own birth and leaving her terribly disfigured, strikingly parallels descriptions of birth typically found in seventeenth-century medical literature:

> Pensive here I sat
> Alone, but long I sat not, till my womb
> Pregnant by thee, and now excessive grown
> Prodigious motion felt and rueful throes.
> At last this odious offspring whom thou seest
> Thine own begotten, breaking violent way
> Tore through my entrails, that with fear and pain
> Distorted, all my nether shape thus grew
> Transform'd (*PL*, 2.777–85)

This birth is grotesque and cruel, but not without foundation in commonplace medical understanding. In other words, the horrific details are not simply poetic extravagances on Milton's part. The following, for example, is a passage describing the onset of labor and birth from Ambroise Paré's *Workes*, one of the most often cited medical texts of the period:

> WHen the naturall prefixed and prescribed time of child-birth is come, the childe being then growne greater, requires a greater quantity of food: which when he

cannot receive in sufficient measure by his navell, with great labour and striving hee endeavoreth to get forth: therefore then hee is moved with a stronger violence, and doth breake the membranes wherein he is contained. Then the wombe, because it is not able to endure such violent motions, nor to sustaine or hold up the childe any longer, by reason that the conceptacles of the membranes are broken asunder, is relaxed. And then the childe pursuing the aire which hee feeleth to enter in at the mouth of the wombe, which then is very wide and gaping, is carried with his head downewards, and so commeth into the world, with great pain both unto it selfe, and also unto his mother.[6]

The belief that the infant was physically active in its birth was prevalent in the period, and almost all of the obstetric literature contains descriptions of birth that are remarkable for the violence they ascribe to the infant.[7] William Harvey, for example, in his *Anatomical Exercitations*, argues that "the assistance of the *foetus* is chiefly required in the *birth*," relating several anecdotes of post-mortem deliveries and ruptured wombs explained by the still-living infant's action. He also tells a story about a woman whose genital tissues were closed off by the scars she had acquired in a particularly difficult delivery, only to have the passage opened again by the action of her next child:

how great furtherance the *foetus* doth conferre to its own *Birth*, several observations doe clearly evince. A certain *Woman* here amongst us (I speak it knowingly) was, (being dead over night) left alone in her Chamber: but the next morning an Infant was there found between her *Leggs*, which had by his own force wrought his *release* …

I also knew a *Woman*, who had all the interiour part of the neck of her *Womb* excoriated and torne, by a *difficult* and *painful delivery*: so that her time of *Lying in* being over, though she proved with Child againe afterward, yet not onely the sides of the *Orifice* of the *Neck* of the *Womb* neer the *Nymphae* did close together, but all the whole *Cavity* thereof, even to the *inner Orifice* of the *Matrix*, whereby there was no entrance even for a small *probe*, nor yet any egress to her *usual fluxes*. Hereupon the time of her delivery being now arrived, the poor soul was lamentably tortured, and laying aside all expectation of being delivered, she resigned up her keys to her Husband, and setting her affairs in order, she took leave of all her friends. When behold, beyond expectation, by the strong contest of a very lusty Infant, the whole tract was forced open, and she was miraculously *delivered*; the lusty Child proving

[6] Ambroise Paré, *The Workes of that famous Chirurgion Ambrose Parey*, trans. Thomas Johnson (London, 1634), p. 899.

[7] See also, for example, Jane Sharp, *The Midwives Book* (London, 1671), p. 168, and Jakob Rueff, *The Expert Midwife* (London, 1637), pp. 75–8. Many held that the infant first began to struggle in the seventh month, failed, and then needed the whole of the eighth month to recover its strength for the final labor (See Paré, *Workes*, pp. 901–2; Sharp, *The Midwives Book*, pp. 173–4; and Rueff, *The Expert Midwife*, pp. 64–6).

the *author of his own*, and *his Parents life*, leaving the passage open for the rest of his Brethren who should be borne in time to come.[8]

The birth of Death is unnaturally violent and a grotesque exaggeration, but it follows the same basic and familiar etiology. In a terrible parody of a normal, healthy infant, Death, "breaking violent way," tears through his mother's pregnant – though presumably still "heav'nly fair" (line 757) – body. His birth is announced by the "prodigious motion" of the monstrous infant and the "rueful throes" of the womb that cannot contain him. His birth goes through the sequence thought normal in the seventeenth century. And in both cases (and in that of the hounds Death later forcibly engenders with his mother), the child emerges hungry.

Like the women in Harvey's anecdotes and Paré's medical account, Sin is also portrayed as entirely subject to the actions of her infant. The child, not the mother (or even her body), is understood as the agent of birth. We will return to the significance of this below, but it is clear that a good deal of the passage's pathos derives from Sin's helplessness. This child not only causes "great pain both unto it self, and also unto his mother," but it causes her to undergo the process of birth, while, like Scylla, she watches helplessly in fear and pain as her formerly "beautiful" body (beautiful at least to her and Satan) is distorted and transformed into something terrible.

Although Sin, from the moment of her birth, is – as the reaction of the rebel angels in heaven shows us (lines 758–63) – both alluring and detestable, her transformation during the birth of Death complicates the allegorical resonance of her narrative by insisting on a physical alteration that, again, suggests certain contemporary obstetric conditions. On one level, the transformation reveals Sin's true nature more clearly (this is the monster, as it were, behind the seductive mask). On the other hand, it allows Sin's experience to figure the painful transformations in childbirth that will later become woman's post-lapsarian destiny. The permanent transformation of the lower half of Sin's body, which Milton adapts from Ovid with some telling alterations, has its correlative in the permanent external disfiguration of the genital area that many women experienced in the seventeenth century. As we saw in Chapters 1 and 2, obstetrical practices that led to such disfiguration were common in the period. While a certain amount of tearing of the perineal tissues is common in normal childbirth, practices among many seventeenth-century obstetric practitioners, mostly deriving

8 William Harvey, *Anatomical Exercitations Concerning the Generation of Living Creatures* (London, 1653), pp. 491–3. This is a translation of *Exercitationes de Generatione Animalium*, which was first published in 1651.

from the recommendations of the single most influential midwifery handbook of the period, *The Birth of Man-kinde*, caused a good deal of extra harm.[9] This was, perhaps, further exacerbated by a sort of "cult of difficulty" among middle-class women who believed that difficult birth was a sign of greater cultural and spiritual refinement, and therefore, perhaps without realizing it, insisted on birthing techniques that insured greater suffering.[10] Many otherwise normal births were, as a result, more torturous and disfiguring than they had to be. On the other hand, for these and other reasons, most abnormal births were simply nightmarish. An obstructed stillbirth, for example, even if handled by a reasonably experienced midwife or surgeon, meant removal of the infant's corpse by surgical dismemberment, and this not only increased the danger of crippling disfiguration and deadly infection, but it was also, as one can well imagine, overwhelmingly terrifying. In addition, most midwives had very light case-loads, were not full-time professionals, and operated on a "rural" pattern even in the city, only attending women whom they knew well. This meant that many never developed the experience necessary to handle emergency cases (safe means of extraction, the ability to tell a dead infant from a live one, etc.). The midwives and obstetrical surgeons who had developed such expertise were few and far between, and were often called upon very late in a difficult labor, sometimes after less experienced practitioners had made the situation much worse, or infection and exhaustion had overcome the mother. In this way, many simple malpresentations escalated into full-blown emergencies that resulted in death or permanent injury.

Accounts of obstetric disfigurements like the one I quoted in Chapter 2 of this study, in which Percival Willughby described how a midwife inadvertently tore "a breach about an inch long into the fundament" of a woman, causing "afterward her excrements [to come] forth from the birthplace," offer us a sense of the kind of circumstances that resonate in Sin's narrative.[11] Such disfigurations, even in milder cases, occasioned no temporary trauma. Injuries suffered in a difficult birth could follow a woman for years as permanent disfigurations that could make subsequent births more frightening and painful. This is why, as I noted, Willughby and other practitioners recommended that if a woman could endure such disfiguration, it

9 See Eccles, *Obstetrics and Gynecology* in Tudor and Stuart England (Kert, OH: Kert State University Press, 1982), pp. 11–12, 88, and the discussion in Chapter 2 of this study.

10 Eccles, *Obstetrics and Gynecology*, pp. 88–90, and Chapter 2 of this study.

11 Percival Willughby, *Observations in Midwifery*, ed. Henry Blenkinsop (Warwick: printed by H. T. Cooke, 1863; rpt. Wakefield: S. R. Publishers, 1972), p. 54. See above, pp. 46–7 for the full passage and references to others.

was better to leave it than to cure it surgically. The state of a woman's perineal tissue was often left in a condition designed, as Willughby put it, to make "the ensuing births…more easy, by reason of the spaciousnes of the breach."[12]

For a reader who lived in Milton's London, such practices and conditions were a part of the texture of everyday life, affecting, perhaps, a minority of women, but in ways that, as we have seen, would have had a powerful effect on the way most people felt about a birth as it neared. For such a reader, Sin's account of the birth of Death and its permanently disfiguring transformation of her lower half could very well have brought to mind the painful and lingering suffering of women like those described in the passages I have quoted here and in Chapter 2, a suffering that was both physical and psychological. Satan's opening address to Sin actually indicates that her transformation has made her unrecognizable and repugnant to the father of her child. In addition, Death tears her open like the child in Harvey's account, preparing the way for his siblings, leaving her subject to a cycle of painful repetitions. After Death rapes his mother, bringing his ghastly siblings into being, they begin to act out a cycle of figurative births and conceptions, "hourly conceiv'd/ And hourly born, with sorrow infinite" (lines 796–7) to their mother, and they are goaded on in this by Death himself. With the historical context I have been describing in mind, Sin's story begins to take on an allegorical significance that runs parallel to the moral allegory that Milton derived from James and St. Basil (about which I will have more to say, below):

> he my inbred enemie
> Forth issu'd, brandishing his fatal Dart
> Made to destroy: I fled, and cry'd out *Death*;
> Hell trembl'd at the hideous Name, and sigh'd
> From all her Caves, and back resounded *Death*.
> I fled, but he pursu'd (though more, it seems,
> Inflam'd with lust then rage) and swifter far,
> Mee overtook his mother all dismaid,
> And in embraces forcible and foul
> Ingendring with me, of that rape begot
> These yelling Monsters that with ceaseless cry
> Surround me, as thou sawst, hourly conceiv'd
> And hourly born, with sorrow infinite
> To me, for when they list into the womb

[12] Willughby, *Observations*, p. 54. See also Eccles, *Obstetrics and Gynecology*, pp. 106–7, and pp. 46–7 of this study.

That bred them they return, and howl and gnaw
My Bowels, thir repast; then bursting forth
Afresh with conscious terrours vex me round,
That rest or intermission none I find.
Before mine eyes in opposition sits
Grim *Death* my Son and foe, who sets them on,
And me his Parent would full soon devour
For want of other prey, but that he knows
His end with mine involv'd (lines 785–807)

The way Death emerges from his mother's torn and transformed body, the way she flees in terror, naming him, the way he rapes her and torments her, sitting "in opposition" and driving the hounds to re-enter her womb, gnaw her bowels, and then burst forth afresh over and over again, all suggest a set of concrete referents that operate alongside the passage's theological abstractions.

In a complex way, the birth of Death, the subsequent rape, and the terrible pain he causes to his mother all combine into a nightmarish allegory of certain core anxieties. Not only does the cycle of painful repetitions suggest the pains and fears that, given the physical risks involved, would attend any birth, it also suggests a fear of incessantly repeated pregnancy, itself an inextricable part of married life for many upper- and middle-class women. The fertility rates among upper- and middle-class London in the period, as we saw in Chapter 2, were relatively high, leaving many women (to use Sin's words) little "rest or intermission." Although parity rates varied, and many women had no more than five or six children in the course of their reproductive lives, some women in the wealthier parishes gave birth as often as every twenty-three months (with some fluctuation), until they either died or entered menopause. That could mean – if we include mid- and late-term miscarriages – as many as ten to fifteen times in the course of their reproductive years (that is, if they survived their own fertility and reached menopause).[13]

And, as we also saw in Chapter 2, surviving that fertility was by no means guaranteed. Chief among the fears that attended birth was fear of death itself. In their repeated regress into Sin's womb and their gnawing at her bowels, goaded on as they are by their allegorical father, the behavior of the

[13] See Chapter 2. Also, as I observed in Chapter 7, Mary Powell, following the conventional pattern, gave birth to all four of her children in the space of about six-and-a-half years. Had she lived and a similar pattern continued, she could easily have given birth more than nine times before she was in her forties.

hounds who are born of Sin's rape evoke the very basic and pervasive fear of painful death that accompanied birth throughout the seventeenth century. The hounds raging around their mother with "ceasless cry" (line 795), the "conscious terrours" (line 801) with which they vex her at Death's instigation, and the howling and gnawing of her insides all suggest the ever-presence of that fear as well as of the physical conditions that inspired it: the fevers, cramps, hemorrhages, and infected lacerations that killed many women in the days or weeks following a birth. The figuration seems particularly apt given that, even if a woman survived a difficult birth, these conditions often followed her for years, each new pregnancy bringing fears of further pain as well as the aggravation of conditions from which she already suffered. The goading on of the yelling monsters by Death suggests, therefore, very directly the role fear of death, disease, and deformity could play in the imaginations of women who, at the higher levels of the fertility spectrum, lived approximately half of their lives pregnant.

Because of Death's shapelessness and voracity, his birth should also, finally, be understood as a monstrous birth (Death is called a monster at line 675; his movements in Sin's womb at the onset of delivery are "prodigious" – the hounds are also called monsters at line 795). The allegorical mode of the passage furthermore ties Sin's account to several Renaissance traditions and discourses about monstrosity. Medical and zoological texts, as well as Broadside Ballads and Wonderbooks, provided an almost endless stream of tales and case studies in the period, a rich and strange literature that itself deserves further study.[14] Despite the fact that the medical literature of the seventeenth century had begun to offer empirical explanations for monstrosity, the popular literature remained moralized and theologically allegorical throughout the period. It is to these traditions that Milton seems most indebted to here, drawing on the popular belief that unlawful or

[14] See Katherine Park and Lorraine F. Daston, "Unnatural Conceptions: the Study of Monsters in Sixteenth and Seventeenth-Century France and England," *Past and Present* 92 (1981), 20–54. For one of the central statements of the period on monstrosity, see Paré's catalogue of causes (*Workes*, pp. 961–2). Relevant broadsides can be found in several large collections, especially *The Pack of Autolycus or Strange and Terrible News of Ghosts, Apparitions, Monstrous Births, Showers of Wheat, Judgments of God, and Other Prodigious and Fearful Happenings as Told in Broadside Ballads of the Years 1624–1693*, ed. Hyder Edward Rollins (Cambridge, MA: Harvard University Press, 1927); *The Roxburghe Ballads*, eds. William Chappell and J. W. Ebsworth 9 vols. in 8 (Hertford: printed for the Ballad society by S. Austin and Sons, 1871–1899); and *The Bagford Ballads*, ed. Joseph Woodfall Ebsworth (New York, NY: AMS Press, 1968; rpt. London: Ballad Society Publications, published in 4 parts, 1876–1878). See also Simon McKeown, *Monstrous Births: an Illustrative Introduction to Teratology in Early Modern England* (London: Indelible Inc., 1991). Further details can be found in Schwartz, "Conscious Terrors," 88, n. 34 and Sauer, *Barbarous Dissonance*, pp. 88–97.

perverse copulation – in this case between Satan and himself (in his idolatrous self-love), later between Satan and his daughter, and then that daughter and her own son – could lead to monstrous issue.

"[R]est or intermission none I find" and "Before mine eyes in opposition sits/ Grim *Death*" (lines 802–4) – these are words that a typical seventeenth-century married woman was likely to find echoed her own sentiments (and those of her husband) given that in the course of her fertile years, if she lived through them at all, she was likely to be pregnant often, often sick, and perhaps disfigured. The passage provides, in the voice of Sin, a position from which a seventeenth-century reader, especially a female reader, could recognize very "conscious terrours" indeed.

RAPE, ABANDONMENT, AND MASCULINE GUILT

I will have occasion later to refer briefly to some of the other matters suggested by the naturalistic elements and concrete referents of Milton's allegory, although there is no room in this chapter to treat them all in detail. Some are, however, worth mentioning in relation to the anxieties we are discussing. The relationships between Satan, Sin, and Death, because they are presented as a set of incestuous sexual acts (one a rape), are associated with certain extremely painful aspects of human experience: those associated with female vulnerability to male sexual violence, and also to widowhood and abandonment. Sin speaks of herself in her narrative as a sort of war-widow and "single mother," abandoned and deformed by birth, until she meets Satan again at the gates of Hell. The episode is a ghastly reunion, and Satan himself – after hearing Sin's story and recognizing who she is – even behaves like an aristocratic libertine confronted with the illegitimate results of some courtly backstair-work. In addition, the rape itself is a complex figure in the context of this passage.[15] Not only does it stand violently and sexually for the negating compulsions of sinful behavior, it also stands as a figure for the compromising of the will a woman experiences in an actual rape, as well as that attendant upon pregnancy and birth, particularly when they are the result of sexual violation. I will have more to say about this particular issue later, but it is important to the overall significance of the passage that pregnancy and birth are understood as processes that sexual congress can set in motion with or without the cooperation of a woman's will.

[15] See Alexander Myers, "'Embraces Forcible and Foul': Viewing Milton's Sin as a Rape Victim," *Milton Quarterly* 28 (1994), 11–16.

It should also be said here that Milton is giving us another echo of his own reproductive experience – this time a truly nightmarish version. For example, the passage, like the passage that describes Eve's creation (although much less directly), contains what may be two significant verbal echoes of Sonnet 23. Sin tells Satan twice that she "fled" from Death, and what she is fleeing are his "embraces" (lines 787–93).[16] The connection may seem tenuous, but it is hard not to feel the psychological resonance of Milton's choosing to frame the first naming of "death," the first experience of its terrors in the created universe, as wound up with a terrible scene of sexual violence, one that is very specifically identified as "ingendering," and in which female terror echoes through the feminized caves of Hell, with an echo of the sonnet in which he expressed a powerful sense of guilt over the fact that men were exempted from such direct suffering. If the echo of the sonnet is there, this is perhaps the darkest version we get of the psychological and theological weight of Milton's sense of his own bereavements. Here, the sense of guilt expressed in the sonnet is given far freer rein, touching, perhaps, on deeply rooted feelings of shame concerning the relationship of reproduction and both violent and lustful impulses. The passage thus ranges beyond its most immediate sources of personal feeling toward an exploration of sexual reproduction as seen as fully as possible from the sin-bearing perspective – and with pointed attention to the difference gender makes in how one sees it.

By cataloguing all of these terrors, I do not mean to imply that Milton's vision of childbirth was unremittingly bleak. The passage, however, is the one place in his work where he seems to have given himself full license to imagine and give poetic form to the worst anxieties, memories, and fantasies that plagued his own experience and that of countless others in the period. Milton's purpose in the passage is not to provide an account of normal childbirth, or to say that all birth was nightmarish, but to provide an elaborate allegory of the worst aspects of birth as it could unfold in the fallen condition. As the next section of this chapter makes clear, his greatest concern is with the *perception* of the dangers involved, and Sin is primarily meant to represent perception overwhelmed by fear. She is rendered by her familiar and justified fears, her "conscious terrours," unable to see the light of divine intention at work in even the most painful experiences, and it is this despair that Milton, like so many of the writers I quoted in Part I, feared even more than the pains that could occasion it.

[16] My thanks to John Shawcross for pointing out the echo.

"WITH FEAR AND PAIN/DISTORTED": READING SIN'S NARRATIVE

In constructing the allegory, particularly in Sin's account of her own life, Milton drew on traditional materials. However, he reworked these materials not only to suggest contemporary conditions, but also to give figures of birth pride of place in his narrative. For the order of events and their details, he used genealogies found in Phineas Fletcher's *The Purple Island*,[17] James, and St. Basil's Sixth Homily on the Hexamera, along with portions of *The Faerie Queene* and elements of Ovid's description of Scylla, which is alluded to by the narrator in one of the passage's epic similes (lines 659–61).[18] Milton uses this set of theological commonplaces and literary allusions to create an allegorical narrative that focuses attention on birth, while adding a complex psychological density.[19] Pregnancies and their effects therefore become central to the function of his allegory in ways not encompassed by the literary sources or by the oft-cited genealogies of Sin found in James:

> Then when lust hath conceived, it bringeth forth sin: and sin, when it is finished, bringeth forth death. (James 1:15)

Or St. Basil's more exact:

> death, which immediately seized upon us and which had been begotten by sin, the first-born offspring of the demon, source of evil.[20]

Milton, for example, draws on Redcross Knight's confrontation with Error in *The Faerie Queene*, 1.1.14–26, altering and refocusing certain Spenserian details. Both Sin and Error are described as mothers. Error is the mother of a brood of nursing, snaky young who creep into her mouth for safety as soon as light shines on them. She later vomits them back up, as a

[17] Canto 12.26–31, where Hamartia, or Sin, is the first to be spewed out of the "stinking panch" of the Dragon, Satan. She is the daughter of an allegorical union between Satan and Eve (in *Paradise Lost*, Sin exists *before* Eve). Fletcher, like Milton, draws heavily on *The Faerie Queene*, 1.1.14–26 (Error) and 1.11–12 (the Dragon).

[18] See Steadman, "Tradition and Innovation" and "Milton and St. Basil: the Genesis of Sin and Death," *Modern Language Notes* 73 (1958), 83–4.

[19] William Kerrigan, *The Sacred Complex: on the Psychogenesis of Paradise Lost* (Cambridge, MA: Harvard University Press, 1983), pp. 187, 240–1, and Lieb, *Dialectics*, p. 163. Both discuss the psychological density of the passage in terms of incest, monstrosity, and cannibalism.

[20] *St. Basil: Exegetic Homilies*, trans. Sister Agnes Clare Way, C. D. P. (Washington, DC: The Catholic University of America Press, 1963), p. 84. The following passage from Milton's *DDC* is marked by the same figure: "God does not drive the human heart to sinfulness and deceit when it is innocent and pure and shrinks from sin. But when it has conceived sin, when it is heavy with it, and already giving birth to it, then God as the supreme arbiter of all things turns and points it in this or that direction or towards this or that object" (*CP*, 6.332).

weapon, along with half-digested food, books, and blind toads and frogs. After she is beheaded by Redcross, they are unable to climb back into her mouth, and so instead drink her blood until they literally burst their own guts. Sin is also a mother, both of Death and of a brood of howling monsters that cry and bark around her, returning into her womb at any sign of disturbance to gnaw at her bowels. Milton's images retain some of the force of perverted nurturing and cannibalism, but he exchanges Spenser's scatology for a focus on obstetrics. Not only does the womb replace the mouth as the place of regress, but the fathering and birthing of the children are described with attention to the physical consequences for the mother of these events, and this expands the possible meanings of the allegory.[21]

It is important that the transformation of Sin's lower half, along with the fear and pain caused by the "conscious terrours" (line 801) that vex her after she is raped by her son and gives birth to the hounds, are the results of her painfully giving birth twice, and that these births alter her original beauty. This is, in fact, perhaps the most striking change Milton introduces. Both Spenser's Error and Fletcher's Hamartia are born in their deformed states. Ovid's Scylla is transformed, but the metamorphosis has no obstetric connection (though this is where Milton may have gotten the idea of the dogs).

Milton's change not only puts birth at the center of his narrative and emphasizes its physical nature, it also brings to the fore the fact that pregnancy is something that happens to a woman as a result of sex with or without her consent. Sin's second pregnancy (and to some extent her first) is an unwanted pregnancy, and she experiences it as a process beyond her control, enforced from without, occurring within, and then exploding out again and repeating the cycle with further pain and mutilation. Even the first pregnancy, which as far as we can tell was not exactly forced upon her, concludes in a birth that she not only must undergo abandoned and alone, but that, as we have seen, deforms her in a way that is terrifying and, again, beyond her control. She is in this sense very close to her model in Scylla, although with another telling difference. In Ovid, Scylla becomes first deformed and then demonic, her physical transformation changing the nature of her personality. Sin's metamorphosis, on the other hand, must be seen as the revelation of an already inherent potential activated by her copulation with her father. At this moment, however (as it is in the first part of Ovid's narrative), the primary effect is of pathos. The effect is meant to be disarming (though not just for Satan), and it is meant to draw us into sympathy and identification with Sin, although this is not, as I will

[21] Quilligan, *Milton's Spenser*, pp. 80–98.

show, simply a guilt-laden, Fishian identification that is meant to be recognized as misguided and then completely rejected.

The passage is, in fact, affectively complex in ways that have not been adequately accounted for in the critical literature.[22] The difference between Sin's own speech and that of the narrator at lines 648–73 (the first to describe her to us) is telling. The narrator focuses on the loathsome appearance of the allegorical pair. He tells of the "foulness" of her "scaly foulds," her "mortal sting," the "hideous" noise made by the hounds both inside and outside of her womb, and he ends with an epic simile that refers both to Scylla and infanticide witches who dance beneath a "labouring Moon" in eclipse. The tone is detached and moralized, meant to provoke disgust, particularly in its attention to obstetric details, which are rendered with simple abhorrence, even down to the witches' sabbath and the eclipsed moon, both compact emblems for the negation of maternity.[23] Sin, on the other hand, delivers an account of her life designed to provoke a very different response. In the following passage she laments her ugliness, tells of her "birth" from Satan's head, speaks with pride of her original beauty and with nostalgia of her dalliance with her father and their subsequent separation by the war in Heaven:

> Hast thou forgot me then, and do I seem
> Now in thine eye so foul, once deemd so fair
> In Heav'n, when at th' Assembly, and in sight
> Of all the Seraphim with thee combin'd
> ...
> All on a sudden miserable pain
> Surpris'd thee ...
> ... till on the left side op'ning wide,
> Likest to thee in shape and count'nance bright,
> Then shining heav'nly fair, a Goddess arm'd
> Out of thy head I sprung: amazement seis'd
> All the Host of Heav'n; back they recoild affraid
> At first, and call'd me *Sin*, and for a Sign
> Portentous held me; but familiar grown,
> I pleas'd, and with attractive graces won
> The most averse, thee chiefly, who full oft
> Thy self in me thy perfect image viewing
> Becam'st enamour'd, and such joy thou took'st
> With me in secret, that my womb conceiv'd
> A growing burden. Mean while Warr arose,
> And fields were fought in Heav'n (lines 747–68)

[22] Although, again, see Thickstun, *Fictions*, p. 65 and *Moral Education*, pp. 45–52.

[23] Sara Van Den Berg, "Eve, Sin, and Witchcraft in *Paradise Lost*," *Modern Language Quarterly*, December (1986), 352–4.

She then goes on to detail a gruesome family romance. The pregnancies and births that resulted from her congress with her father and her subsequent rape by her new-born son, Death, are described carefully and with a pathos that is surprisingly affecting, given the identity of the speaker and our awareness of her present rhetorical need to move Satan. In lines 785–9, Hell – here feminized and full of womb-like caves – echoes Sin's naming of her son and the fear he inspires as he lunges at her in lust and forcibly engenders on her a generation of "yelling Monsters." The echoing caves suggest a community of witnessing women who confirm this terrible naming, a revelation of this offspring's true nature rather than a loving parental or communal gesture.[24] Death, rather than life, and violent threats, rather than love, are revealed as the outcomes of this birth, outcomes that will, as we have seen, continue to torment. As I argued earlier, the ensuing descriptions she gives of her rape and the subsequent cycles of birth and cannibalism that she then experiences – and continues to experience – take on a painful psychological weight, expressing deep horror not only at sexual violence, but at the violence of birth itself, its compromising of the will and the pains and dangers it brings. In the last half of Sin's speech, from lines 790–809, the allegorical and the dramatic are tightly woven together. Along with the extravagant and grotesque rendering of James' and St. Basil's genealogies and the almost absurd allegorical stalemate of Death's inability to eat Sin, we have details very much at odds with the program of the moral allegory as it has been traditionally read: the sheer horror of the oedipal rape, the physical specificity of phrases like, "howl and gnaw/ My Bowels, thir repast; then bursting forth" with their stressed repetitions of diphthongs and consonant combinations ("howl"/ "Bowel-"; "respast"/ "burst-"), also the references to extreme emotional states ("sorrow infinite," "conscious terrours," the weariness expressed by "rest or intermission none I find"), and the horribly ironic suggestiveness of puns like "dismaid," whose connotations conflate loss of maidenhead with "dismay" and "unmaking."[25] These are all affecting, to say the least.

[24] My thanks to Alice Berghof for her comments in private conversation.

[25] Milton may have known that the word is derived from the Old High German, *magan* ("to be powerful or able" [*OED*, "dismay," v[1]]), which suggests that "dismaid" primarily means "disempowered." This fits well with the description of a rape. My thanks to John Shawcross for pointing out the etymology. The *OED* also lists relevant instances of related words: in his 1603 translation of Montaigne, Florio used the verb "dismaiden" to mean "to deprive of maidenhood," and Giles Fletcher in *Christs Victorie* (1610) used "dismayed" to mean "stripped of May-blossom" (*OED*, "dismay," v[2]). Perhaps even more interesting is a usage Milton may have come upon in Spenser, and which the *OED* quotes for "dismayd," meaning "mis-made, mis-shapen." The lines are part of the description of the assault on the "fort of smell" during the battle at Alma's castle: "Likewise that same third Fort, that is the *Smell*/ Of that third troupe was cruelly assayd:/ Whose hideous shapes were like to feendes of hell,/ Some like to houndes, some like to Apes, dismayd" (*FQ*, 2.11.4). See

Her lines pull us in two directions. On the one hand, we are presented with an unfolding moral allegory that reveals to us certain things about the nature and origins of sin as it tempts and confronts the individual will. The description is hellish, and we are invited to distance ourselves as the narrator has done. On the other hand, we are confronted with a highly affecting dramatic voice, one that expresses pain in language that is poetically rich and allusive and which foregrounds a woman's experience of birth. Lines 762–4, for example ("attractive graces" and "thy self in me thy perfect image viewing"), anticipate what we will hear in idealized form about the original love between Adam and Eve in Books 4 and 8. In addition, Sin's later words at lines 861–2 ("in perpetual agonie and pain,/ With terrors and with clamors compasst round/ Of mine own brood, that on my bowels feed") are echoed by Milton's narrator in the invocation to Book 7, where he complains – in one of the most starkly autobiographical passages in the poem – of his vulnerability and isolation: "In darkness, and with dangers compast round" (*PL*, 7.27), a clear evocation of Milton's own condition just following the Restoration.[26] Sin's narrative as a whole also tells us, on one level, what is in effect a straightforward and familiar story of illicit sex (here made awful by its being incestuous) followed by abandonment – the stuff of a thousand ballads and love complaints. It would be a mistake to understand this narrative separately from its allegorical significance, but Milton seems bent on delivering his allegory in a form that suggests in dramatic fashion the prodigious etiology of what is both familiar and pathetic for himself and for others. Given what we have seen of contemporary obstetric experience, it should be clear that the pathos of the passage is an invitation to an uneasy and complex form of identification with its figures.

The passage, in fact, suggests to us how we are to read it. Look again at lines 777–85. The syntax of the second sentence in the passage is knotty, but it seems best paraphrased as follows: "At last this odious offspring…tore through my entrails, so that, distorted with fear and pain, my nether shape thus grew transformed." This paraphrase makes the force of the phrase that

Edmund Spenser, *The Faerie Queene*, ed. A. C. Hamilton, (London: Pearson Education, 2001), p. 263. The episode's anatomy of temptation would certainly have been relevant to Milton in his description of Sin. The close incidence of "houndes" and "hell" in these lines may also have helped bring the word to his mind. Also, five stanzas later, Alma herself is described as "dismayed" in the more usual senses of the word.

[26] Rumrich also discusses this connection (*Milton Unbound*, pp. 99–100). In her discussion of God's later description of Sin and Death as "Dogs of Hell" (*PL* 10.616–20, 629–40), Mary Ann Radzinowicz (*Milton's Epics and the Book of Psalms* [Princeton, NJ: Princeton University Press, 1989], pp. 184–7) argues that Milton derived the dog imagery from Psalm 22:16 ("For dogs have compassed me, the assembly of the wicked have inclosed me" [*KJV*]). The dogs in the first part of the verse's parallelism connect it with the hounds that torment and surround Sin. The "wicked" of the second part suggests the situation of the imprisoned Milton in Book 7. It may be relevant that Psalm 22 was sometimes recommended to women for recitation during difficult childbirth: See above, pp. 69–70.

modifies the second clause more explicit. It is significant that Milton did not write: "so that, with fear and pain, all my nether shape thus grew transformed," which is much simpler, telling us only that an experience of fear and pain accompanied the transformation. Instead, Milton complicates matters by adding the seemingly superfluous participle "distorted" to the prepositional phrase. The additional word does more than just emphasize the physical change (certainly the main thing on Sin's mind) by giving us two words for it. The effect is to momentarily reify the physical and emotional experience of fear and pain, which is properly experienced by Sin herself and not just by her lower half (even if we allow that pain might be said to be "experienced" by one part of the body, the same cannot be said of fear). In addition, if "distort" etymologically denotes the twisting of something from its original or natural shape (a meaning very dear to Sin at this point), here it also suggests a common figurative usage as a term to describe perception. Milton actually uses the term this way in *The Reason of Church Government* and in *Tetrachordon.*[27] In the poem, Milton's syntax and diction suggests that, from Sin's perspective, her being was not only changed in a manner that inspired fear and pain, but was "distorted" by the experience. That is to say, she is not simply altered physically, but altered in her self-perception. Sin seems to know what she was and what she has now become; she watched it and felt it happen, and, as we have seen, her language suggests that her emotional and physical states are woven together. The reader is, in fact, asked to see this weaving together as a central reality of her nature.

Sin's perception of herself at any point may be properly considered a distorted one (she might even be said to have arrived at her true form only now) but a specifically obstetric fear and pain together constitute the astigmatic lens through which she comes to look at herself and through which she expresses an odd, but very important, allegorical self-consciousness. This self-consciousness in an allegorical figure produces a circular process of reference, like a serpent with its stinging tail in its mouth. Sin is an allegory of a particular theological condition, but we are invited to view her, to some extent, as a self-aware subject, one who is immersed in the very condition she represents as an allegory. When she looks at her lower half, she sees not that she is changing into something she recognizes as not

[27] Speaking in *The Reason of Church Government* of the revelation of God's power and wisdom in Christ, Milton says, "this is one depth of his wisdome, that he could so plainly reveale so great a measure of it to the grosse *distorted* apprehension of decay'd mankinde" (my italics) (*CP*, 1.750). In *Tetrachordon*, Milton claims that rigidity in biblical interpretation only appeals to those who "are fain to stretch & *distort* their apprehensions, for feare of displeasing the verbal straightnesse of a text, which our owne servil feare gives us not the leisure to understand aright" (my italics) (*CP*, 2.636).

herself, but that she is changing into what she actually *is*, and she is overwhelmed in the process by the pain and fear that are her own attributes. In other words, she sees from within the distorting condition that she herself represents. In this way, "subjectivity" is, in effect, accommodated to allegorical figuration, and the subjectivity is that of a suffering mother.

It is through such a distorting lens, or in such a distorting mirror, that Milton here requires us to gaze. He is, in fact, suggesting – because the perceiver here is *Sin*, and Sin is speaking as a mother – that our gaze, the gaze of a subject in a condition of sin, is always distorted, conditioned as it is by the general sin of post-lapsarian existence of which birth pain is a key manifestation. The naturalistic and dramatic aspects of this allegorical passage therefore function like the ripples or distortions in the glass in which we now see darkly. And the key to the complex working of the allegory is that those ripples, and the precise ways in which they distort our view of ourselves, come in the shape of the commonplace pains and fears of post-lapsarian reproductive life.

It has been traditionally assumed, because Sin is beautiful from the waist up and a stinging serpent from the waist down, that she signifies temptation to what Milton calls "individual sin" with a strong emphasis on sexuality. However, if we take the gender and appearance of Sin as signifying a temptation to immoral, dissolute, and destructive behavior with a strong emphasis on sexual immorality, the only solid subject position the allegory provides is one for a man who might be allured by the fair upward appearance. The gender of Milton's figure in the reading I am suggesting, however, comes to have a wider significance, providing subject positions for both men and women in a complex figurative tableau with childbirth at its center. Milton's birth imagery here functions rhetorically to include the male and the female reader in the allegory, therefore suggesting that human birth itself must be read allegorically. This forces the female reader to see herself, when she sees herself as a mother, as a living allegory of the consequences of original sin and of her own fear and pain in confronting those consequences. It no less forcefully functions in this way for the male reader, though for the male reader it is his mother, lover, wife, or victim whom he sees transformed into one part of the allegory, while he plays the ultimately destructive role of Death or the originally responsible role of Satan. In other words, it provides a poetic figure designed to draw readers into contemplation of childbirth along most of the major lines of thought I described in Chapter 3 of this study. It also provides a position for further contemplation of the male grief, guilt and anxiety that Milton also explored in the epitaph for Jane Paulet, in Sonnet 23, and in Adam's account of Eve's nativity. In light of what is suggested by the obstetric content of her narrative, Sin should be seen not merely as a figure expressive of misogyny, whether Milton's own or that of the theological traditions or social systems that identified woman as the source of sin. She is, instead, a figure for the fallen state itself, one in which birth plays the part of a complex metonymy for a set of experiences that compromise the free exercise of the will by presenting it with a strong temptation to despair.

The episode constitutes a stark revision of the allegorical representation of the reproductive cycle that Milton created for the tableau of *A Mask*. Here, his imagination opens to a vision of what that cycle might be like to an entirely sin-bound imagination, never giving way to a vision of an end to the cycle of suffering in the realm "farr above." Sin is given no vision of herself as an "eternal bride," and her "fair unspotted side" is merely a memory (*A Mask*, lines 999–1011). Indeed, the poet's hopeful vision of Lady Jane "clad in radiant sheen," and the shining vestments of Mary Powell and Katherine Woodcock in their restored physical and spiritual integrity are here only recalled in Sin's memory of herself "shining heavn'ly fair" in heaven before the war (line 757). Even the husband's condition in Sonnet 23 (enduring and darkling, but holding on to a trust in a restoration to come), and Adam's brief, proleptic moment of darkness in Book 8 here give way to a general and unrelieved darkness, one that is faced more fully and directly, and with no end in sight.

Milton has designed Sin's account to inspire a more complex and difficult engagement with the nature of sin-bound reproductive suffering than any of his other, earlier poems or passages suggested. It also forces us to a more complex and difficult engagement with the sinful condition itself than most traditional readings of the allegory have allowed. For Milton in *De Doctrina Christiana*, all post-lapsarian human life, mired in "the sin common to all men" (as opposed to "the sin of each individual"), is in its essence turned away from God unless choice amends it (*CP*, 6.383–92). All fallen human life, irrespective of personal morality or faith, therefore manifests a process of decay that – as Milton puts it, speaking about the "spiritual death" that came with the Fall – occasions "loss or at least extensive darkening of that right reason, whose function it was to discern the chief good" (*CP*, 6.395).[28] Sin signifies the terror that comes between human kind and God in a universe degraded by an original disobedience from its original perfection.

[28] Milton understands the Sin of Adam and Eve (their "individual" but our "common" sin) as consisting of four kinds of "death." These are: (i) "the evils which tend to death" (particularly guiltiness), (ii) "spiritual death," (iii) "the death of the body," and (iv) "eternal death, the punishment of the damned" (*CP*, 6.393–414). It is, of course, this last, eternal death that despair in the childbed risks.

And here, Milton has made the key distorting experiences violent, incestuous sexuality and painful, disfiguring, and dangerous childbirth.

The allegory of Sin and Death becomes, therefore, a horrific but sustained and sympathetic allegory of the way we saw (in Chapter 3) many women were desperately afraid they might come to see (and see through) their own pain. Those women saw their own bodily experiences as trials in allegorical terms, and this is precisely the way Milton presents Sin's failure to see herself in other than distorted ways. Such an interpretation has important implications for how we read the extravagance of Milton's allegorical passages. For example, some have found the episode darkly and satirically funny. But is it? I would grant that the relations of Sin and Death are a parody of divine relations within the Godhead, and that there is a good deal of satiric grotesquery and irony in the passage. If we hold that these elements alone should dictate our interpretive framework, then we are, of course, free to laugh ruefully. But when we begin, as I think we must, to imagine the allegorical narrative as a parody of human relations with concrete contemporary resonances, laughter falls away, and *our* dismay should become very real. The contemporary references in the passage collapse the distance that would otherwise make such laughter easy. There may be an irony, for example, in the "deflowering" of Sin, who is no virgin in any number of ways, but the humor of the pun is severely delimited by the context I am suggesting.[29] And the irony itself takes on a different character than it might otherwise. This is especially true when one considers that any maid, even the most innocent, is subject to the pain referred to here, even when, as Milton's own experiences and the other poems and passages we have examined should remind us, it is the chaste marriage bed that brings about the deflowering. The passage is a parody of divine relations, yes, but a parody that names something very dark and urgently immediate for men and women in seventeenth-century London.

Given that its abstractions are meant to be imagined into the bodies and family ties of its readers, the affective ambiguity of the episode, especially of Sin's speeches, presents a trial for the reader of a different kind than, for example (as I noted earlier), a Fishian reading might suggest. This trial calls out a charitable impulse, not to reveal it as idolatrous or fallen because it is aimed at the wrong object, but to force us to make a finer, more difficult judgment, one that redeems and allows us to experience the redemptive power of our own pity, even our self-pity.[30] The interpretive trial presented

[29] Lieb, *Dialectics*, p. 163.

[30] Rumrich offers a related argument about Milton and charity, with its own approach to birth and the maternal (*Milton Unbound*, pp. 73–4).

by the passage is, therefore, complicated by our willingness to risk, not reject, the possibly bewildering affective response it invites. It is easy to see the truth clearly if we react to Sin the way the narrator does at lines 648-66: she's horrible, witch-like, and evil, flee from her! It is harder to do so when we recognize that just because we are commanded to reject sin does not mean we are absolved of feeling charity toward those who suffer sin's consequences. The passage forces us powerfully in both directions.

Milton has the Archangel command Adam in Book 12 to "add Love,/ By name to come call'd Charitie, the soul/ Of all the rest" to his other virtues (*PL*, 12.583–4). It is the last, best, and most comprehensive virtue, but also the most potentially bewildering. Instances like the allegory of Sin and Death, in my reading at least, ask us implicitly "how are we to obey this commandment and weep over the suffering of this world (our own and that of others) without tipping over into either despair or a righteous indignation that leads to rebellion?" (what Fish calls imagining oneself impaired).[31] It also asks how Milton risked giving us opportunities to obey this commandment while we are reading a poem that is also supposed to help us learn to regulate the responses it itself inspires. I believe that, at his best, and I think the allegory of Sin and Death is one of the best things Milton ever wrote, he is trying to be equally rigorous in both directions, inviting us to weep uncontrollably and pity unreservedly, while at the same time admonishing us to dissolve our weeping in joy, and quell our pity with zeal.

"FRUIT OF THY WOMB": CHILDBIRTH IN THE STRUCTURE OF BOOKS 10 TO 12

Milton's examination of the problematics of childbed suffering in *Paradise Lost* does not end with the allegorical episode in Book 2. It extends through his brief return to his personifications in Book 10, in the reconciliation scene between Adam and Eve in that book, and in the long biblical paraphrase of the final books. In this larger figurative and narrative arc, which is created by the repetition of particular motifs, images, and allusions, Milton suggests how birth-pain, as a part of Eve's legacy, arrives in the world along with Death, and makes its home in the female body, which, by the end of the epic, becomes a central matrix of human emotional, generative, and spiritual experience. The obstetric focus of Sin's narrative serves to tie Sin

31 Stanley Fish, *How Milton Works* (Cambridge, MA: Harvard University Press, 2001), pp. 511–12. For Fish's own approach to the allegory, which concerns a different matter than the one I am discussing, see pp. 97–9 and 492–3.

proleptically to Eve, who will, upon her fall, become subject to the very fears, pains, and dangers to which Sin's nightmarish experience refers. Through Eve, of course, these difficulties are then bequeathed to womankind as a whole, including, most immediately, the female readers of the epic. The process by which these connections occur in *Paradise Lost* in counterpoint to the arguments for Christian consolation in the later books is worth examining. What the reader witnesses, beginning with the Fall in Book 9, will draw the allegorical details of the end of Book 2 into the texture of human life. The Fall will, to put it simply, make those figures real. As the narrator starkly notes at 10.585–90, Sin had been an "actual" presence in the garden since the Fall itself (a matter of Adam and Eve's actions), but only now does she arrive there "in body" along with her terrible son. Then in the last two books the full human and theological significance of the imagery of childbirth found in the epic is brought into relation with the Nativity, the master figure of a birth that will make possible the redemption of all human suffering, including, of course, the suffering that has attended all births from Cain's on down.

Let us examine how this pattern unfolds. In Book 10, when the Son proclaims sentence on Adam and Eve, and when Sin and Death arrive in Paradise, birth continues to function as the tangible mark of the changes that occur in creation.[32] The statement of Eve's childbed curse is followed only some thirty lines later by Sin's motherly promise to finally feed her ravenous son (10. 193–6, 229–63). The sudden sympathy that Sin says draws her to the earth (*PL*, 10.243–9) is in some sense the widening of her scope of reference as an allegorical figure "authored" by Satan (whom she calls "our great Author" [line 236]). In tempting Eve, Satan has enlarged the role of his daughter/lover and son/rival in the morality play he is writing, and their allegory expands to encompass the natural conditions of the created world, the sudden mortality of which is described in detail. Given that this pair and the hideous potentials they represent have now become aspects of the experience of Adam and Eve, there is something both correct and yet overwhelmingly naive about the comforting words that Adam utters near the end of the book in which all these figures and implications have dovetailed:

wee expected
Immediate dissolution, which we thought
Was meant by Death that day, when lo, to thee
Pains onely in Child-bearing were foretold,

[32] Lieb, *Dialectics*, pp. 170–9, 206–21.

And bringing forth, soon recompenc't with joy,
Fruit of thy Womb: On mee the Curse aslope
Glanc'd on the ground, with labour I must earn
My bread; what harm? (*PL*, 10.1048–55)

What harm indeed. These words are part of the consoling conclusion to a conversation in which Eve has suggested sexual abstinence and suicide as ways of avoiding the derision of future generations for having brought them into a world of misery. Since they are going to bring children into a fallen world, and since they also cannot imagine living with each other without making love, she proposes that they kill themselves. Adam, his "more attentive mind/ *Labouring*" (my italics) (lines 1011–2), remembers the prophecy about Eve's seed bruising the Serpent's head, and reasons instead that this must mean revenge against Satan himself, "which," as he says to Eve, "will be lost/ By death brought on our selves, or childless days/ Resolv'd" (lines 1036–8). In other words, he recognizes the centrality of childbirth in the working out of the consoling plan of providence. He remains blissfully unaware, however, of just what childbearing is going to cost in terms of suffering and loss.[33]

Adam's words about the compensatory joys of bringing a child into the world begin a key reversal of the meaning of childbirth in the rhetorical strategy of the epic. Though he is unaware of this, Adam's remark unconsciously and ironically evokes not only a host of painful conditions about which he has not been told, but through its echo of Christ's eschatological analogy from John 16:21–22, it evokes the Resurrection and Second Coming as well. As we saw in Chapter 3, according to John, Christ tells the disciples not to worry about his coming death:

A woman when she is in travail hath sorrow, because her hour is come: but as soon as she is delivered of the child, she remembereth no more the anguish, for joy that a man is born into the world.

And ye now therefore have sorrow: but I will see you again, and your heart shall rejoice, and your joy no man taketh from you. (*KJV*)

The allusion to this biblical passage has tremendous resonance at this moment, particularly coming from an author whose first two wives had come to childbed in that same sorrow, but neither of whom lived long enough to feel that sorrow drowned in the joy of raising the daughters they

[33] Although they miss the allusion to John 16 (see below), Lieb and Sauer both discuss the regenerative and reproductive aspects of the episode at length (see Lieb, *Dialectics*, pp. 208–12, and Sauer, *Barbarous Dissonance*, pp. 125–7).

had just borne.[34] These words were, of course, among the most commonly quoted in all of the consolatory childbirth literature of the age, and had, in that context, powerfully consoling Christological resonances. It is surely also no coincidence that the allusion should come just one hundred lines or so after Eve's decisive moment of *imitatio Christi* at lines 930–6, where her offer to ask God to allow the entire punishment to fall on her so as to remove it from Adam finally draws Adam into commiseration and forgiveness.[35] Milton clearly chose the words carefully, and their effect at this moment is both painfully ironic and hopeful. However, the immediate needs of the consolatory rhetoric of the rest of the epic will necessitate a muting of the irony inherent in the allusion, driving it well below the surface of the text in favor of the allusion's more hopeful implications. Milton suggests two things here, but if the consolatory purposes of his epic's conclusion are to be effected, he knows that he can only follow through on one of them fully.

The realities of death and the difficulties of life itself, as well as the full difficulty of accepting as effectual the consolations of God's grace, will hit home for Adam after he is sent into a fit by the vision of human history provided by Michael in the course of the next two books. However, in neither the above passage nor in the later vision or narrative will the full fatal connections of those "Pains onely in Child-bearing" with death (a connection so familiar to Milton himself) be articulated for Adam in the epic.[36] This connection had already been articulated both in the descriptions of the terrible mother and child who just a few hundred lines earlier – and just thirty-three lines after the initial utterance of the Curse of Eve – arrived to devour and corrupt, snuffing "the smell/Of mortal change on Earth" (*PL*, 10.193–6, 229–414, 585–609), but the treatment of birth from this point on and into the last books of the epic is marked by a strong and rhetorically strategic avoidance.

34 Scholars have long been aware of the allusion, although no one has connected it with the childbirth discourses before. See, for example, James H. Sims, *The Bible in Milton's Epics* (Gainesville, FL: University of Florida Press, 1962), p. 269, which also notes the reference back to Genesis 3:16 and the echo of the hailing of Mary (Luke 1:42) in *Paradise Lost*, 10.1053.

35 This is something that, had it occurred to Adam when he saw that Eve had fallen, would have, by the logic of substitution that God proclaims in Book 3, effected her redemption. Adam's rhetoric at the Fall in Book 9 is Christ-like, but in the wrong way. Eve's in Book 10 also falls short, because she is indeed guilty at that point, and cannot provide an innocent sacrificial substitution, but her imitation is far more Christ-like than Adam's, which was motivated not by a desire to save Eve, even at the cost of his own life, but by a desire to avoid losing her, which he thought he could only do by falling with her. (Where was his "more attentive mind" then? Probably, as I noted in Chapter 7, remembering her sudden disappearance when she was first created.)

36 I argue, below, that they may be articulated for Eve, although "off stage."

The darker aspects of childbirth find no place, for example, in the visions and narratives of Michael's instruction. Set against Adam's general horror (and finally annulling its terror), we experience instead a crescendo of gradually clarifying (and increasingly celebratory) reiterations of the miraculous birth of Christ as the woman's seed. The first of these is at 11.148–61, where Adam, with an echo of "Mee thougt I saw my late espoused saint" at line 151, describes his sense that his and Eve's prayers have been, in some sense, answered. Here, again, he remembers the Son's prophecy about Eve's seed bruising their foe, and in another proleptic echo of a key reproductive passage from the Gospels, hails her as "Mother of all Mankind,/ Mother of all things living" (lines 158–61). A few lines later, Eve reiterates the formula: "I who first brought Death on all, am grac't/ The sourse of life" (lines 168–9). The prophesy of the seed, and with it references to birth, appear again at 12.327, when the Nativity itself is finally foretold explicitly, and at 12.379–85, where Adam hails the future Virgin Mary directly, remarking – in a way suggestive of the function she had for women in the childbed – on how the fact that she will come from his loins makes it possible for him to refer to his own reproductive function again with joy. The crescendo of reiterations of this formula continues up to within twenty-five lines of the end: "thy Seed" (*PL*, 12.395); "his [Abrahams's] seed" (lines 449–50); "The Womans seed" (line 543); "her Seed to come/ (For by the Womans Seed)" (lines 600–1); and, finally, Eve's proclamation of what she has learned in her dream while Adam was with the angel: "By mee the Promis'd Seed shall all restore" (lines 623–4). At the epic's conclusion, birth is purely an occasion for celebration, and is inextricably wound up with the promise of redemption.

Both Lieb and Shawcross have gone so far as to argue that the concluding episode of the poem, especially the expulsion from Eden, is itself a great, concluding birth-figure. Its alchemical imagery, as well as its rich evocation of the Exodus (which Shawcross treats as itself "an archetype of birth"), combine with archetypal womb and birth images concerning the Garden, its gate, its waters, and Adam and Eve's passage to the "subjected plain" of subsequent human experience to suggest all that humankind will suffer, as well as all that God, in the end, will offer. For Shawcross, "the graphic delivery of Adam and Eve from the *hortus conclusus*, or enclosed garden" combines with the "presage of the Promised Seed (that which brings forth repentance and hope in the poem), and it is that Promised Seed that will lead man out from bondage to Satan."[37] One birth, in other words, expels mankind out into the difficulties of life, among which birth will

[37] John Shawcross, *With Mortal Voice: the Creation of Paradise Lost* (Lexington, KY: University of Kentucky Press, 1982), pp. 136–8, and Lieb, *Dialectics*, pp. 205–21.

figure prominently, but the figure of birth also contains the promise of Christian *re*birth. One exodus leads to wanderings and trials that will, however, end in another exodus. Birth, presented both as a sign of sin-worn mortality and as a way out of it, is the poem's crowning and culminating image.

The terrors of childbirth's actual individual unfolding in time, however, seem to have been largely and deliberately forgotten. For example, it is odd that childbed death makes no appearance in the catalogue of disease in the vision of the Lazar House at 11.477–99. This is particularly striking given that, as I noted in Chapter 2, pregnancy and morbidity were very closely associated in the period. Not only did women suffer more disease during their reproductive years, but many of the symptoms of pregnancy itself were similar to the signs of humoral imbalance familiar to practitioners and described at length in the medical literature.[38] At the moment in *Paradise Lost* that catalogues the conditions of humoral disease, however, there is no explicit mention of childbirth. But birth does maintain an oddly and subtly allusive presence. For example, we glimpse it in the description of Adam's tears at the sight of disease: he cries despite the fact that he was "not of Woman born" (that is to say, in an unmanly but understandable fashion). The line easily fits with renaissance commonplaces about the way men and women should or should not express emotion, but it is also interesting that the lines should recall the phrase used to describe Macduff's birth in *Macbeth*, that he is not "of woman born," having been untimely ripped from his mother's womb in perhaps the most famous figure for caesarian birth in English literature.[39] The repression of disastrous birth in the catalogue seems to return in the poetic echoes of the language, quietly suggesting to an attentive reader what is being kept from the surface.

Other negative images of birth reappear only intermittently in the final books: for example, in Adam's proclamation that, given such suffering as he is witnessing, it were better for his offspring not to be *born* at all; in Michael's brief reference to the "prodigious Births" produced by the ill-mated marriages of the Sons of God and the Daughters of Men (11.683–7);[40]

[38] Gail Kern Paster (*The Body Embarrassed: Drama and the Disciplines of Shame in Early Modern England* [Ithaca, NY: Cornell University Press, 1993], pp. 182–3) even goes so far as to suggest that pregnancy itself was sometimes thought of as a disease, although this perspective is not as widespread in the literature as her comments suggest.

[39] See *Macbeth*, 4.1 and 5.8. The passage did not have the same fame then as it does now, but Milton almost certainly read the play, which appears in the second Folio, to which he contributed "On Shakespear." The evocation of the gendered commonplace about tears also recalls Macduff's reaction in *Macbeth*, 4.3 to the news of his family's death.

[40] Milton's account of the episode from Genesis 6:1–4 stretches from *Paradise Lost*, 11.556 to 718. The section is rich in references to sexual behavior and marriage, but beyond the reference to prodigious

and in the way that the narrator figures the flood in terms of a cosmic abortion.[41] Such passages are as close to the problems of post-lapsarian childbirth as we get in the last two books of the epic, and many of them, along with much of the final two books (especially the allegorical visions and perhaps some of the material that paraphrases biblical narrative) are probably among the earliest that Milton wrote. They may therefore date from the original dramatic form he envisioned, or from his earliest plans for the epic. It seems likely that much of what he finally did with the epic's conclusion entailed adaptation of these earlier materials to his final consolatory scheme. He planned to end the work on a consolatory note as early as the first sketches in the Trinity Manuscript (in the earliest drafts, Faith, Hope, and Charity were to comfort and instruct Adam after an allegorical pagent of human ills). The idea, however, of making birth so centrally important probably did not occur to him until the later stages of composition, after the deaths of Mary and Katherine.[42]

It is possible to read the submergence of explicit allusions to childbed suffering as a failure, a failure of Milton to be Milton (that is, a failure to provide us with a tensely balanced confrontation between diametrically opposed visions of a thing that then asks us to choose or somehow maintain the balance). In other words, in composing or adapting his final epic materials, Milton failed to make them fully express the terror he figured in the Book 2 allegory because he wished to confine the implications of his references to birth so as not to disturb the mixed, but carefully balanced, affective quality of the poem's *consolatio*, in which he had decided birth had to bear the burden of redemption. It is possible, however, that something more complicated is going on in these last, tense books of the poem. Indeed, I have become more and more convinced that, as he adapted and composed the final books, Milton did know what to make theologically of childbed

offspring, no mention is made of reproduction. Milton concentrates here on an etiological account of illicit sexual behavior that hearkens back to the critique of harlotry in the narrator's epithalamic praise of "wedded Love" (*PL*, 4.750–70).

41 See *PL*, 11.738–62 and 824–9, where the firmament that divides the waters above and below of the womb-like creation are broken, aborting the monstrous creatures it had, in a sense, been gestating. Another interesting figure appears in the description of old age, where Adam is told that if he keeps the rule of temperance, he may live undisturbed by disease "till like ripe Fruit [he] drop/ Into [his] Mothers lap" (11.535–46). This comes after Michael, in line with seventeenth-century medical opinion, blames disease on incontinence and the sin of Eve. A possible echo of Milton's *An Apology Against a Pamphlet* perhaps also suggests that the incontinence Michael speaks of here is sexual. Both Michael and the younger Milton speak of incontinence (in Milton's case, unchaste sexual acts) as defacing the image of God in man and woman (*CP*, 1.892). On Milton's habit of associating images of birth with images of devouring, see Lieb, *Dialectics*, pp. 165–72.

42 See Allan H. Gilbert, *On the Composition of* Paradise Lost (Chapel Hill, NC: University of North Carolina Press, 1947) and Shawcross, *With Mortal Voice*, pp. 173–7.

suffering and death, and that he worked very hard in Books 11 and 12 to delineate its redemptive form in a manner appropriate to his epic theodicy – a matter of working out the typological implications of the way Eve's curse is characterized in 1 Timothy 2:15 (as it was understood, at least, by some commentators).

In other words, Milton perhaps didn't simply repress the ugliness he figured earlier in the text. On the contrary, the poem does lay out a schema for dealing with that ugliness. Beginning with the allegory of Sin and Death and moving on to the birth of Eve, the pattern of references to that ugliness is maintained. It picks up again, also, with reminders of pain provided by the reappearance of Sin and Death (10.229–414) and the metamorphosis of Satan (10.509–90, especially 529–31), then in the heartbreaking irony of Adam's unconscious quotation of John 16:21 (10.1048–55). These lines indicate Adam's naivete about what he and Eve and we are in for, but they also point to the eventual solution of the problem in the person and actions of Christ, the original speaker of those words (although he had yet to speak them). This positive typological figuration is further emphasized by the echo in the middle of the passage (line 1053) of Elizabeth's inspired praise of Mary at Luke 1:42. From there, it moves through the reiterations of the oracle, gradually revealing that the ongoing process of human reproduction will lead to the advent of that very speaker. Eve's suffering womb (this schema implies) will be healed in Mary's because all the pains of all the women who came before her and made that birth possible will be taken on by the child born from it, just as they each took on, in proleptic, typological imitation of Christ, their own individual pains. All female reproductive experience becomes an ages-long labor, a collective female labor, relieved at the central point of its history by the nativity it made possible. From that historical middle-point on, women who suffer and die in childbirth can be seen not as the meaningless dead swallowed up by what Milton called in "Lycidas" "the monstrous world," but instead, to draw again on "Lycidas," as the geniuses of the human shore, guardians of the liminal space between the dry land of physical security and the whelming tide of physical suffering under sin. Only they can – and only then can they – embrace in their large recompense all who embark on the perilous passage of the birthing chamber, both as victims and witnesses. The suggestions return us, with a complicating and enriching difference, not only to "Lycidas," but also to the typological symbol that, as a young man, Milton thought could carry the weight of consolation in "An Epitaph on the Marchioness of Winchester" (hereafter "An Epitaph") There, Milton had drawn on Dante to suggest a female line ending in Mary that both distinguished and united the two sides of the heavenly rose and the two dispensations they represented. Milton again places a line of suffering women in the larger narrative of human revelation and redemption, and identifies the crucial role women play in its unfolding.

People will still drown in the Irish Sea and die in childbirth, but Milton's typology suggests that, if we can remember the example of figures like Eve, Mary, Rachel, Lady Jane, and Lycidas (not to mention women like Mary Powell and Katherine Woodcock) correctly, we can attain a higher understanding of what happens to us. As it is in the passage from John that Adam unknowingly quotes, the ongoing suffering of women is given the Christological meaning and the comedic narrative shape we explored in Parts I and II of this study. Just as Milton was led to the final figuration of "Lycidas" by a sudden remembrance of the story of Christ's walking on the water, and in "An Epitaph" by Dante's allusion to the story of Rachel, he is led in *Paradise Lost* to the redemption of childbed suffering by the remembrance of the Christological discourses that made childbirth an instance not just of individual trial, but of *imitatio Christi*. In both the elegies and the epic, he suggests a resolution to what troubles consolation by poetic recourse to a common figurative use of the Bible.

I do think it is true, however, that in the epic, Milton deliberately shied away from doing what he *might* have done at certain points in the unfolding of this schema to make clear the full nature of the struggle. The resolution in *Paradise Lost* is both marked by the epic's earlier treatment of the pain and horror that attended childbed trial, and by the deliberate refusal to fully recollect these problems in the last two books. The turn at the end of Book 10 is not an abrupt reversal like the one in "Lycidas." An abrupt turn was acceptable in the elegy, I think, because the issues there were less personal, and the genre, in any case, allowed for it. The same was true in a different way, as we saw earlier, with the epitaph for Jane Paulet. It is one thing for a young man to make a symbol of his own anxieties out of the death of another young man or woman, to resolve them in a structure designed to, above all, demonstrate poetic skill and power, and then to use them to make a general point about the nature of Christian consolation. As moving as they are, the purpose of poems like "Lycidas" and "An Epitaph" is not to represent a man facing a great personal loss – their impersonality is, in fact, part of what makes them work so beautifully on behalf of others or on behalf of ideas. It is quite another thing, however, for an older man to truly and without any quivering in the voice say that he is contented with the deaths of two women he lived with, had children with, and loved intimately. This is why Sonnet 23 projects the solution of grief to a future not yet fully or stably grasped (though trusted in) by the speaker. It is not that the speaker does not believe that the future holds good things for him (he does, after all, tell us that he does believe this), but the poem ends with a very painful reiteration of the "not yet" that first appeared in Milton's work in the Nativity ode (line 150) and then echoed through it for at least three decades.

When he comes to the final consummating moment at the end of *Paradise Lost*, where we expect the knots of human grief to be finally untied, Milton does keep some of the harder ordeals of fallen life at bay for Adam and Eve. However, the way he sets up the conclusion shows that he is aware of the fact that they will have to fall from the naive optimism that Adam consciously expresses in his allusion to John 16, and into the rueful irony with which we – who know more about the human future – take that allusion. He also knows (or hopes) that they will then be able to move on to a reaffirmation of their original optimism in a more experienced key. Adam and Eve will have to face each of their future trials afresh. Even the instruction that they receive in the last two books will only do them so much good in the face of actual trial (just think about how much good Raphael's patient instructions did them on the morning of the Fall). In his reflection back on his earlier poems, Milton reenacts this same story with its still uncertain conclusion. As a young poet, he was able to wait, like the angels at the end of the Nativity ode, "in order serviceable," but then he imagined he waited in an illuminated space, not in the darkness of "day brought back my night," or at the start of what he knows will be a long, uncertain journey for the first two human wanderers. In the intertext of the epic and Sonnet 23, he suggested the distance between what we know abstractly of consolation and what we need if we are to actually feel it with any security. This is also the subject of Sonnet 19 ("When I consider…"). Patience can prevent murmuring, but not always and not securely (it's always likely to start up again while you wait – and, in any case, just when you think you've made some peace with going blind, your wife and child die). We and the poet know more than Adam does because we have experienced more, and one of the things we know is that all the knowledge and experience in the world may not be enough for the next trial. That, at least, is one more possible reason for Milton's not having had the Archangel educate Adam directly in the matter of just what childbirth could cost, despite the fact that he did take time in Book 2 to make sure the poem did instruct or remind its readers. At this late point, it may not have seemed worth the risk of reminding those readers again, and it may not have seemed likely to do enough good anyway. One question remains, however: just what did he imagine Eve might have learned?

EVE'S DREAM

In the end, I believe Milton did not so much fail or give up as he, in a kind of relieved act of the deepest humility, refused to make any final claims about how to make clear and consoling sense out of childbed loss and suffering. He lays out some of the materials, but refuses or is unable to show us the trial itself actually overcome. As I have argued, he gives the sense of it over to the mysteries of divine love and justice, framed by, but not fully articulated by, the logic of the typological traditions (Christological and Mariological) found in the childbed discourses – the ones surrounding the passages from Timothy and John, and that find expression in the devotional texts he may have come across or overheard in use.

By way of offering a reading of one of the more interesting anomalies of the epic's final episode, however, I would like to suggest that Milton finally, after so much – but by no means exclusive – concentration on male perspectives (his own and Adam's), gives the burden of turning the raw experience of birth into a good and affirming trial over to the women who continue to bear the brunt of it. This is, indeed, I believe, a final explanation for why there are so few explicit references to childbed suffering in the final books. As I have said, Milton always kept his eye on the prize of Christian consolation. However, how women themselves were to wrestle with the wounding angel of their own suffering is not something he could attest to himself. I would suggest, by way of conclusion, that the wrestling he wanted us to imagine takes place off-stage, away from the prying eyes of men, not in the visions and narratives that Michael provides for Adam, but in the secluded space of Eve's final dream.

When Michael announces to Adam that he is taking him up a hill to show him a vision of the human future, he associates this vision with the internal sight that Adam had of the nativity of Eve. He also distinguishes between what he will now offer Adam and what will happen to Eve, who is left behind in her own trance (11.366-9, 411–22). It is also interesting that the first vision he gives to Adam is of his first two children, Cain and Abel, who are referred to by the angel as "some to spring from thee" (11.425), and that the visions finally become too much for Adam, giving way to angelic speech, after the depopulating and aborting vision of the flood (12.8–12). The period of Adam's dream-like visionary experience is, in other words, framed by tragic reproductive figures. Eve's eyes have themselves been "drenched," the Angel tells us, but nothing in his language suggests that she will do anything but sleep. At the end of his long instruction to Adam, the Angel's last command to him is, in fact, that he go and instruct Eve about all that he has learned. There is no explicit indication in what he says that she has been given any instruction of her own.

That Eve, however, *has* been given instruction, therefore comes as a surprise. Milton, indeed, seems to have gone out of his way to sequester the space of her dreaming, as though it took place in a realm only for Eve, a space cut off from the open, referential space of the rest of the epic, the way the lying-in chamber was cut off from the rest of ordinary social space in traditional birthing practice. At this point in the narrative, Michael reveals that Eve has been given a dream designed to calm her and compose her spirits to "meek submission," but if Michael had known about the actual content of the dream, he would not have felt the need to instruct Adam not just to wake her up, but to share with her what he has learned, naming in particular "what may concern her Faith to know,/ The great deliverance by her Seed to come" (12.594–605). An important irony at the expense of Adam's pedagogical role therefore attends what happens when Adam descends the hill to wake Eve. He finds her already awake, and her words prevent him:

> Whence thou returnst, and whither wentst, I know;
> For God is also in sleep, and Dreams advise,
> Which he hath sent propitious, some great good
> Presaging, since with sorrow and hearts distress
> Wearied I fell asleep: but now lead on;
> ...
> This further consolation yet secure
> I carry hence; though all by mee is lost,
> Such favour I unworthie am voutsaft,
> By mee the Promis'd Seed shall all restore. (12.610–14, 620–3)[43]

"So spake our Mother *Eve*," the narrator tells us, underlining the significant maternal self-awareness that Eve now carries forward into her future (and that of all womankind). The first few lines of the speech suggest that the instruction was only of some vague comfort, "some great good" whose specific outlines remained unclear. However, the final lines, reinforced with a ghostly ABBA set of slant-rhymes, suggest something much more specific, something that has, in effect, been taken out of Adam's hands and given to

[43] Milton may have at one point forgotten this discrepancy himself, given that the "Argument" to Book 12, printed in the second edition of the poem, says that Adam "wakens Eve." It was first noted by Thomas Newton, *Paradise Lost: A Poem in Twelve Books*, vol. 2 (London, 1749), p. 423, and has not been commented upon as much as it should. See, however, Joseph Wittreich, "'John, John, I Blush for Thee!': Mapping Gender Discourses in *Paradise Lost*," in Laura Claridge and Elizabeth Langland, eds., *Out of Bounds: Male Writers and Gender(ed) Criticism* (Amherst, MA.: University of Massachusetts Press, 1990), pp. 22–54, especially 35–41. He argues that Eve's dream and final speech carry the weight of prophesy. See also Sauer's pointed rebuttal (*Barbarous Dissonance*, pp. 135, 184 n23).

her directly. Of course, we cannot know any more than the narrator just what she was told of or what she saw in her dream (that is, I believe, a deliberate reticence on Milton's part). The language here allows us to imagine, however, that some difficult lesson may have been imparted, some answers to questions that would have plagued anyone who had thought hard about birth under seventeenth-century conditions: how did women do it? how did they find the strength to bear up under their trials and maintain faith in the process and hope for the future?

Milton said all he could about failure and despair in the face of such trials in the allegory of Sin and Death, and about his own struggles as a witness to such trials in Sonnet 23 and in Adam's dream of Eve's nativity (a dream of which, in contrast, we are given a full account). In the sonnet and in Adam's dream, he clearly declared that he was himself in ongoing pain, but that he, at least, had a vision of a consoling future in which he would re-embrace the women he had lost and have a chance to again express his love and his sorrow to them, and perhaps confess his guilty conscience to them, face to face. Meanwhile, he remained in the dark, committed to remembering the feeling of hope along with all of his guilty ambivalence and sorrow and yearning – all of this laid bear and confessed to anyone who can read, but not to the two people most concerned. This is why he wrote the sonnet and echoed it in the epic (or vice versa): not to get through to his dead wives, but to stand as a repeatable point of engagement with what is hoped for but not yet experienced. It is at once the embrace of Creusas's ghost, the admonishing apparition of Dido's face in the dark underworld crowd, and a trust that someday he will see his own wives again, and they will not turn away as Dido did, will not flee as the dream-vision did, but will instead listen and understand – and that he will be able to do the same (and neither woman will be lost again or have anything to fear). The grace of the sonnet, what little it does attest to, inheres in its repeatability. Furthermore, its dark conclusion is not a conclusion, but a period between iterations that each, over and over again, offer a glimpse of the light to come, a light learned of in a lesson given at the start of fallen life and (like the sonnet) in a dream. In this sense, *Eve's* dream and whatever lesson it taught her (presumably, the way through and out of the despairing self-apprehension represented by Sin's experience) had been carried, so Milton might have imagined, by all the women who had entered and emerged since the Fall from the enclosed space of their suffering. It might be learned by the men excluded from that space too, he hoped, in the end. The glimpse of that lesson, only gestured at by the poetry, offers, in any case – without self-justification and with sorrow and remorse intact – an affirmation devoutly to be wished, and in which he did place his trust.

CHAPTER 9

The "womb of waters" and the "abortive gulph": on the reproductive imagery of Milton's cosmos

At this point, I hope I have convinced most readers that allusions to contemporary obstetric conditions and to Milton's own biographical experience of them are of central importance to *Paradise Lost*. There is, however, one aspect of the epic that requires further comment in this respect: Milton's cosmology. This is a difficult and contested area of study, and comprehensive conclusions about it lie outside the framework of this book, but the reproductive images that Milton used to describe his cosmos have long been recognized as important, and it has been rare for scholars to pay much attention to contemporary obstetric contexts in interpreting them. I would therefore like to conclude with some suggestions about how attention to such contexts, especially to anxieties attendant upon maternal mortality, might help us to better understand some of the stranger aspects of these images.

Milton's descriptions of the physical layout of his universe have caused a good deal of confusion over the years, and his seeming failure to be clear about particular details has been attributed to a number of causes.[1] Some

[1] Debates began as early as Hume's 1695 commentary, and a consensus about how the seeming inconsistencies might be resolved has developed only slowly. Of chief importance early on were the comments of the Richardsons (1734) and Newton (1749), and later, the detailed accounts offered by Keightley (1859) and Masson (1874). Thomas N. Orchard is crucial for modern readings, although not all aspects of his account have met with acceptance. See Orchard, *The Astronomy of Milton's* Paradise Lost (London: Longman's, Green, and Co., 1896; rpt., New York, NY: Haskell House, 1966) (2nd edn. revised and retitled *Milton's Astronomy: the Astronomy of* Paradise Lost [London: Longman's, Green, and Co., 1913]; Allan H. Gilbert, "The Outside Shell of Milton's World," *Studies in Philology* 20 (1923), 444–7; Grant McColley, "The Astronomy of *Paradise Lost*," *Studies in Philology* 34 (1937), 209–47; Harry F. Robins, "The Crystalline Sphere and the 'Waters Above' in *Paradise Lost*," *PMLA* 69 (1954), 903–14 and "That Unnecessary Shell of Milton's World," in *Studies in Honor of T. W. Baldwin*, ed. Don Cameron Allen (Urbana, IL: University of Illinois Press, 1958), pp. 211–19; Kester Svendsen, *Milton and Science* (Cambridge, MA: Harvard University Press, 1956); Walter Clyde Curry, *Milton's Ontology, Cosmogony, and Physics* (Lexington, KY: University of Kentucky Press, 1957); Marjorie H. Nicolson, "The Discovery of Space," *Medieval and Renaissance Studies* 1 (1965), 40–59; and Harinder Singh Marjara, *Contemplation of Created Things: Science in* Paradise Lost (Toronto, ON: University of Toronto Press, 1992).

have said that he was himself confused in the face of the various debates of his day concerning astronomy, and that this led him either to self-contradiction or to an unsuccessful attempt at reconciling the traditional Ptolemaic scheme (in its later Alphonsine elaboration) with the cosmologies implied by Genesis and by various classical, medieval and contemporary authors. Others have, more simply, blamed the confusion on various forms of poetic expediency or on Milton's lack of interest in the concrete consistency of his cosmos. Most at this point agree, however, that despite the occasional anomaly, the cosmos of the poem is consistent enough to achieve its primary purpose: creating the impression of a vast construction that testifies to God's glory as well as to His intimate attention to every detail.[2]

Among these details are features and processes that Milton describes using figurative language derived in striking ways from the living and breathing bodies of the creatures that inhabit this cosmos. Alastair Fowler, for example, has noted that Milton makes his universe seem "instinct with life" in every part: "Like the universe in Plato's *Timaeus* it is alive: animate throughout, it moves, engages in metabolic exchanges… and exhales, transpiring fragrant spirit to God in prayer."[3] What Fowler does not mention is that it also *reproduces* life; it conceives, gestates, and gives birth, and these processes are essential to its function as the great embodied stage upon which Milton has the human drama play itself out.

As we have seen, reproduction organizes an important network of images in the epic, and that network is comprised of two chains of association: one connecting idealized images, the other images of perversion, monstrosity, or abortion. These chains, we should also note, link several important cosmic vistas in the poem.[4] The positive or "light" chain begins with the description of creation in the invocation to Book 1. It appears again in the invocation to Book 3 and the cosmological descriptions that accompany Satan's arrival at the outer realms of the creation and his transit to the sun and the earth.[5] The chain of positive associations then weaves its way through the descriptions of Eden's fertility and of human sexuality in Books 4 and 5, through the full creation narrative of Book 7, and reaches its climax in Adam's description of the nativity of Eve at the end of Book 8,

[2] See Alastair Fowler's comments in John Milton, *Paradise Lost*, 2nd edn., ed. Alastair Fowler (New York, NY: Longman, 1998), pp. 33–6.

[3] Fowler, *Paradise Lost*, p. 33.

[4] The general structures of these chains of association were first worked out by Michael Lieb, *The Dialectics of Creation: Patterns of Birth and Regeneration in* Paradise Lost (Amhearst, MA: University of Massachusetts Press, 1970).

[5] On the invocations see Lieb, *Dialectics*, pp. 37–55.

where Adam identifies human sexuality as the sum of his earthly bliss. After the Fall, as we have seen, human procreation becomes a matter of deep ambivalence. Its redemptive powers, encapsulated in the figure of the Nativity and in Eve's submission to motherhood, battle with the negative associations brought into the poem by the dark chain, which dovetails fully with the light in Book 10, creating the tense, although ultimately positive and redemptive, reproductive figuration of the epic's final books.

Before Book 10, the dark chain also weaves its way through the poem from the start. Dark, parodic images of reproduction first appear at the building of Pandemonium (in the maternal mining / rape simile of 1.684–90).[6] They then play an important role in the council scene that takes up the first half of Book 2, where the fallen angels speculate about chaos and their own possible destructibility (Belial and Satan both evoke womb imagery to characterize chaos and the anxieties it inspires – 2.146–51, 138–41). As we have seen, of course, a strong sequence of dark reproductive images then extends through the description of Hell's landscape and the allegory of Sin and Death. These continue and are intensified in the descriptions of Satan's passage through chaos, which is described as "The Womb of nature and perhaps her Grave," where "embryon Atoms" do battle and "pregnant causes" mix "confus'dly" (2.899–900, 910–14). The dark images largely retreat in Books 3 and 4, although they are there in a muted way in the description of the area of chaos that surrounds the globe of creation, and in the account of the Paradise of Fools (3.74–6, 418–539). Negative images reappear again briefly in Satan's final retort to Abdiel at the end of Book 5 (his idea that he and the other angels were born directly from the material of Heaven at 5.853–63) and in the passage on the invention of artillery in Book 6 (6.470–91, 507–20).[7] As we saw in the previous chapter, Milton wove some disquieting allusions into the otherwise idealized description of the birth of Eve, and a number of darker reproductive images also attend the temptation and the Fall in Book 9.[8] The dark chain, however, arises again in full force in Book 10, with the articulation of Eve's curse at lines 193–6. Key reproductive images can then be traced in the following sequence of events: the departure of Sin and Death from Hell, their building of the bridge, their meeting with Satan, their arrival on the Earth (10.229–410, 585–609),

[6] See John Rumrich, *Milton Unbound: Controversy and Reinterpretation* (Cambridge University Press, 1996), pp. 112–17 on the reproductive resonances of the scene and its connections with the nativity of Eve.

[7] On the reproductive resonances of the artillery passage, see Rumrich, *Milton Unbound*, pp. 114–16.

[8] Lieb discusses the temptation and the Fall at length in *Dialectics*, pp. 184–201, also detecting such resonances in Eve's dream in Book 5.

Satan's return to Hell (the epic simile that associates his serpentine metamorphosis with the Python engendered from the slime left behind by the flood at 528–32), the destabilization of the creation's cosmological order at God's command (649–714), and the long complaint that Adam utters as he witnesses these changes and their terrestrial effects (720–844).[9] The reemergence of this dark valence is central to the complex effect of the reproductive images and allusions that Milton wove into Adam and Eve's reconciliation scene (10.909–1104), Adam's response to the vision of the Lazar House (11.477–99), the account of the flood (11.738–901), and the epic's ambivalent final consolation.

Of the cosmic vistas that make up important links in these two chains, two are particularly important for an understanding of the way anxiety over maternal mortality may have affected Milton's descriptions of his cosmos: the descriptions of the globe of the prelapsarian creation (3.72–6, 416–742) and the description of chaos (2.890–920). Both provide – one before the Gate of Heaven, the other before the Gate of Hell – vantage points from which we can take in not just what Satan sees at two points in his journey (both scenes end with parallel leaps forward on that journey), but also important aspects of Milton's larger cosmic reproductive symbolism. The two parallel scenes provide descriptions of two great wombs: in Book 3, we see the great, fertile womb of creation that serves as a central metonymy for the bright side of Milton's reproductive vision (a cosmic womb full of potential, but also, in important ways, fragile and uncertain); in Book 2, we get a dark and profoundly disquieting vision of a paradoxically "abortive" womb, the gulf from which the other emerged, and the grave to which it might someday return.

If I am right that Milton's and his immediate audience's perceptions of reproduction were filtered through a pervasive anxiety, then it should be possible to read these two great parts of the cosmos of *Paradise Lost* – its two great wombs – as bearing the marks of that anxiety. The two cosmological regions form, I believe, a dyad offered for our difficult contemplation. On one side, the anxiety is expressed indirectly by a series of fragile idealizations. These can console, and they claim for human reproduction a divine beauty and mystery, but they also tell a story of lost perfection, of a fall from a state of free, creative choice to one of painful and uncertain trial. In this sense, they function much like Adam's vision of the birth of Eve. On the dark side, however, we see a more direct expression of pain and fear. Some passages, like the allegory of Sin and Death and the account of Hell's prodigious and

[9] Lieb, *Dialectics*, pp. 161–83, 204–7.

perverse fertility, are aspects of the poem's imagination of damnation, a cycle of unrelieved pain that goes nowhere and gives birth to nothing but more of the same. The associations inherent in chaos, however, are different. These, like the descriptions of the brighter precincts of creation, express a tension between consolation and fear, and they are therefore closely associated with the ambivalent reproductive discourse of the final books. A mistaken apprehension of them could lead to damnation. Right apprehension, on the other hand, could mirror God's own acts of creation from disordered potential.

CREATION AS A WOMB

Let me begin by explaining the grounds we have for imagining the created universe as a great womb – in fact, as a series of concentric wombs. As I noted earlier, the consensus position on the structure of Milton's creation, which has developed over the past century or so, suggests that the globe of the creation, which in Book 3 we first see along with Satan from the outside, is surrounded by what looks and feels like and functions as a shell (the narrator calls it a "firm opacous globe" at 3.418). The shell is firm enough for Satan to walk upon, although its surface is vexed by the storms raging in chaos, to which we are told it is "exposed" (line 425). This outer surface will later become the location of the Paradise of Fools (lines 440–97). It is never precisely said just when the shell was created, but its position suggests that it follows the curve of the circle drawn by the outer leg of the golden compass that, according to Raphael, the Son wielded on the first day of creation (7.224–31). It was perhaps – although this is by no means clear – established at the time the Son drew that circle. In any case, the sphere clearly encloses, and is itself a part of, the segment of chaos that was circumscribed on that day and then transformed over the following five days into the vast, light-infused, clockwork universe that Adam and Eve inhabit before the Fall.

Somewhat oxymoronically, an earlier passage describing Satan's approach to the shell from the perspective of God and the Son (3.56–79) describes it as "imbosomed without firmament" in the element of chaos – that is to say, both embraced or immersed, on the one hand, and exposed on the other as a "bare outside." Unlike the earth, which emerges during the creation itself below a sea of "waters above" (Genesis 1:6–8 and *PL*, 7.261–75), the surface of the shell has no firmament to keep the "Illimitable Ocean" of chaos (*PL*, 2.892) away from its surface. Indeed, its purpose is itself to enclose the luminous orbs within it, the nine concentric spheres of the created universe and the earth itself, "From Chaos and th' inroad of

Darkness old" (3.420–1). It is a protective shell for the inner spheres, not one of those spheres, and as a protective shell, it seems to work perfectly. Although it is itself vexed and exposed on the outside, everything within it is peaceful, bright, and – at least before the Fall – in perfect alignment.

Earlier in Book 2, we had also been told that the globe of the creation is attached in some unspecified way by a golden chain to the bottom of Heaven (2.1051–3), and later we discover that it actually hangs somewhere very near Heaven's gate (3.501–25). It therefore hangs in a somewhat tamed area of chaos – its upper reaches – where the influence of Heaven calms the warring elements, making Satan's flight, as well as the protective work of the shell, easier. Only the very top is entirely calm. The rest is "exposed" to chaos, and this sense of exposure is intensified by the ease with which Satan lands upon its surface and then later infiltrates it.[10] He does so through what Milton refers to as "a passage wide" (3.526–39), in which a bright, calm sea or lake of pearly, crystalline liquid flows. The opening leads down into the very center of the creation's womb.

This sea flows not only within the opening, but between the inside surface of the shell itself and the outermost surface of the region of spheres the shell encloses. As what I said before suggests, this sea is what Raphael refers to in his paraphrase of Genesis 1:6–8 as a "crystalline ocean" of circumfluous waters, Milton's version of the "waters above" of the biblical account. The association of this ocean with the "waters above," and its position in relation to other parts of the cosmos, are less clear than we might wish, but the consensus holds – I believe, correctly – that the region specified by Raphael in *Paradise Lost*, 7.261–75 as the "firmament" – itself made up of the nine Ptolemaic spheres – is below these waters and holds them up. The highest of the nine spheres is the *primum mobile*. Many accounts of the Ptolemaic system also included the *empyrean* as either a tenth sphere or as a heavenly realm outside the spheres themselves. Milton lists the seven planetary spheres and the two outer spheres (the former without giving their order, but the latter – the *crystalline sphere* and the *primum mobile* – in their conventional places) at 3.481–3. However, in what is generally recognized to be a revision of the conventional scheme, he places the "crystalline ocean," rather than the *empyrean*, at the outside of the ninth sphere. He then adds the outside shell, places chaos outside and around it, and positions Heaven – his version of an *empyrean* realm – both outside and

[10] John Leonard, "Milton, Lucretius, and 'the Void Profound of Unessential Night,'" in *Living Texts: Interpreting Milton* eds. Kristin A. Pruitt and Charles W. Durham (Selinsgrove, PA: Susquehanna University Press, 2000), pp. 198–217, especially 212.

above the whole configuration. It seems clear, therefore, that he wished to distinguish between his cosmos and that envisioned by the conventional astronomy of his day in order to produce just this configuration: a globe that hangs in the vexed, oceanic element of chaos, but that contains within it an ocean of exceptional calm in which floats another globe, one formed and upheld by the nine-fold firmament of Ptolemaic spheres.[11] These nine spheres fill the space between this ocean and the surface of the earth, which is itself at first "englobed" in "the waters *below*" (my italics) of the Genesis account, what Milton calls in his description of the third day of creation as the "Womb as yet/ Of Waters." At that point, the earth floats in this womb as an "Embryon immature involv'd" (7.276–7), and it is out of *that* womb that dry land emerges on the third day. The land and sea are then, on later days, made themselves to give birth to the various plants and animals.

This description suggests we imagine the "firm, opacous globe" surrounding the whole of creation as a kind of uterine wall. It gives form to the entire creation as a womb suspended within the upper reaches of chaos, protecting what is inside it, allowing the creation to gestate peacefully in the waters of the crystalline ocean and to bring forth whatever potentials God's commands make possible. Moreover, it suggests that the creation, with its firmament dividing its internal waters, is itself a womb within a womb, or more exactly a womb that sits within a womb as though the inner womb were itself a developing fetus. That firmament holds within it the earth, which is, again, itself both fetus and womb, and the figure extends in Chinese box fashion down to all the wombs that are later born from the womb of the earth, including those of the animals, and most importantly those of Eve and her daughters, especially, in the eventual event, that of Mary.

Like the human womb, as we meet with it in the medical and anatomy texts of the period, the womb of creation is described as having a protective function. Also, like the human womb, it contains areas both hollow and filled with fluid, separated by membranes, and, as we shall see, an opening capable of dilation and contraction. It may not, however, be possible to go so far as to argue that Milton was influenced directly in the creation of his elaborate figure by contemporary medical descriptions of the womb, and of

[11] For some different approaches to these and other cosmological questions, see the studies by Robins, Curry, Svendsen, Gilbert, and Marjara, cited above. On the deliberate, consistent, and functional nature of Milton's revision, however, I believe that Orchard got it right almost a century ago (*Milton's Astronomy*, p. 74).

the disposition within it of a developing fetus.[12] It is important, however, to recognize that, especially in its prelapsarian state, the figure of creation as a womb does abstract certain characteristics of the human womb, idealizing them rather than faithfully reflecting them. Furthermore, the manner in which it does so was influenced by Milton's own experiences of pain and uncertainty, and approaching the figure with this comparison in mind can help us to understand some of its more puzzling aspects.

Consider, for example, the description of the exposed part of the crystalline ocean that fills the opening at the top of the creation (3.518–22, 526–39). The pearly liquid of the sea in this scene might refer, in a wide sense, to three fluids associated with human reproduction in seventeenth-century accounts: uterine waters, male semen, and female ejaculate, the latter of which was believed to come forth from a woman's body (from the ovaries into the uterus) in response to sexual stimulation.[13] The "liquid Pearl" (3.519) is not any one of these things in a consistent way, but the scene is so suggestive of an embodied religious eros that it invites the imagination in that direction. It is as if the fluid were welling up as a response of fullness to the creator, the womb of the creation opening itself at the gate from which He first emerged to circumscribe her disordered material from the rest of chaos, and then to infuse her with His creative warmth. It may be thinking too precisely on the event (and I have to admit to a certain embarrassment as I write), but we must assume that Milton made love often enough with his first two wives to be familiar with the post-coital behavior of bodily fluids. Given what he would have read in the anatomy books, he would have imagined a mixture of both male and female seed, and there is no reason to discount the possibility that he is here providing us with a cosmic and divinely idealized figure for matters that writers like Paré described, in any case, with striking candor.[14] Milton would never have thought to write about such matters explicitly, but he may have given himself unconscious liberty to infuse his highly idealized description of this symbolic vista – one of the poem's most beautiful symbols of the relationship between God and His unfallen creation – with such an idealized (and idealizing) eros. In their

[12] For good examples of such medical descriptions, however, see the 1649 edition of Thomas Johnson's translation of Paré's works: Ambroise Paré, *The Workes of that Famous Chirurgion Ambrose Parey*, trans. Thomas Johnson, (London, 1649), pp. 99–103, 593–7, and Jane Sharp, *The Midwives Book* (London, 1671), pp. 34–40, 133–7.

[13] See, for example, Paré, *Workes* (1649), p. 592.

[14] Paré goes into remarkable detail in his description of how a husband is to sexually stimulate his wife (*Workes* [1649], p. 593).

divine aspect, after all, the human powers to love and to procreate were for Milton matters of both physical pleasure and high seriousness and mystery.

The relationship between the opening and the gate and stairway, the latter two of which together suggest both phallic and womb-like forms, also echoes the hermaphroditic nature of God's brooding over and impregnating the "vast Abyss" in the invocation to Book 1 (1.19–22). The chain from which the pendant world hangs furthermore suggests – although, again, not with any strictly logical consistency – an umbilical cord. Suspended from it, the fetus/womb of the creation develops in the half embrace of Heaven's light and warmth, precariously suspended over chaos and waiting to give birth upward to creatures who will later, we are told, pass at will between both realms, both living in creation and repopulating Heaven. The passage also echoes other reproductive tableaux in the epic: for example, the relationship between the "Sun's fervid rays" and "earth's inmost womb" (5.300–3) (which responds with the overflowing fertility of the garden) and, of course, the sexual union of Adam and Eve in Book 4 before the Fall.[15]

The idyll, however, is quickly broken. Satan is too diminutive in the sublime scene to compete with the divine relationship between Heaven and unfallen creation. He does, however, violate the open and passive womb upon which he gazes, literally plunging into it, and this will eventually alter for the worse the relationship implied by the delicate balance of the scene. As a result, the womb of creation will be turned into a more imperfect vessel, one much like the fallen human womb in its vulnerable uncertainty.

The fact that, at the time of Satan's arrival, the opening at the top of the globe is widely dilated furthermore suggests one last echo of a contemporary reproductive belief. In the midst of his description of the opening, Milton's narrator, projecting forward into our uncertain future, tells us that it will later contract – at one point to the size of the Holy Land, later to the size only of Mount Zion. The past tense of his description in fact suggests that, at even later ages of history, this opening will perhaps be completely shut (3.528–37). It is possible that this closing of the womb of creation and the way its processes of gestation are rendered unpredictable with the Fall is based in Milton's reimagination of the common belief that, upon fertilization, the uterus shut tightly to retain the coagulating seeds of both the man and the woman.[16]

[15] I am not alone in reading such imagery this way. See James Grantham Turner, *One Flesh: Paradisal Marriage and Sexual Relations in the Age of Milton* (New York, NY: Oxford University Press, 1987), p. 201. See also Mary Adams, "Fallen Wombs: the Origins of Death in Miltonic Sexuality," *Milton Studies* 29 (1992), 165–79.

[16] For descriptions, see Paré, *Workes* (1649), p. 594, and Sharp, *The Midwives Book*, pp. 35, 102–3, 133–4.

The image, as Milton would have encountered it in the medical literature, is one of exclusion of the man as the woman withdraws from him in a physical process that is hers alone, as well as into a period of life whose rituals and customs are likewise exclusively female. The period of a pregnancy is a period of anxiety as to outcome, and the woman recedes almost fully from the presence and influence of her husband in the later stages. Perhaps, therefore, behind the open, reciprocal situation at the top of the universe before the Fall lies Milton's imagination of the grateful and expectant state of a married couple who have just discovered a pregnancy but who have yet to face the crisis of the coming birth. It might also suggest a fantasy of how a man might have approached his wife's childbirth before the Fall (before it became a source of so much worry). Here in Book 3, as Satan, with all his malice, gazes down at an entirely innocent universe, Milton imagines him gazing into what would later become the secret space of woman's reproductive function, as well as the enclosure of her reproductive body itself. In doing so, he can imagine it himself and do so without shame or present fear, although not without a tragic sense of foreboding. Satan's subsequent plunge is therefore a profound violation not only of the creation itself, but also of a moment of profound intimacy, echoed again in his later violation of the bower and of Eve's "Organs of…Fancie" (4.800–09). In light of the figurative copulation Satan later achieves with Eve (the "easie entrance" he wins to her heart at the point of the Fall itself), the strange description of the contraction of the opening at the top of the world suggests the world's gradual estrangement from its creator. And it is, of course, significant that the reversal of that estrangement will be effected in the Incarnation, another act of spiritualized physical procreativity (a descending, in that case, of God himself, rather than Satan, into the wombs-within-wombs of creation). Until that point (and even, as we have seen, well after it) human beings will not be spared the suffering that comes with the punishment for original sin. However, the form that the reunion took in Mary's womb offered humankind a way to imagine its way through such suffering, connecting the poem's earlier cosmic vistas to the logic of the ambivalent consolation that frames the last two books.

THE MATTER OF CHAOS

When Milton describes Satan's first view of the other great cosmic womb in the poem, however, we see something quite different from the poised, bright enclosure of the creation, although this vision too suggests ambivalence about fallen reproduction, not merely horror. The womb of chaos, unlike that of the creation, represents a state of pregnant potential that cannot actualize itself and that contrasts with, and at times seems to rage against, God's creative order, although with a paradoxical impotence. God's commands forced a circumscribed part of it to realize its disordered potentials in particular directions, but in its original, uncreated essence, it stands for a state of existence that has no particularity or direction at all. In general, I accept the arguments of critics like Dennis Danielson and John Rumrich, who see chaos as providing the *essentially* good substance from which God forms his various creations (and I agree that it therefore has its own positive creative and reproductive resonances).[17] I would argue, however, that the reproductive elements that Milton made use of in his descriptions of the material of chaos and the space within which it exists (as well as the gendered language he uses to create the corresponding allegorical characters, Chaos and Old Night) have a largely negative function in Milton's handling of reproduction. These do not suggest a kind of evil or the consequences of any coherent principle of opposition to divine will (these are, I believe, more properly figured in Satanic, hellish, or simply sin-worn modes of reproduction, as found in the allegory of Sin and Death or the descriptions of Hell's landscape or the Paradise of Fools).[18] They do not, however, suggest a primal cosmic fertility that can be easily or consistently associated with Milton's ideas about the freedom of the will, or the reader's freedom of interpretation.[19]

[17] For Rumrich's argument about chaos, which includes his influential idea that it constitutes "God's womb," see "Milton's Concept of Substance," *English Language Notes* 19 (1982), 218–33; "Uninventing Milton" *Modern Philology* 87 (1990), 249–65; "Milton's God and the Matter of Chaos," *PMLA* 110 (1995), 1035–46; *Matter of Glory: a New Preface to* Paradise Lost (Pittsburgh, PA: University of Pittsburgh Press, 1987), pp. 53–69; *Milton Unbound*, pp. 140–6 and "Of Chaos and Nightingales," in *Living Texts: Interpreting Milton*, eds. Kristin A. Pruitt and Charles W. Durham (Selinsgrove, PA: Susquehanna University Press, 2000), pp. 218–27. Dennis Danielson's classic argument for the theological basis of this sort of approach to chaos can be found in *Milton's Good God: a Study in Literary Theodicy* (Cambridge University Press, 1982).

[18] The bibliography on this side of the question is a long one. See, in particular, Robert M. Adams, "A Little Look into Chaos," in *Illustrious Evidence: Approaches to English Literature of the Early Seventeenth Century*, ed. Earl Miner (Berkeley, CA: University of California Press, 1975), pp. 71–89; Regina Schwartz, "Milton's Hostile Chaos: '…and the Sea Was no More,'" *ELH* 52 (1985), 337–74, and her fuller argument in *Remembering and Repeating: Biblical Creation in* Paradise Lost (Cambridge University Press, 1988), pp. 18–30; and Leonard, "Milton, Lucretius, and the Void."

[19] On this way of reading chaos, see Rumrich, *Milton Unbound*, pp. 140–6; see also Catherine Gimelli Martin, "'Pregnant Causes Mixt': the Wages of Sin and the Laws of Entropy in Milton's Chaos," in *Arenas of Conflict: Milton and the Unfettered Mind*, eds. Kristin McCoglan and Charles Durham (Selinsgrove, PA: Susquehanna University Press, 1997), pp. 161–82, which appears in expanded form as part of *The Ruins of Allegory*: Paradise Lost *and the Metamorphosis of Epic Convention* (Durham: Duke University Press, 1998), pp. 162–200.

Despite the fact that, from a theological standpoint, we do have every reason to think of chaos as substantially good, the terror expressed by these passages is very real. So the important question is: why the ambiguity? In an award-winning essay published a few years ago, John Leonard has suggested an answer that, I think, leads in the right direction. Although he is not concerned with reproductive images, in arguing that the ambiguity of the descriptions is expressive of an ambivalence Milton had about cosmology itself, Leonard suggests a way in which these passages may be linked to Milton's reproductive anxieties.[20] He argues that Milton was deeply affected by his reading of Lucretius and by some of the speculations of the new astronomy (especially the works of Galileo and Bruno). He was then, in a sense, scared of his own power to imagine an infinite and disordered cosmos, and he could not keep that vision in permanent imaginative exile as he tried to describe a universe ordered by God's good will. John Rumrich, on the other hand, in a response to Leonard, has suggested that we might associate Milton's feelings about the dark and night with his epic project itself, which is, after all, an attempt to make sense of what he is afraid might not indeed make sense. The overlap in what both of these critics are willing to allow each other suggests to me at least one other source for Milton's manifest ambivalence about this realm, and I would like to conclude this study by suggesting that he was also afraid of his own reproductive imagination. His need to confront that fear drove him, I believe, to create the great double figure we are exploring in this chapter.

In Leonard's reading, the outer shell of our universe is, unlike Lucretius' wall of fire, an impermeable barrier that completely divides our world from the realm of chaos. It is a figure for the strenuousness of Milton's struggle to drive away a cosmological vision that disturbs him. Leonard, however, points out a few strange places where that vision creeps back in (for example at 3.724–32, where "night" is briefly characterized by Uriel as something that might threaten to "invade" creation, and the several strange moments where Milton seems to suggest that chaos is both infinite and co-eternal with God). Moments like these are, to extend Leonard's figure a little further than he does himself, unconscious chinks in the impermeable barrier Milton had set up as a figuratively dividing line between two realms of the universe – indeed, two ways of imagining a universe. One realm is ordered, finite, and enclosed not only in an outer protective shell, but within the narrative logic of a providentially willed process of procreation. Its extension in space is

[20] See Leonard, "Milton, Lucretius, and the Void," which won the James Holly Hanford Award from the Milton Society of America for 2000.

strictly determined. Its extension in time is somewhat less so, but still it moves through time teleologically – toward an end that might delay in a way determined by the freedom granted to its creatures, but that remains a determined end nonetheless. The other, described not only as a womb but as "perhaps [a] grave" (2.911), is, as Leonard puts it:

> a thing of darkness that Milton sees clearly but is reluctant to acknowledge. He tries to expel it from our universe, but it creeps back in his despite. The void is threatening because it raises uncomfortable questions about our importance, and about the creator's power and even his existence.[21]

The vision of this realm offered at the Gate of Hell is one that Danielson described vividly as a "fine picture of any world without God."[22] Strictly speaking, it is undetermined. For Leonard, this suggests a vision of the universe that a theodicy can barely entertain – and must, in any case, reject – one without any meaning or order. It is, however, a vision that Milton did allow into his poem, though perhaps reluctantly.[23] What Leonard does not note, however, is that Milton took the Lucretian image of "*moenia mundi*," or "walls of the world," and made them function not only as a barrier between creation and chaos, but also as a wall between two realms imagined as wombs. It is, in fact, the wall itself of one of those wombs. In doing so, he created a vast, double figure, and Leonard's treatment of the way the darkness "creeps" back into his brightly lit creation crucially suggests that Milton may not have been completely successful at maintaining the distinction at the heart of his figure. If the chaos we meet with at the open gate of Hell is "a fine picture of any world without God," then the "womb" of chaos can be said to provide a vision of a *womb* without God, or by extension, *a female body* without God – in other words, the dark twin, of the womb we meet with at the open gate of Heaven. In the larger context of the epic's network of reproductive images, the description of chaos suggests a locus of powerful anxieties about reproduction, possibly suggesting childbed itself as an instance of experience that threatens to undermine theodicy, a moment of abandonment – or seeming abandonment – by God.[24]

21 Leonard, "Milton, Lucretius, and the Void," p. 213.

22 Leonard quotes the phrase ("Milton, Lucretius, and the Void," p. 214). See Danielson, *Milton's Good God*, p. 50.

23 Leonard, "Milton, Lucretius, and the Void," pp. 213–14.

24 Gardner Campbell has suggested to me in conversation that God's withholding of his goodness from chaos (*PL*, 7.165–73) can perhaps be thought of as a type of God's abandonment of Jesus on the cross. If that is so, the Christological resonances of the figure would certainly fit with the Christological resonances that childbed suffering had in the period, especially for those who might recite Psalm 22 as they faced it.

Rumrich's response to Leonard's argument provides me with a concluding observation that, however, recuperates an important positive valence of chaos as a reproductive figure. Rumrich has acknowledged that Leonard and others are right to note that Chaos, Night, and their tumultuous realm can be terrifying, but he also continues to insist on the positive nature of the reproductive imagery that appears in the passages that describe them.[25] In "Of Chaos and Nightingales," he clarifies his approach to the distinction between the two allegorical figures of Chaos and Night, reminding us of his contention – central to his arguments as far back as 1982 – that Chaos, described in his allegorical form by the narrator as an "Anarch," is a figure for "God's *voluntary* absence from Night's realm…the absence of God's goodness – his creative, ordering will."[26] This means that chaos is "good," in the Augustinian sense that anything that exists must partake of divine goodness (and chaos came forth from God *ex deo* in Milton's conception of creation), but it lacks His active, *creative* goodness.[27] Rumrich also points out that Night, at least in the form in which we find it/her *within* the creation, is also at times represented as pleasant, making possible, for example, the "grateful" vicissitude that gives creation its variety, something often acknowledged as a major source of its beauty.[28] Even more provocatively, however, he suggests that such darkness is a source of Milton's own impulse toward beauty, and of his creative powers as a poet.

I would add that these impulses can be said to be rooted in both a love of and a terror of darkness. Rumrich suggestively reminds us that, in the invocation to Book 3, Milton characterized himself as a nightingale, "the wakeful Bird" that "Sings darkling, and in shadiest Covert hid/ Tunes her nocturnal Note."[29] The image suggests Milton's physical blindness, his experience of having parts of the poem come to him at night in dreams, as well as the more general benightedness of all fallen human experience, and it, in turn, reminds us that poetry is, after all, often a sort of whistling in the dark. As Rumrich beautifully puts it, "perhaps darkness is the price to be paid for Nightingales." This captures one of the resonances of the myth of Philomela: that beauty often has its source in great pain, deprivation, and

25 Rumrich, "Of Chaos and Nightingales," pp. 219–20, and Leonard, "Milton, Lucretius, and the Void," p. 207–8.

26 "Of Chaos and Nightingales," p. 220.

27 The claim is central to Rumrich's argument, and has not been fully addressed in print by his critics. Gardner Campbell has, however, offered a suggestive alternative reading of *Paradise Lost*, 7.165–73 in a conference paper entitled "Milton Bound," delivered at the Conference on John Milton, Murfreesboro, Tennessee, 1999. I thank Professor Campbell for making the paper available to me.

28 "Of Chaos and Nightingales," pp. 224–6.

29 "Of Chaos and Nightingales," pp. 226 and *Milton Unbound*, pp. 107–8.

disability.[30] Rumrich hastens to assert that Milton does not present "his affliction as desirable." "[Y]et," he continues, "he does seem to register it as the condition of his epic inspiration."[31]

I agree with Rumrich that Milton's creative power was closely associated with darkness. It is rooted in darkness, emerges from it, and, in that sense, it can be said to be inspired by it. It has, of course, been my assertion throughout this study that Milton's inspiration was inextricably tied-up for him in images of reproductive suffering. The "shadiest covert" of the Book 3 invocation is yet another enclosed wombic space, a lying-in chamber of a kind, although one inhabited by a solitary man rather than the female community of the childbed rites. When Milton retired into his bedchamber on all those nights during the long gestation of *Paradise Lost*, the fruits of his labor there were as uncertain to him as those he worried about back in 1630 when he tried to frame an adequate praise of Shakespeare's genius. They were also as uncertain as those of any woman who retired to her own chamber to give birth. He felt strongly enough about those uncertainties, in fact, to express them explicitly in the invocations, especially in the very fraught one to Book 7, which is not only a prelude to his stunning evocation of God's creative power, but also contains that strange personal echo between his present political suffering and the reproductive suffering he imagined in the allegory of Sin and Death (see Chapter 8). As in any birth under seventeenth-century circumstances (perhaps under any circumstances), that chamber could only be deemed a place for celebration or known as a place of mourning in the wake of its final outcome. In the creative process (as it unfolds in the course of the epic's framing narrative of its own creation), it is also a place of uncertain but conscious terrors. Just like the terrors of the childbed, these had to be faced with faithful prayer and meditation, as well as with full spiritual and imaginative engagement. A woman might produce prayers, laudable acts, and hopefully a living infant. Milton produced a poem with chaotic, perfect, and fallen wombs at its center, a poem he hoped might bear, like his earliest compositions, certain signs that it would live both to adulthood and to aftertimes. As he lay there in bed, in the "birthing" chamber that might also have been the room in which his second wife died, impregnated in the imagination by his "Celestial Patroness," he was

30 On this aspect of the myth and its relationship to traditional self-reflexive figures in Western poetics, see Allen Grossman, *The Long Schoolroom: Lessons in the Bitter Logic of the Poetic Principle* (Ann Arbor, MI: University of Michigan Press, 1997), pp. 18–38.

31 "Of Chaos and Nightingales," p. 226.

haunted by fears of incompletion that took the form of fear of a more physical kind: of abortion, monstrosity, and maternal death.

Taken together, the passages in the poem that evoke such fears show Milton enacting the basic dynamic of his great argument at its highest pitch. Far more complex and consequential than his early, more self-involved allusions to women's anxieties and creative powers, the images in the epic suggest, in a new way, that the actions of the poet and of the suffering mother – or those of the suffering witness to a mother's suffering – are not absolutely different. Both the poet and the laboring woman must confront a condition that seems to deny the existence of a benevolent God and yet apply frames of reference that can bring Him to light – give "birth" to Him in two significant senses: as the believer is born anew when grace manifests itself in his or her actions (birth-actions included), and as grace itself was born into the world through Mary's womb. All three births make manifest the existence of that God Milton believed was there all along, although He sometimes hid. The imagery Milton used to describe creation invites us to see the suffering that attends the process of reproduction in the wake of original sin as a circumscribed, though terrifying, realm of disorder over which God gave the human mind and spirit dominion. As we hover over that space, or lie within it (the poem tries to argue), we can redeem it if we exercise our wills against despair, and, as Michael puts it in Book 12, if we can add deeds of love. The poem, produced in the dark night and in the wombic enclosure in which the "wakeful bird" sang darkling, is such a deed. It is a response to the fear and terror that such darkness *could* inspire, but finally, in this case, did not, or did not merely. The experience of such suffering "wraught" from Milton a "commiseration" like the one the narrator tells us turned Adam back to Eve in their reconciliation scene (*PL*, 10.939–41). That Adam's response should have been inspired by a woman's invention of *imitatio Christi* once again shows how closely Milton associated the pains of childbirth with his poem's central purpose. In justifying the ways of God to sinful humankind, he himself – as he has Eve put it in that crucial, self-sacrificial passage – returned again and again to "the place of judgment" (10.932), a place created in his imagination by the Christ-like suffering of women, and there he made his offering.

Index